Lynda Brown, one of the country's most respected food writers, has had a life long passion for, and commitment to, organic food and gardening. She describes this book as the most important she has yet written, which she hopes will help consumers bring about the eating revolution that everyone wants.

A familiar face and voice from her TV appearances and her contributions to radio, especially Radio 4's celebrated 'The Food Programme', she has written extensively for all major national newspapers and journals over the last ten years and is a winner of the prestigious Glenfiddich Cookery Writer award.

Her previous book, *Modern Cook's Manual*, published by Michael Joseph, won the Jeremy Round award for the most innovative work of 1995. Her other books include *The Cook's Garden* and *Gardeners' World Vegetables for Small Gardens*. She is a life member of the organic gardeners' association, HDRA, and the Soil Association.

Also by Lynda Brown

the shopper's guide to organic food

Lynda Brown

FOURTH ESTATE • LONDON

For Charlotte, with love

First published in Great Britain in 1998 by
Fourth Estate Limited
6 Salem Road
London W2 4BU

5 7 9 10 8 6 4

A catalogue record for this book is available from the British Library.

ISBN 1-85702-840-6

Printed on natural and renewable fibre from
environmentally controlled and managed forests;
it is totally chlorine-free and contains no optical brightening
agents. Recyclable and biodegradable.

Designed by Blackjacks, London
Typeset by Rowland Phototypesetting and Blackjacks
Printed in Great Britain by Clays Ltd, St Ives plc

Contents

With every meal, we are intimately affected by the quality of the food and water we consume. The complex mix of chemicals we eat and drink may include both nutrients essential for life and other chemicals that may jeopardise our health. Just as individual choices about food influence one's personal health, aggregated choices about what we eat influence agricultural practices, the use of technology, and environmental quality wherever food is produced.

John Wargo, *Our Children's Toxic Legacy*

We tend to think of revolutions as being noisy, rather public events. There is, however, another kind, where the change is undramatic, though the results are just as far-reaching. The organic revolution is one of these. Time was when organic farming was thought of as a kitchen-garden affair, producing misshapen carrots to be sold in health-food shops. The reality nowadays could not be more different.

Michael Wynn Jones, editor,
Sainsbury's *The Magazine*, October 1997

Acknowledgements

It is impossible to write a book of this nature without drawing heavily on the expertise, advice, guidance and help of many people – indeed, it is they who have made this book possible. I should like to acknowledge my heartfelt debt to them, and to thank everyone most sincerely for their patience and unstinting generosity.

First, my particular thanks to the staff at the Pesticide Safety Directorate, who could not have shown more consideration; my thanks also to the Pesticide Usage Survey Group, the Veterinary Medicines Directorate and to all the other Ministry of Agriculture personnel whom I have consulted.

My special gratitude to Lucy Atkinson, Sally Bagenal, Francis Blake, Eric Booth, Mike Brook, Helen Browning, Lee Castle, Jan Deane, Gaye Donaldson, Tim Finney, Jackie Garfit, Patrick Holden, Chris Johnson, Tim Lang, John Lister, Suzanne Rees, Charlotte Reynolds, Julian Rose, Alan Schofield, Peter Segger, Iain Tolhurst, Andrew Whitley, Alan Wilson, Thoby and Josa Young; Peter Beaumont and David Buffin of the Pesticides Trust and Dr Douglas Parr and the staff at Greenpeace; many of whom took the trouble to read and comment on draft sections.

I should also like to acknowledge Lisa Saffron for drawing my attention to nitrate studies in vegetables and for allowing me to read her own unpublished report compiled for the Bristol Cancer Centre; Dr Vyvyan Howard of Liverpool University for his paper on chemical mixtures and synergism; Dr Jean Munro for various papers and her book, *Chemical Children*, written with Dr Peter Mansfield; Dr Dick van Steenis for his work on toxic substances and cancer clusters; John Reeves for his correspondence on minerals and animal health; and BBC News for providing a transcript of their bulletin on sperm counts.

My thanks as well to Sarah Jane Evans of the BBC *Good Food Magazine* and Keren Williams of the *Daily Mail You Magazine*, for their co-operation in my request for readers' views. And to the many people who responded, telling me why they buy organic food, what they buy, and where, my most profound thanks; your letters and cards were an inspiration to me and gave me constant encouragement. My thanks, too, to the many wholesalers and suppliers who provided me with their catalogues and answered many questions; and to Sainsbury's *The Magazine*, Out of this World, *Radio Times*, Top Quali Tea and Yale University Press for permission to use their quotes.

My grateful thanks to my publishers, Fourth Estate, for taking me in their stride and for giving me their wholehearted support; to Sue Phillpott for her painstaking copy editing; and, especially, for tuning into its voice and listening to its heartbeat, to my editor, Louise Haines, who has worked tremendously hard on the book and has been a beacon of light throughout. We are both organic shoppers and her experience, especially in feeding two small children, has been invaluable. For having faith in me again, and for guiding me through with unerring gentleness and thoroughness, my affectionate thanks for ever.

The following have helped me on specific subjects, and I thank them all. My apologies to anyone I have omitted to mention.

Alternative supermarkets: Richard Adams, Jonathan Dwek, Renée J. Elliott, Andy Haughton, Jon Walker; *baby food*: Baby Organix, Boots, Cow & Gate, the Food Commission, Lucy Grammer, Hipp, Dr Vyvyan Howard, Janette Marshall, Dr Jean Munro, Lizzie Vann; *box schemes*: Eric Booth, Isabel Davies, Jan Deane, Alan Schofield, Ronny Smith, Iain Tolehurst; *brands*: Brewhurst Health Foods, Country Organics, De Rit, Infinity Foods, Meridian Foods, Nordex Foods, Suma, Whole Earth Foods, Windmell Foods; *chocolate*: Josephine Fairley, Women's Environmental Network; *dairy foods*: Sally Bagenal, Malcolm Gliddon, Hergest Farm, Marilyn James, Lotte Kjergaard Larson, Mark Measures, Nick Rebbek, Peter Redstone, Julian Rose, Gareth Rowland, Gillian Stone, John Svensson; *dried foods*: Community Foods, Bill Henry, Infinity Foods, Grahame Man, Paul Smith; *eggs*: Martin Pitt, Will Taylor, David Woolley; *farm shops*: Pam and Bill Beaumont, Andrew Carnegie, Jane Faulkes, Sue Gerard, Henrietta Green, Elizabeth Rose; *fish*: William Blake, Bob Kennard, Dr Brian Scott; *flour and cereals*: John Lister, Claire Marriage, Bill Starling; *fresh produce*: Kevin Benson, Simon Brenman, Paul Burgess, the Food Commission, Harold Linfield, Geoff Mutton, Kerry Rankine, Suzanne Rees, SAFE Alliance, Lisa Saffron, Alan Schofield, Pete Segger, Thoby and Josa Young; *genetic engineering*: Greenpeace, Dr Doug Parr, Ian Taylor; *game*: Julian Murray Evans; *health*: Teresa Hale, Dr Peter Mansfield,

Janette Marshall, Dr Jean Munro; *herbs and spices*: British Herb Trade Association, Mike Brook, Gaye Donaldson, Martin Gill, Stephen Lunn, Mike Secretan, Peter Turner; *honey*: De Rit, Peter Jacobs, New Zealand Natural Food Co.; *ice-cream*: Peter Redstone; *juices*: Andrew Jedwell; *labelling*: Peter Crofts, Philip Pridoe; *mail order*: Jackie Garfit, Louise Unwin; *markets*: Jenny Usher; *meat*: Jane Brodie, Helen Browning, Lee Castle, Clare Druce, Farm Animal Welfare Network, Tim Finney, Juliet Gellatley, Alison Glennon, Richard Guy, Bob Kennard, the Meat and Livestock Commission, the Ministry of Agriculture, Fisheries and Food, Peter J. Onions, John Reeves, Charlotte Reynolds, Dr Dick van Steenis, Mary Weston, Richard Young; *olive oil*: Joachim I.F. Blok, Charles Carey, Andrew Jedwell, Judy Ridgway; *organic farming*: Alan Gear, Bernward Geier, Patrick Holden, Pete Segger, the Soil Association, Lawrence Woodward; *organic standards*: Nigel Agar, James Anderson, Francis Blake, Peter Crofts, Robert Sculthorpe, Valerie Watts; *pesticides*: Josie Armes, Peter Beaumont, David Buffin, Vera Chaney, the Food Commission, Greenpeace, Teresa Hale, Caroline Harris, Lindsay Holmes, Tim Lang, Alan Long, the Pesticide Trust, Diane Ward, Women's Environmental Network; *retail shops*: Julie Allbeson, Jackie Garfit, Ray Hill, Chris Johnson, Charlotte Mitchell, Jill Turton, Simon Wright, Shelia Wye; *supermarkets*: Booths, Safeway, Sainsbury's, Tesco, Waitrose; *tea and coffee*: Equal Exchange, David Henry, Ian Henshall, the International Coffee Organisation, Simon Parkes, Sam Roger, Kiran Tawadey, Martin Warttam, Anthony Wild; *wine*: Lance Pigott.

I should also like to acknowledge *Thorsons Organic Consumer Guide*, a pioneering book, and the first of its kind, written by David Mabey and Alan and Jackie Gear, published in 1990.

Finally, I should like to pay tribute to Derek Cooper and Radio 4's *The Food Programme*, who have given me much needed encouragement throughout my career and who have done so much to campaign for and raise awareness of good food.

Foreword

Farming has undergone a revolution since the Second World War. Science and intensive farming methods have been applied as never before, and now we take for granted a huge range of cheap, plentiful food, available whatever the season. Well, at least we did. Over the last few years, concerns about food and farming have increased. We started with good intentions, but somewhere along the way we took a wrong turn and we now need to find a new way forward, and with some urgency. So we are in the middle of another revolution in food and farming – the organic revolution. No longer on the fringes, organic food is here to stay and to increase its share of the market as fast as it can be grown.

Lynda's book is timely. It is a comprehensive and indispensable source of information about organic food. It tells you what it is, where you can get it, and it shows how much is already happening. It rightly points to the real drivers behind the new revolution – the consumers making small, positive choices that will benefit themselves, the environment and the wider world.

We warmly welcome Lynda's book. Having invested solidly in organic food and farming for more than twenty years, we are delighted to see how the sector has grown and matured. We were convinced of its future when it was the concern of only a few lonely voices. Now there is no shortage of initiative, ability, and demand for organic food and farming.

This book will arm you, the shopper, with all you need to know to make the choices which will carry a new revolution in food into the next century.

Glen Saunders
Triodos Bank
Brunel House
11 The Promenade
Bristol BS8 3NN
Tel 0117 973 9339
Fax 0117 973 9303

Triodos ⊛ Bank

Preface

have written this book because I feel that organic food should be for everyone, and that everyone ought to be able to buy it when they want to. I want to dispel some of the myths about organic food, to give some practical guidance about its quality, availability and cost, to explain why most organic food tastes better, and to encourage as many people as possible to include some organic food in their regular shopping basket. Organic food is accessible to all. My hope is that the book will promote a better understanding of what organic food is and why it is worth buying; and, most importantly, where and how to buy it.

Writing this book has changed my life in many ways. When I began, though I had eaten organic meat, bread, dairy and fresh produce for several years, I had no idea how much organic food is available, nor of the huge variety of foods that now exists. Indeed, such is the tidal wave of new organic foods coming into the shops that it has been almost impossible to keep track; and by the time this book is printed, there will be many more. I have come gradually to realise, too, that the more organic food you eat, the better, happier and healthier you are likely to feel, physically, emotionally and mentally. After all, organic food is man's and animals' natural diet, the one best suited to our nutritional needs. It is natural to eat it and natural to want it.

The 'feel-good factor' cannot be overestimated. Eating an organic meal whose ingredients you have bought and cooked yourself is satisfying beyond belief – and is easier to achieve than you may think. Not only does the food taste better, but you have the satisfaction of knowing exactly how it has been produced, that it has been produced in an environmentally enhancing way, and that it is as pure as possible.

I also had little idea of how deeply so many people feel about what is happening to our food and our environment, and how strong is the desire for something better. The many letters and cards that I have received from people of all walks of life, who buy or who want to buy organic food, all testify to this. For the organic food revolution – and this is what it is – has been a consumer-led revolution. As someone confided to me, the real heroes of the organic food movement are the shoppers. The reason, he said, why the Ministry of Agriculture and the National Farmers' Union, for example, are finally getting enthusiastic about organic farming is that the food industry is being harangued by shoppers. That the organic food sector is beginning to thrive is a victory for and testament to all those who love food and who care about what they eat.

The particularly difficult issue for me personally is pesticides. The more I read, the less reassured I feel about official statements that they are 'safe', and the more effort I put into trying to buy more organic food. It saddens me that so much money and energy (well over £2.5 million of public money per year) are spent on monitoring pesticides, which should not be present in our food in the first place, yet so little is spent on encouraging farmers and food-producers to switch to organic means of production. The savings in pollution costs alone would make organic food the cheapest, in real terms, to produce. I ask myself, too, would the world have collapsed and would we all be starving if pesticides had not been invented? I seriously doubt it. At the moment few people feel they can afford to eat a totally organic diet, but I do believe this will change. What it requires most is political will – and only mass shopping demand will persuade politicians. As long as we continue to say loudly and clearly what we want, and support organic food when we can, the change to organic farming methods will, I believe, be unstoppable.

The organic food revolution is part of the good food revolution. As we approach the millennium, I can think of nothing better than for everyone to be able to feed themselves with healthy and delicious food that leaves the environment in better shape. I hope you will enjoy its fruits as much as I do. I know you won't be disappointed. Good luck, and happy eating!

Disclaimer

The organic food sector is developing at a rapid pace, and though every endeavour has been made to provide accurate information, no responsibility can be held for any changes occurring after the time of going to press. I would be grateful for any suggestions or comments for possible inclusion in future editions.

Abbreviations

The following abbreviations have been used:

ADI	*acceptable daily intake*
EBDCs	*Ethylene Bisdithio Carbamates*
FAO	*Food and Agriculture Organisation*
FAWN	*Farm Animal Welfare Network*
GM	*Genetically modified*
GMOs	*Genetically modified organisms*
IFOAM	*International Federation of Organic Agricultural Movements*
IOFGA	*Irish Organic Farmers' and Growers' Association*
MRL	*maximum residue limit*
OCs	*organochlorine pesticides*
OF & G	*Organic Farmers & Growers*
OPs	*organophosphate pesticides*
SA	*Soil Association*
SOPA	*Scottish Organic Producers' Association*
UKROFS	*UK Register of Organic Food Standards*
VMD	*Veterinary Medicines Directorate*
WPPR	*Working Party on Pesticide Residues*
WWF	*Worldwide Fund for Nature*

chapter one

organic food and farming

What Is Organic Farming?

Organic farming works with nature to produce healthy, nutritious food economically and in a manner that is beneficial to man and planet alike. As one Swiss expert has put it, organic farming is 'practising ecology'. Before the introduction of industrial techniques into agriculture in the 1940s, all farming was carried out along organic lines. Today, organic farming combines the best of traditional farming practices with the kind of scientific research that produces a system both sustainable and environmentally benign.

When you buy organic food you are buying much more than food grown 'naturally', 'without artificial fertilisers' and 'not sprayed with chemical pesticides'. In organic farming systems, food production is viewed not as the supplying of a commodity, but as a holistic enterprise where sustainability and health, each as important as the other, are interlinked, and where healthy food can be produced only on healthy soils and from animals reared on a natural diet.

The first objective of an organic farm is to be able to sustain itself; in other words, to buy in as little as possible. Organic farms aim to provide their own fertility, raise their own animals and grow their own feed. This makes for a fundamentally cost-effective, low-energy system. The second objective is to be sustainable in the wider context; that is, to use farming practices that encourage the balance of nature and that nurture and sustain the environment. With the best will in the world, it is impossible to achieve this by means of conventional agricultural practices; though the worst excesses can be avoided – and much publicity is given to environmentally friendly farming practices – regrettably, such measures are fundamentally cosmetic. By the same token, you cannot convert a chemical farm into an organic one merely by not using chemicals.

People often ask, can organic farming sustain the world's population? As the many thousands of successful organic farmers worldwide will testify, the short answer is yes. As Cuba, which has experienced an organic farming revolution, has shown, organic farming methods can easily produce enough food to feed people. The problem is that, to apply this worldwide, it would be necessary to engage in a radical rethinking of farming practices and priorities, food production would need to become primarily home-based, and it would require massive political and economic upheaval. Although this is unlikely to happen for some time, as environmental issues become more pressing, so organic farming will acquire an increasingly high profile.

Is organic farming perfect, and is it completely natural?

The answer to both questions is no. For example, organic farmers use sprays, although, save in exceptional circumstances, they use only those based on natural compounds which biodegrade quickly and do not leave residues. All sprays have unwelcome side-effects, which is why organic farmers do everything possible in order not to use them. Derris, for example, an organic spray used to control pests, also harms beneficial insects. Organic farmers may also use natural mineral fertilisers. Growing organic crops or raising animals organically, for commercial purposes, involves compromises. For example, there is insufficient organic feedstuff, straw or manure to support the industry at the present time, which means that a small amount of conventional stuff is allowed to be bought in if necessary; this is known as a 'derogation' (see p. 23).

Though the principles and guidelines of organic farming are firmly established, organic certification standards vary, both here and within Europe. This is as much a headache for organic producers as it is confusing to the customer, and efforts are being made internationally within the International Federation of Organic Movements (IFOAM) to improve the situation. There are inconsistencies, and, occasionally, standards that are debatable. For instance, though I know of no organic poultry producer who practises it, debeaking is allowed under the UK Register of Organic Food (UKROFS) standards and is condoned by the RSPCA, as is the use of certain antibiotics for a limited period in chick feed if – and only if – it is deemed necessary. Standards are constantly evolving and being updated, and, as anomalies are ironed out, will become uniform both here and in Europe.

The organic movement is experiencing a period of rapid development, which brings another set of challenges, and there is still much to learn and improve upon. What is indisputable is that organic farming can no longer be considered a niche market, that standards of professionalism in organic farming and food manufacture have progressed enormously in the last five years, that supplies are much more reliable and that consumers can look forward to a very bright organic future.

Converting to an organic system

In the UK, conversion from a conventional to an organic farming system takes a minimum of two to three years, and can take longer, depending on individual circumstances or on the crop, the prime objective being to 'clean' the land and build natural fertility. During this time, produce from the farm may not be sold as organic. At the end of the conversion period, the farm will be inspected by an independent certifying body. If it has fulfilled the necessary standards, it will then be registered and, after the first harvest, its produce may be sold as organic. Thereafter it will be inspected annually.

Is organic food guaranteed free from pesticide residues?

No. Pesticides are endemic in water, soil and air. Because of the general high level of pollution, background contamination and, for example, spray drift from surrounding farms, it is impossible to guarantee that organic food is free from pesticide residues.

Nevertheless, extensive monitoring tests conducted in Europe show consistently that organic food has either no or minimal residues. In the UK, the Working Party on Pesticide Residues (WPPR) has now begun to monitor organic food. The latest report, of 1996, found residues, for example, in organic bread samples. As part of their remit, the WPPR investigates such findings in order to determine whether any such residues are unavoidable or the result of malpractice, which is a welcome development that should further help to check potential fraudulent activity.

Why do people buy organic food?

Consumers throughout Europe buy organic food for the same reasons – namely health, fewer pesticide residues, taste, the belief that organic food has a higher nutritional value, and concern for the environment and for animal welfare. It is natural food that people most feel they can trust. As time goes on, the environmental benefits are likely to play the biggest role in people's food choices. In Britain, even conventional companies now include the organic factor in their market research, and are finding the same pattern emerging.

The health issue is an interesting one. It has been proved, for example, that organic produce contains fewer nitrates, has a higher dry-matter content (good for flavour) and minimal concentrations of pesticides, and sometimes has higher vitamin C and mineral levels. Conventional scientific studies comparing standard nutritional values, however, are ambiguous, and it is not possible to deduce that there is a clear nutritional difference between organic and conventional food. But how much notice we should take of this is questionable. Such studies, done in experimental rather than real-life situations, are fairly meaningless. Also, food is a biological entity. To measure its value as nutrient ash in a laboratory is largely futile. On the other hand, the overall health and vitality – a much more difficult thing to capture in a test tube – of organic produce is undoubtedly one of its most important attributes. People who eat organic food, including many scientists, are convinced of this (see p. 15). Sophisticated techniques such as those looking at photon emissions have shown that organic food 'radiates' more vitality, and studies that examine people rather than nutrients (see p. 126) point the way forward.

Quality and flavour

Time was when all you had to do to judge the quality of a food was to be guided by its taste. Other obvious factors are freshness in fresh produce, tenderness and flavour in meat, and absence of artificial or cheap ingredients in manufactured foods. Appearance has also come to assume enormous importance. However, none of these factors takes into account how the food is produced or how animals are treated, or what effect it has on the environment, or directly or indirectly on our health. The advent of BSE (bovine spongiform encephalopathy) has changed all that. In future, as the rising demand for organic food shows, how food is produced will be as important as the traditional benchmarks of 'quality'. This is where organic food scores best.

In terms of the conventional benchmarks, though the quality of organic food improves constantly, it does not necessarily always match up to what people have been used to. Standards do vary. Organic foods have their own characteristics, fresh produce is rarely cosmetically perfect and though some taste similar to their conventional counterparts, others taste different because they *are* different. Because organic produce is closer to nature and grown in different ways from conventional food, its taste varies with the season, and so on. Also, people's preferences are conditioned by the tastes they are used to: for me the perfect organic cornflake is a wholegrain cornflake such as Whole Earth's, because it's nutty and crunchy and not in the least bit sweet or salty; for some it's Evernat's, because they say it looks and tastes most like conventional brands, while others rave about Doves Farm, which manages to achieve both.

I believe that, as it becomes the norm, it will be organic food that sets the benchmarks for quality and flavour, and not the other way round. In the meantime, there is already plenty of choice and enough suppliers to please everyone and cater for all tastes; and in a rapidly growing market this means more and better choices for the foreseeable future.

what they say . . .

'We describe food in terms of chemistry, yet the methods of chemistry do not imitate nature. The separate molecules of fat or protein bear no resemblance to food. A chemist could never hope to make a cabbage. Also, for all we know about genes, we have no idea how a human works.

'Organisms have an invisible energy-map that contains vitality as well as a design. We can measure this vitality scientifically, through chromatography, for example, but we do not yet take it seriously. These measurements show very clearly that vitality and structural harmony are the defining characteristics of organic food – many times larger than that of equally fresh food grown chemically.' – *Dr Peter Mansfield, Director, Templegarth Trust*

'I buy organic food mainly because of the wider implications of non-organic production for the countryside, the environment, animal welfare, and – not least – those involved in food production . . . I hardly look at the price of food nowadays, because I assume that cheap food in this country equals a countryside empty of human reason and full of machinery and chemicals (for which we are paying the price somewhere else, anyway), while the Third World is on a runaway roller-coaster of international cash-crop competition with a disastrous outcome for all.' – *Kate Midgley, Somerset*

Organic versus Conventional Farming

Organic and conventional farming systems differ in ways that have far-reaching consequences. The major factors are:

The environment Organic growers are guardians of the environment. Caring for the environment, maintaining biodiversity and providing for and protecting ecological habitats are factors that are built into standards and are fundamental to the organic farming creed. Everything possible is done to encourage ecological balance, including maintaining hedgerows, walls and existing habitats, planting trees and allowing for greater field margins. Removing hedges and exploiting peat bogs are both prohibited. The use of artificial fertilisers and synthetic pesticides means that it is impossible to achieve environmental stability via conventional agriculture.

Pollution Organic farming systems are designed not to pollute the land, the atmosphere or watercourses; as a fundamental requirement, polluting practices including the burning of plastic waste are banned.

Soil Nothing is more important to an organic farmer or grower than the soil. It is the foundation on which the organic farming system is built. Produce is grown in healthy, 'living' soils enriched with organic matter to provide natural fertility, biologically high in microbial activity and other soil life, providing a mine of complex nutrients that plants can tap into and animals can feed off. In conventional agriculture, the soil plays a far less important role and soil improvement is not a priority. The artificial fertilisers used do not improve the soil, which gradually becomes impoverished, and the extensive use of insecticides, fungicides and fumigants severely depletes soil life.

Fertilisers Organic growers do not use artificial fertilisers. Instead, soil fertility is maintained by crop rotations, compost, and animal manures. Non-organic sources of manure are restricted and sources documented; manures from intensive or factory farming are prohibited. Conventional farming systems primarily use artificial fertilisers, which provide plants with the main elements needed for growth – nitrogen, phosphorus and potassium – only; crop rotation is more limited, or non-existent; such systems do not make or use compost.

Scale Though there are exceptions, herd and field sizes are smaller, the excesses of monoculture are avoided and most farmers operate mixed farms.

Extensive versus intensive Organic farming systems are extensive, aim to be self-sustaining and are relatively low energy-users. Conventional farming systems are mainly intensive, usually highly specialised and high energy-users, dependent on external inputs. They are thus incapable of being self-sustaining.

Growth A guiding principle of organic farming systems is that neither produce nor animals should be forced beyond their natural capabilities. Since no artificial fertilisers are allowed on crops, or growth-promoting agents, including antibiotics, for livestock, both crops and livestock grow and develop more slowly, thus maximising the potential to develop more flavour.

Health Organic farming systems aim to maximise health rather than yields.

Varieties Organic growers favour and promote biodiversity. Though modern varieties and breeds do play a part, those suited to organic growing, rather than those bred only for high yields and intensive monoculture, are of particular importance. Traditional breeds best suited to our climate are a feature of organic livestock husbandry.

Genetic engineering The use of genetically modified (GM) seeds, crops, feedstuffs, animals or any genetically modified organism is banned in organic farming systems.

Breeding and rearing Livestock form an integral part of most organic farms. Though it is permitted to buy in up to 10 per cent of stock per year, the aim is to maintain closed flocks and herds by breeding and rearing all replacements, to provide as much home-grown feed as possible, and to use farm manure as part of the ongoing fertility-building of the soil. All animals slaughtered for meat must be born and raised on an organic holding.

Animal welfare Intensive farming practices, including those to do with housing and feeding, are banned. In addition, the purchase of animals through livestock markets and the export of livestock for slaughter are forbidden.

Calving and weaning A fundamental aspect of organic livestock management is that newborn stock are suckled naturally for as long as possible to enable them to develop natural immunity and to give them the healthiest start in life. Weaning times are twice as long as in conventional systems, and may be considerably longer. Organic calves are not allowed to be sold for veal export, and may not be sold through livestock markets at less than one month old.

Diet Organic livestock are fed a natural diet suitable to their species, and which mainly comprises organic feedstuff, most of which is usually grown on the farm. The feeding of animal proteins to herbivores was banned in 1984.

Green manures These are an essential part of organic production. Up to 25 per cent of organic land is taken out of cash production every year to grow nitrogen-fixing legumes, which are turned back into the soil to break down and enhance its fertility.

Rotations These are at the core of organic crop production and organic farming systems. Monoculture – namely, the production of the same crop continuously on the same land – is not practised.

Weeding Organic growers use no herbicides. Weeds are controlled by manual or other physical means, by blow-torching and by mulching.

Pest and disease control Organic growers use no synthetic chemical pesticides. Emphasis instead is on producing a healthy soil and healthy plants using crop rotations, resistant varieties and strategic planting dates, greater diligence and physical inspection. They encourage natural predators in both the micro and macro environment through the use of hedges, ponds and so on, and through scientific measures such as biological control whereby predator species are introduced to control pest populations. A small number of permitted insecticides are used when absolutely necessary.

Post-harvest treatment Organic produce receives no post-harvest treatment of insecticides or fungicides.

Medication The prime concern of organic farming systems is to raise animals which are naturally healthy and robust. This is achieved by raising them in non-intensive ways, giving them high-quality feedstuffs and ensuring that they lead stress-free lives. Illness is rarely a problem, and vet bills are minimal. Routine antibiotics are banned, though they must be, and are, used when necessary to prevent suffering or where there is no other effective treatment.

Records In order to qualify for certification as an organic farm or holding, detailed records of every aspect of the farm, crops and livestock must be kept for inspection purposes and may be examined at any time by the certifying body concerned. Every farm is inspected annually, and may also receive unannounced visits to check that standards are being upheld. No similar regulatory procedures are enforced in conventional farming systems.

Counting the Cost of Industrial Agriculture

Industrial agriculture and modern farming practices enable food to be produced more cheaply but generate many hidden costs that are not apparent when we pay for food at the till, but are paid for elsewhere. There are three examples that affect everyone: BSE, pesticides in drinking-water, and nitrates in drinking-water.

BSE

Mad cow disease, bovine spongiform encephalopathy, has been the worst food crisis in living memory and has affected the whole nation. The costs involved are astronomical.

- Government action to eradicate BSE first began in 1988. By early 1996, 190,000 cattle had been destroyed, and £237.6 million of tax-payers' money had already been spent.
- The official estimate of public expenditure for 1996/7 was a further £1.2 billion – over one hundred times that originally predicted. This includes £9.6 million in compensation to farmers, £57 million in agricultural inspection and enforcement costs, £130 million in aid to abattoirs and £81 million in aid for beef producers.
- The budget for 1997/8 for BSE-related matters has been set at a further £789 million. This excludes the cost of the selective cull.
- In addition to animals suspected of having BSE, all cattle over the age of thirty months have had to be destroyed, including organically raised cattle. Currently

over 1.3 million cattle have been destroyed in this way. The average compensation paid is £386 per animal – a total cost of over £5 billion.

- By the end of 1996 over £56 million had been spent on research into transmissible spongiform encephalopathies, of which the MAFF spent £30 million on BSE research.

Pesticides in drinking-water

An increasing number of raw drinking-water sources contain pesticide concentrations in excess of the EU standard of 0.1 microgram/litre. The need to reduce these has triggered a huge investment in treatment plans by twenty-one UK companies, which users pay for in rising water bills.

- Estimates of capital investment since 1992 aimed at combatting pesticides in drinking-water range from £799 million to £1,000 million. Annual running costs are estimated at a further 10 per cent of capital expenditure, or from £79 million to £100 million.
- The estimated cost of monitoring and analysing pesticides in water supplies is at least £1 million per year for each water company, or a total of £121 million a year.

Nitrates in drinking-water

The major source of the nitrogen applied to crops as a soil fertiliser for boosting growth takes the form of nitrate compounds. These are highly soluble, and any excess not taken up by the plants leaches into the surrounding water supplies. An increasing number of raw water sources exceed the EU maximum allowable nitrate concentration of 50mg/litre, and water companies have been required to introduce water-blending and -treatment programmes.

- Estimates of capital investment to deal with nitrates in water supplies range from £148 to £200 million, with an estimated running cost of £10 million a year.
- Since 1989 total government expenditure on nitrate

control programmes in England and Wales has been £74.9 million. The annual running cost for 1996/7 amounts to £13.4 million.

Source Counting the Costs of Industrial Agriculture, Soil Association, 1996; the Ministry of Agriculture.

Organic Farming Facts

Scale

- There are currently only 30,000 certified hectares, 900 producers, and 20,000 hectares in conversion to organic farming in the UK. This is set to increase by 50 per cent a year, with the aim of having three times more producers by the year 2000.
- The amount of land farmed organically in the UK, 0.3 per cent, is one of the lowest in Europe, and one quarter of the EU average. Scandinavia, Germany, Denmark, Holland and Austria all exceed the UK. Austria aims to be 50 per cent and Denmark aims to be 20 per cent organic by 2000. The UK aims to be 1.5 per cent.

Subsidies

- In comparison to conventional farming, organic farming is very poorly subsidised. For a 2,000-acre arable farm, switching from conventional to organic methods would mean a loss of more than £50,000 a year in direct support payments alone.
- The UK subsidy level for voluntary set-aside land – land where the farmer is paid to grow nothing – is over six times that of the average given to farmers in conversion. Subsidies for set-aside are received indefinitely as long as the scheme lasts; conversion subsidies last for five years only. In 1994, just over half set-aside land received

applications of herbicides. The subsidy figures are
£338.03p per hectare for set-aside, and an average of
£50 per hectare for conversion.

● The Ministry of Agriculture, Fisheries and Food
currently spends twice as much testing for pesticides as it
does on R&D into organic farming, and almost half as
much monitoring pesticide usage as it does on support
for farmers in conversion through the Organic Aid
Scheme every year. The figures per annum are £2 million
for monitoring pesticide residues, £1 million for organic
R&D, £375,000 for monitoring pesticide usage and
£846,000 for the Organic Aid Scheme.

Economic and environmental benefits

● A new three-year government study into organic farming
at Prince Charles' Home Farm, Highgrove, has
confirmed that organic farming is better for the
environment and more profitable than conventional
farming using chemicals. A long-term study of fourteen
successful organic farms conducted by the US National
Academy of Sciences found that some farms had corn
yields 32 per cent higher and soya bean yields 40 per
cent higher than local conventional farms.

● Organic farms support more wildlife, bird species and
butterflies. Oxford's Wildlife Conservation Research
Unit found twice the number of non-pest butterflies on
organic farms than on chemical farms. To help
counteract the decline in bird species, the Royal Society
for the Protection of Birds has called for 5 per cent of
UK land to be farmed organically within the next five
years, and substantially more thereafter.

The market

● The market for organic produce in the UK has increased
more than fivefold since 1987, from £40 million to an
estimated £225 million-plus, and is expected to increase

by 30 per cent every year until 2000.

- The UK production of organic food, currently expanding by 50 per cent per annum, cannot keep up with the demand for it.
- Most consumers would prefer to buy organic food. Given the choice, only 4 per cent would choose non-organic. Over half consumers are recent converts, and one-quarter or more households now buy some organic food.

what they say . . .

'I think buying and eating organic food is a positive step that will bring us all forward to a healthy life and a better environment for everyone. It's sometimes more expensive to buy, but you are buying the best of food when it comes to organic. It's a change for the best.' – *Martha Reid, Dublin*

'My wife and I shop organic and have done so seriously for the past ten years. As we learn more and more about conventional farming and the processes used, the reasons for shopping organic continue to multiply. Organic products reflect a true economy, whereas conventionally farmed goods never include the price to society of pesticide regulation and testing, hazardous waste disposal and clean-up and environmental damage.

'If you look at shopping organic in a cost/benefit framework, the benefits seem to far outweigh the costs: better overall quality, better taste, better soil, no genetically engineered products, less ground water pollution hence better drinking-water, fewer pesticides used and consequently produced, better animal husbandry, significantly reduced usage of antibiotics, better farm health, better working conditions, sustainable agriculture, reduced energy consumption and more locally produced products – together with all of the benefits this brings to the local community.' – *William Lana, Greenwich, London*

'One day research will show the extra money we pay for organic foods reflected in good health. I am sorry for the farmers who have a difficult time changing to organic farming methods, but I am convinced polluted food, water and air ruin your health. Farmers

should be financially assisted to change, and pensioners helped to buy wholesome food. How can you put a value on good health?'
– *Pam Campbell, Chaldon, Surrey*

Organic Food and Our Health

Irrespective of whether science can prove it, people eating organic food believe that they enjoy better health and are safeguarding their future health. Alternative practitioners and health food gurus such as Leslie Kenton who recommend organic food do so because they believe it is healthier and significantly reduces the toxic load on the system. This seems to be borne out by the many cards and letters I have received from those who have changed to organic food for health reasons.

what they say . . .

'Organic food/good nutrition is one of the essential building-blocks for good health. It prevents illness from occurring and aids the treatment of illness with complementary medicine. In fact, many complementary treatments will only be fully effective if patients are prepared to adjust their dietary habits. A saying from Ayurvedic medicine puts it very succinctly: without proper diet medicine is of no use; with a proper diet, medicine is not needed. Organic food offers, I believe, the best chance of optimum nutrition.'
– *Teresa Hale, founder, Hale Clinic, London*

'Within my daily work as a practising herbalist, I see the consequences of poor diet. I am also an allergy therapist, and the most common chemical sensitivity is to phenol, which is found in pesticides. I and my family choose organic food wherever possible. For two adults and one seven-year-old I think our food bill is probably high. However, when I open my fridge what I see is our own private health insurance scheme. My daughter has never had to see a doctor; we enjoy good health and well-being.'
– *Jules Miller, Chester*

'I buy all kinds of organic food ranging from yoghurt to fruit and vegetables . . . I believe it is a real investment in health and well-being and think that it is well worth paying a bit extra to guarantee the safety of my food. My health has improved considerably since my new eating regime and I have much more energy than I used to have, even when well.' – *Rachel Wilson, Wolverhampton, aged twenty-three*

'Some eight years ago I suffered from arthritis . . . A friend lent me a book which put me on the road to buying organic food . . . With the help of organic food wherever possible, avoiding certain additives and processed foods, I have beaten my arthritis and although I find organic food more expensive, it is well worth it.' – *Mrs E. Trevethick, Surrey*

'I buy organic because I think chemical pollution of non-organic food is one of the major reasons for the breakdown of our immune systems. I think the cumulative effect is a huge strain on the liver and kidneys (detoxifying organs), leading to the breakdown of various bodily systems according to individual weakness. I also think this happens because of mineral imbalances caused by wrong treatment of the soil. For example, putting potash on the soil depresses uptake of cobalt. Chemical fertilisers upset the natural balance and health of the soil, leading to the use of chemical pesticides. It's like flogging a dead horse. We should return to respect for nature's wisdom.' – *Helen Jarvis, Ilkeston, Derbyshire*

'I have been buying organic food for about fifteen years now, as I believe in it so strongly. I am never ill and put it down to the food I eat . . . Although organic food is dearer, in some cases nearly double the price of non-organic, I make savings in other areas so I can give my family organic food, as I know it is so much better for us.' – *Mrs V. Smith, Berkshire*

The Wider Picture, Europe and Beyond

Less than 1 per cent of British agriculture is farmed organically, but this gives a false impression of the importance of organic agriculture elsewhere in the world. It also explains why about 75 per cent of the organic food you buy in shops is imported.

So buoyant is the worldwide organic market that statistics and predictions are difficult to keep up with. In the last seven years, for example, there has been an almost explosive rise in organic agriculture globally, including developing countries in the southern hemisphere and in Eastern Europe, while Japan is rapidly becoming a world leader. The International Federation of Organic Agricultural Movements (IFOAM) now has over six hundred member organisations and represents organic agriculture movements in a hundred countries worldwide.

In the EU the number of certified organic farms has increased eightfold in the last decade to over 55,000, and acreage has risen from 0.12 million to 1.3 million hectares, an annual rise of 25 per cent. The boom country is Austria, where 20,000 farms are now organic. Sweden, which has reduced its use of pesticides by three-quarters in the last ten years, aims to be 10 per cent organic by the year 2000, as do several other countries. During 1995–6 organic agriculture in Greece rose by 50 per cent, and the number of organic farmers there has increased from 165 in 1993 to 1,109 at the time of writing. In Denmark, there is a consumer boom for organic food – every supermarket stocks a wide range of products. Comparable developments can be seen in Germany, whose baby food industry is on its way to becoming entirely organic. Meanwhile, Europe's meat and dairy market, currently worth US$1.10 billion, is expected to triple in the next five years.

Those countries where government support is strongest, such as Austria and Denmark, are showing the most rapid growth. The Danish environment minister has predicted that 20 per cent of the Danish food market will be organic by the year 2000, and some forecasts predict that they will be 100 per cent organic in some foods soon. The Danish government has also recently commissioned a study on the feasibility of the country becoming entirely organic – the first to do so. Switzerland is another pro-organic country, and Swissair the first company to commit themselves to an all-organic catering service.

America is another major player. It is already the largest global exporter and consumer of organic products. Home sales have increased more than 20 per cent a year for the last six years and now stand at $2.8 billion, and the USA is expected to dominate world trade in the not too distant future. The organic movement there is the first to place advertisements in the press about organic food and distribute leaflets to retailers.

Organic food is growing steadily in South America: in Mexico, an estimated hundred thousand small farms are involved in organic farming, producing mainly coffee, while in Cuba organic farming and biological control are official policy. In the Pacific, in Australia and New Zealand, the momentum grows and exports of organic kiwi fruit are expected to quadruple in the next four years.

Organic farming methods are successfully practised by hundreds of thousands of farmers all over the world. As Bernward Geier, Executive Director of the IFOAM, has put it, 'We know it works worldwide. In Germany we too say, "You are what you eat!" If you have healthy soil, plants and animals then you can be healthy. The number one safeguard for health is to have organic food. It's time every shopper had a fair choice. That is now happening in Europe, and it could happen in Britain just as easily if organic farming was given the same kind of official commitment and aid that is happening everywhere else.'

Organic Standards, and What the Symbols Mean

The organic food sector is controlled by law and highly regulated by officially recognised organic certification authorities. All organic farmers, food manufacturers and processors are registered with one of these authorities, are inspected annually, and may also be inspected at random. It is the only food sector to have such a comprehensive and co-ordinated self-regulatory system. Producers, manufacturers and processors each pay an annual fee to be registered, and are required to keep detailed records ensuring a full audit trail from farm to table, any infringement of which results in suspension and withdrawal of products from the market. The result is a unique system of checks and guarantees for the consumer. In addition, the organic food system complies with the same stringent regulations as does the conventional food sector.

The overall governing body is the independent UK Register of Organic Food Standards (UKROFS), which sets the basic standards to which all the various organic bodies and producers adhere. UKROFS standards in turn conform to the European Community directive on organic production, EC 2092/91. The standards are stringent and cover every aspect of registration and certification, organic food production, permitted and non-permitted ingredients, the environment and conservation, processing, packaging and distribution. These standards are regularly updated and are then enforced by the six certification bodies recognised by UKROFS, set out below.

Each certification body has its own symbol and EU code number. These are the symbols and codes you will find on organic products, and are visible proof that they have met the required UKROFS standards *and* any others set by that certification body.

NOTE: Standards provide minimum codes of practice.
In reality, most organic farmers and food producers do
more and operate higher standards than are required.

The certification bodies

All the certification bodies are organic organisations in their own right, with their own members. The main difference between them is that either they represent a particular sector of the organic market, or they have a specific philosophy – for example, Demeter. All adhere to UKROFS standards. Some have their own additional ones, though in practice this makes very little, if any, difference to the quality of the food you buy.

 UKROFS An independent body set up to regulate the production and marketing of organic foods. Largely funded by MAFF, this is the government authority responsible for the approval and supervision of the other inspection bodies. Any organic foods bearing the UKROFS logo will have been produced to UKROFS standards. Producers registered with the following certification bodies may also use the UKROFS logo if they so wish. All except the Organic Farmers and Growers (OF&G) and the Scottish Organic Producers' Association (SOPA) are members of the International Federation of Organic Agricultural Movements (IFOAM).

Demeter The Greek goddess of agriculture and protector of all the fruits of the earth is the logo for the Bio-Dynamic Agricultural Association (BDAA), an international educational charity, founded in 1924 by the Austrian philosopher, Rudolph Steiner. It operates in thirty-eight countries, including the UK, and is an international trademark. There are currently around ninety-five symbol-holders in the UK. Bio-dynamic agriculture has been described as organic-plus. Central to the bio-dynamic philosophy is that man, earth and universe are bound together; that cosmic forces have an effect on soil, plants and animals; and that each farm or garden is a unique entity in which the personality of the farmer or gardener shines through. Foods grown under the bio-dynamic system are said to be in tune with the whole universe, and samples of Demeter food that have undergone crystallisation procedures show remarkable form and harmony at the cellular level compared to conventional food. Bio-dynamic farms actively support low external-input sustainable agriculture (LEISA). Wherever possible, farms are mixed. They grow as much of their own feed as possible and depend on their own manures and composts for fertility. Unique to Demeter is that sowing and planting times take account of cosmic forces such as the moon's cycle, and they use specific bio-dynamic herbal preparations on crops and on the soil to promote vitality, well-being and harmony. Many wine-makers are now converting to bio-dynamic methods.

The Irish Organic Farmers' and Growers' Association (IOFGA) Founded in 1982, the IOFGA promotes organic production and consumption in Ireland and comprises farmers, growers, consumers and others interested in organic food and in the protection of the environment; it currently has 530 registered producers. It operates its own inspection scheme and publishes a bimonthly magazine, *Organic Matters*, and has recently published its own organic directory, *The Irish Consumer*

Guide to Organic Food, listing producers, farms and guest-houses (tel: 00 353 1830 7996). It has its own standards, additional to those laid down by UKROFS.

 Organic Farmers and Growers (OF&G) Formed in 1975 by a group of leading organic farmers as a specialist co-operative to encourage organic food production on a commercial scale. The second-largest organic organisation, it has close links with the Soil Association and its members are primarily larger farmers and growers, but also include wholesalers, packers, processors and manufacturers. Its standards conform to those of UKROFS.

The Organic Food Federation (OFF) A trade federation set up in 1986 primarily to help its members, who comprise producers, manufacturers, importers and some retailers, to market organic foods. Its standards conform to those of UKROFS.

The Scottish Organic Producers' Association (SOPA) A charitable society founded in 1988 by Scottish producers to provide a central focus, advice and promotional activities for organic producers in Scotland. Its standards conform to those of UKROFS.

The Soil Association (SA) Founded in 1946, this is the country's leading campaigning organic organisation and the one whose symbol is most familiar. A registered charity, it has over six thousand members including producers, wholesalers, packers, manufacturers, retail outlets and ordinary consumers. It publishes a wide range of briefing papers and its own journal, *Living Earth*. It is the major certification body in the UK and operates its own set of standards, which are more specific and in some cases stricter than those laid down by UKROFS.

The standards for manufactured organic foods

Manufacturers must adhere to strict standards and must ensure organic integrity of products at all times. Manufacturers are required to supply and keep for three years proof of authenticity for all ingredients used, as well as processing records. To prevent substitution, all organic products must be transported either in their own packaging or in sealed containers. If a manufacturer produces both organic and non-organic food, the two must be kept separate at all times and the processing plant thoroughly cleaned down between operations to avoid any possibility of cross-contamination. In these cases, the organic production is normally the first run of the day.

The standards for imported organic foods

Each EU country has its own national organic certification authority which conforms to EU standards. Within each member state there are various independent certification authorities. Germany, for example, has fifty-nine, including Naturland, which is international, Austria twenty-one and Denmark over thirty-five. Holland, by contrast, has only one, SCAL. As in the UK, they may each include additional specifications – for example, to take into account different growing conditions – so will vary slightly from country to country.

The major difference between organic standards in the UK and those that apply in the rest of Europe is that the EU directive does not yet cover organic standards for animal husbandry or for foods composed essentially of animal ingredients; it is hoped that these will be in place by the end of 1998. Instead, most countries either have national organic standards or use those laid down by the International Federation of Organic Agricultural Movements.

For food imported from outside Europe into EU countries, the situation is slightly more complicated, but it is subjected to the same rigorous checks and guarantees. It can be imported only if it has come from a country recognised as applying equivalent standards and regulatory procedures, or if the importer concerned can provide proof to the organic authority of the member state that the product meets its standards, including inspection measures, and if the organic authority has subsequently granted an authorisation for it to be sold as organic. In practice, this means that either a whole country may apply for EU recognition of its organic standards, or, where national standards do not exist, importers may apply on behalf of specific organic producers, who will then be inspected in situ by one of the recognised certification bodies and subjected to annual inspections thereafter in the usual way.

Storage facilities for any imported food must be open to inspection at all times.

> **WATCHWORD: 'Fair-trade'** goods may or may not be organic. First introduced in 1988, fair-traded products guarantee a fairer deal for workers in less developed countries, particularly as regards wages and living conditions. Fair-trade organisations are now active in fifteen countries and work with small communities, providing comprehensive social and welfare packages including education and medical aid. Tea, coffee, cocoa, chocolate, honey and bananas have all become successful fair-traded commodities. Each fair-trade organisation, such as Fairtrade or Traidcraft in the UK and TransFair in Germany, has its logo, which usually appears on the products. Because of the natural affinity of organic and fair-trade ideals and their organisations, increasingly fair-trade products are becoming organic. All those currently available can be found in the relevant sections of the book.

European organic brands

Foods imported from Europe constitute one of the fastest-growing sectors of the market, and we can expect to see many more European organic foods on our shelves. Many different labels and logos exist; a brief description of some of the major organic brands can be found on p. 268.

Derogation

This is the term applied when, because there is insufficient organic material to meet farmers' or manufacturers' needs, they are allowed to use the non-organic equivalent for the time being – be it straw for bedding, or a particular ingredient. This is a temporary measure, which ceases as soon as sufficient organic material can be sourced. In some cases, such as the supply of day-old chicks for the poultry industry, there is currently no organic equivalent, so the organic industry has no alternative but to use conventional sources.

Fakes

No system is infallible, and though the vast majority of people who produce organic food are dedicated to the practice and philosophy of organic farming, there are those who see organic food merely as a way of making money by cheating consumers with conventional food sold as organic. This happens in a tiny minority of cases, and the way to prevent it from happening to you is very simple: *Ask to see the certification, or ask for confirmation of the audit trail.* Anyone selling organic food must be able to provide proof, either direct or indirect, of its authenticity if required; and everyone selling genuine organic food can do this. If in any doubt, consult your local Trading Standards officer, who has responsibility to enact the Organic Products Regulations, drawn up in 1992, amended in 1994, under Statutory Instrument 211.

Reading the Labels

All organic food sold in shops must be clearly marked with the appropriate certification body. Labelling regulations are strict. They are the same for all organic certification bodies, are governed by the EU standards and also apply to imported EU and other prepacked organic goods. There are currently, in addition, two grades of manufactured organic foods:

Fully organic These contain 95–100 per cent certified organic ingredients and are the only products entitled to be called 'organic' on the label. Non-organic ingredients must come from a permitted list of food ingredients for which there is no organic equivalent, and from a small number of permitted additives and processing aids if used; the label will state clearly what these are.
70 per cent or more organic These products must be made with at least 70 per cent certified organic ingredients. They cannot be labelled organic, but must be labelled 'made with X per cent organic ingredients'.

The easiest way to tell if a manufactured product is organic is to look for the symbol of certification on the packaging. This takes the form either of a logo, as mentioned earlier, or, more recently, of one of the certification code numbers listed below. It is now compulsory for every organic product to have one or other on the packaging.

> **NOTE:** Occasionally you may find a product that has not yet changed its packaging to meet the new requirements, though it has been certified, and its organic status will therefore appear on the label.

The UK code numbers are:

UK1 UKROFS
UK2 Organic Farmers and Growers (OF&G)
UK3 Scottish Organic Producers' Association (SOPA)
UK4 Organic Food Federation (OFF)
UK5 Soil Association/Soil Association Organic Marketing Company (SA/SAOMCo)
UK6 Demeter/Bio-Dynamic Agricultural Association (BDAA)
UK7 Irish Organic Farmers' and Growers' Association (IOFGA)

Each European certifying body also has its own code number.

To avoid any confusion with non-organic produce, most organic food is sold prepacked. Where there is no equivalent conventional produce being sold, or it is easy to differentiate between organic and conventional produce, for example, in the case of different varieties of mushroom, produce may be sold loose, though proof of certification must be available.

As already mentioned, manufacturers must be registered. Some shops pay the certification fee to register as organic in their own right. This gives an added assurance to customers. Any shop that repackages goods out of sight of customers, or cooks its own food and labels it 'organic', must have its own licence also.

> **NOTE:** Occasionally, products made with organic ingredients are not certified by the producer, and so are not entitled to be labelled organic. Whether to buy them is your own decision.

Some shops also sell, for instance, take-away foods, or bread made for them locally using organic ingredients. These are not entitled to be labelled organic, though the shopkeeper will be able to tell you what organic ingredients have been used.

The Price of Organic Food

At the present time organic food is often more expensive than conventional food, though there are many instances in this book where it costs the same or, in some cases, less. Organic farming itself is an efficient, cost-effective system. The single most important reason why organic food costs more to buy is because often it costs more to produce.

Crops

It is easier, quicker, less labour-intensive and therefore cheaper to tip out a bag of nitrogen fertiliser than to spread manure or make compost; to spray with a herbicide than to weed by hand or other mechanical means; to spray with a pesticide than to spend time inspecting plants, encouraging natural predators or investing in biological preventative measures. It is easier, instead of growing a green manure to provide natural soil fertility, to grow more crops. It is more economic to grow one crop (mono-cropping) intensively than to grow a mix of crops in smaller fields and rotate them so that pests and soil diseases do not build up and the soil does not become impoverished.

Animals

Animal welfare also comes with a considerable price tag. It is more labour-intensive and therefore expensive to raise animals extensively than intensively. Organic husbandry also incurs an extra financial penalty. Subsidies are paid on headage per hectare – fewer animals mean fewer subsidies and therefore less income. It is more expensive to give them natural feed, most of which must be organic and which therefore costs more than conventional feed;

it is more expensive to keep them longer and not to force their natural growth, instead of feeding them animal by-products and high-protein mixes which include antibiotics and growth-promoting agents to ensure that they grow to saleable weight in the minimum of time. It is more humane but more expensive to suckle calves naturally and keep them with their mothers or foster-mothers for twice as long, not to repeatedly squeeze as many piglets out of a sow as possible, and to give chickens more room to move around and freedom to graze.

Also:

- The price of organic food is usually compared unfavourably with food produced industrially in huge quantities. But you will find that, compared to other foods produced, like organic food, with care and dedication and in small quantities, not only are the prices comparable but, in many cases, organic food is cheaper.
- Organic food is still produced in very small quantities; in the UK, for example, it constitutes less than 0.5 per cent of all crops. This means more work and hence more expense for the retailer, who must source from several small suppliers instead of one. The organic food manufacturer also has to track down his or her certified ingredients from often diverse sources. And there is little room for manoeuvre as far as bulk buying or cost-cutting are concerned, and no cushioning for either retailer or shopper.
- The price you pay for organic food reflects what the food costs to produce and to get it to your table. Organic food producers spend little on advertising and do not use unnecessary packaging.
- The organic food sector bears additional annual costs of registration and certification, which give the consumer a farm-to-table guarantee.
- Organic foods are the only foods guaranteed to be free from genetically modified ingredients. To ensure this, the organic food sector bears the further cost of sourcing and buying non-genetically engineered foods and feedstuffs.

The prices of organic food can, however, be frustratingly erratic. The conventional food sector is a sophisticated market, relatively immune to seasonal changes and to unpredictable supplies and quantities, and because of the sheer volume of food processed it is able to guarantee stable prices or price ranges. When prices go up, they stay up. With organic food, on the other hand, we often don't know how much we should be paying. Organic products are sometimes on the shelves when we want them and sometimes not, prices are sometimes up and sometimes down. This is because the organic food sector is less well developed, because demand far outstrips supply, and because supplies are more seasonal.

But as anyone who buys organic food regularly will tell you, things are improving fast. The organic food market is getting bigger, better and more sophisticated daily. As organic food makes ever-greater inroads on to the supermarket shelves, as more growers and producers convert to organic methods, both supplies and prices are becoming more stable. And the more organic food there is, the more competitive prices will be. This is already happening in some sectors – organic yoghurt, for example, has been the same price as its conventional equivalent for over two years now. Organic vegetables are another sector where the gap has narrowed considerably and where promotional offers are a regular feature. Also, the more organic food grown, the lower the premiums will become, so that falling rather than rising prices can be expected.

For the shopper, meanwhile, the message is clear: be diligent, scour the shelves, compare prices when you can and take advantage of any bargains. Enjoy seasonal produce again, and accept that products may not always be available. Buying organic food when you can, even if only the occasional item, is the first significant step towards achieving a stable and thriving organic food sector – which, economists agree, will lead to affordable prices all of the time.

How Much It Costs in the Shops: Quashing the Myth

During the course of writing this book, I made repeated shopping trips to my local supermarkets, and compared the cost of each organic food item with its nearest equivalent conventional high-quality product. Every time, I found not a single item but several – on occasion up to half a dozen or so – that were the same price, or very close, and in some instances cheaper than their conventional counterparts. Here's a general idea of how my shopping basket worked out.

The same price Yeo Valley organic plain yoghurt, and Doves Farm large organic wholewheat loaf and organic full milk (compared to breakfast milk) were always the same price as their conventional counterparts. Other items recorded were Harmonie organic butter, lemons (4-pack), kiwi fruit, avocados, bagged new potatoes, and cauliflowers (which were about half the price of a pack of two conventional mini-cauliflowers).

Very close The prices of a wide range of fresh produce and other items, organic and conventional, were very close – that is, to around 10p or less – including white cabbage, prepacked carrots, Little Gem and Iceberg lettuce, Ellendale clementines, chilled Florida orange juice, organic pine forest honey, Lye Cross cheddar, Baby Organix yoghurts and Yeo Valley crème fraîche, and, occasionally, apples. Organic eggs worked out at 3p more each than the best free-range brand.

Cheaper Waitrose organic ice-cream is much cheaper than Häagen-Dazs. Loose organic chestnut mushrooms are consistently cheaper than ordinary boxed chestnut mushrooms, and boxed organic chestnut mushrooms often cheaper than ordinary boxed white mushrooms; 6-pack organic kiwi fruit are usually cheaper than conventional kiwis sold loose. Other items recorded as cheaper were onions, Mornflake porridge oats, 4-pack organic tomatoes, pears, Landsby Brie (compared to French Rustique) and Percol organic filter coffee.

Promotional offers Usually available on organic items, in the form of money off – for example, a 20p reduction on fruit yoghurts, a 35p reduction on organic coffee; or in the form of special offers – for example, organic flour, potatoes and kiwi fruit; or a pack of six for the price of four – for example, kiwis and tomatoes.

Bulk goods

Out of This World (p. 73) also track prices. The list below for bulk dried foods shows their own-label prepacked items, which they now stock only as organic because the price differences between organic and conventional have become marginal. The chart opposite is a useful guide to the kind of prices you should be paying for similar own-label prepacked dried foods, and indicates how price differentials are narrowing.

Barley flakes	Muesli base
Brown rice	Deluxe muesli base
Jumbo oats	Popcorn
Porridge oats	Quinoa
Rye flakes	
Wheat flakes	

		old selling price £	new selling price £	% down	non-organic selling price £	% difference organic/ non-organic
brown basmati	500g	199	149	25	139	7
white basmati	500g	249	179	28	149	17
bulgur wheat	500g	129	129	0	113	12
chick-peas	500g	140	129	8	87	33
couscous	500g	199	159	20	111	30
green lentils	500g	121	109	10	76	30
green split peas	500g	135	109	19	69	37
haricot beans	500g	128	119	7	89	25
pinto beans	500g	216	135	38	99	27
red lentils	500g	144	129	10	95	26
red kidney beans	500g	174	169	3	109	36
sesame seeds	250g	121	89	26	74	17
sesame seeds	500g	211	149	29	119	20
LWP cashews	250g	349	229	34	176	23
pumpkin seeds	250g	303	199	34	165	17
sunflower seeds	250g	139	99	29	79	20
sunflower seeds	500g	234	169	28	119	30

Source: *Out of This World, June 1997.*

Falling, falling, falling . . .

Finally, these prices, taken from the Better Food Company's (p. 121) newsletter, give an idea of how organic fresh produce prices fell from 1996 to 1997. Prices are per 450g.

	1996	1997
Carrots	70p	48p
Potatoes	38p	30p
Calabrese	£1.60	£1.35
Onions	56p	50p
Garlic	£4.81	£2.70
English apples	£1.05	98p
Bananas	£1.57	99p

what they say . . .

'The organic market has now reached critical mass, and prices are beginning to fall. A couple of years ago volumes were so small that most UK suppliers bought tiny amounts, usually through a UK importer, and often had to add large mark-ups as they sold so slowly (and because organics were seen as a speciality market which could take higher mark-ups). Now most suppliers are importing directly, and this combined with a more competitive market is bringing prices down dramatically. A year ago, Out of This World own-label organic prepacks were 50–100 per cent more expensive – now they are around 20–30 per cent.

'It's all very encouraging. Bulk prices are falling all the time and there are lots of new branded goods. Our sales of fresh fruit and veg and meat continue to grow steadily. Even *Vogue* magazine now has articles on Mick Jagger eating organic food and saying how great it is. It all seems to be moving in a positive spiral towards a bigger market, better prices, more organic farmers, lots of new products. Eventually the myth that organic food is far too expensive will vanish. We are looking forward to 100 per cent organic or fair-traded food within the next five years.' – *Jon Walker, buyer, Out of This World*

'Sometimes it can be more expensive, but not always. I have seen people choose *non*-organically grown food instead of organic food of the same price and quality . . . Hopefully more people will turn to organically grown food, and we will all be a lot healthier and the balance of nature will be as it should be.' – *Angela Duriez, Walkden, Manchester*

chapter two

pesticides and all that

Though pesticides have been in use since the ancient Egyptians and Greeks, synthetic pesticides are a modern phenomenon; before the 1940s they had hardly been heard of. Since then, over 1,000 active ingredients have been invented, and over 300 active ingredients and 3,500 pesticide products have been approved for use in the UK.

Pesticides are designed to kill. Many are highly hazardous, toxic and complex substances; though some biodegrade, others are persistent. Their use has had profound effects on the environment, on biodiversity and on wildlife, and they are a major pollutant. Pesticides in drinking-water are a fact of life, as is the accumulation of pesticides in seas. They are carried long distances in the atmosphere. Certain kinds, organochlorine pesticides (OCs) in particular, persist for many years and collect in the body fat of animals and humans; DDT, for example, was first found in human tissues in 1944 and continues to be present today. Responsible for thousands of farm workers' deaths from poisoning worldwide every year, pesticides – at least 168 at the last count – are also linked to major diseases of the immune system, cancer, allergies, infertility, and problems in foetal development. Though there are many who defend their efficacy and safety, and the agricultural benefits they bring, I have not found a single document that says they are good for the environment or for your health.

Though crop yields have increased, so have damage and loss due to heavier and more frequent pest attacks, exacerbated by the use of monocultural farming techniques. Pesticides have drastically reduced the numbers of natural predator species. Lack of natural control means that pest populations recover more quickly, requiring ever greater use of pesticides. Increased resistance to pesticides is a major problem, not just for agriculture but for public health, as in the case of malarial mosquitoes, for example. Resistance occurs very quickly – as little as five years after a pesticide has been introduced. As far back as 1985 nearly 450 insect species had developed resistance. More than 80 weed species have developed resistance to over 100 different herbicide strains, and 260 insect and mite species have already developed resistance to organophosphate pesticides (OPs). The result is the 'pesticide treadmill' – a cycle of resistance and secondary pest resurgence now experienced in major crops from bananas to cotton. So great is the problem that diseases such as barley yellow mosaic virus and potato blight are becoming difficult to control. Nor are pesticides effective always: up to 90 per cent of some applications is wasted, disappearing into the air or the environment.

It takes eight to ten years of research and £40–£60 million to develop a new pesticide. Testing procedures are more extensive than those for medicines, yet every year major pesticides once declared safe are banned. The EU list, for example, currently contains 21 banned pesticides. The World Health Organisation (WHO) has a 52-strong and a 78-strong list of pesticides classified as 'extremely hazardous' and 'highly hazardous' to operators and users, respectively. The EU Black and Red Lists of the most harmful chemicals that pollute the environment include OP and other pesticides; and the International Agency for Research on Cancer and the US Environmental Protection Agency have lists of pesticides thought to be probably or potentially carcinogenic to humans.

It is said that safety limits determining pesticide application rates are so strict, and residues, should they occur, so minimal, that they could never be a danger to anyone. To quote from the section on organophosphates in a booklet entitled *Pesticides: the Myth and the Facts*, published by the Fresh Fruit and Vegetable Information Bureau and endorsed by Sir Colin Berry, chairman of the Advisory Committee on Pesticides, 'It is the dosage which makes any chemical compound poisonous – not the substance itself' (a belief, incidentally, that dates back to the sixteenth-century German alchemist, Paracelsus, and which still remains the foundation of modern toxicology). Yet it is estimated that in the UK alone around 120g of active ingredients per head of population are used every year, and in fifteen years of UK monitoring the number of residues exceeding permitted levels, around 1 per cent, has remained approximately the same.

> **WATCHWORD: 'Pesticides'** is the general name given to any chemical used to control a pest or disease. It includes insecticides, herbicides, fungicides and various other '-icides' – such as acaricides (used to kill mites), molluscicides (to kill snails and slugs), nematicides (to kill eelworms) and rodenticides (to kill rats and mice). Desiccants, defoliants, fumigants, insect-repellants and -attractants and insect and plant growth-regulators are all pesticides. It should also be remembered that they are used extensively to control pests in the home and garden, on timber, in parks and other public places, in industry and on railway lines as well as on crops.

Definitions

Maximum Residue Level (MRL) and Acceptable Daily Intake (ADI), expressed in milligrams per kilogram (mg/kg), are the terms quoted whenever pesticide residues are discussed, and it is important to understand the difference between them. These definitions are taken from WPPR (Working Party on Pesticide Residues) reports:

Maximum Residue Level (MRL) The maximum concentration of a pesticide residue legally permitted in or on food commodities and animal feeds. Based on Good Agricultural Practice (GAP) data, it represents the maximum residue permissible when a pesticide has been applied in the correct dose and at the correct rate, in or on food when it leaves the farm gate. MRLs are thus the legal standard against which residues in food are measured. Though the MRL is the figure usually referred to, it is not a safety standard and has nothing to do with health.

Acceptable Daily Intake (ADI) The amount of a chemical that can be consumed every day of an individual's life in the practical certainty, on the basis of all known facts, that no harm will result, expressed as milligrams of chemical per kilogram of body weight (mg/kg). This is a safety standard, with very wide built-in safety margins, set at one hundred times less than the No Effect Level (NEL).

NOTE: MRL figures are set well below ADI figures. In practice, pesticide residues exceeding MRLs are common; those exceeding ADIs are very rare.

Pesticide Residues in Food

Residues are legally permitted to persist in or on food and hence at the dinner table. Tiny traces probably exist in most of the food we eat. It has been calculated that nearly one-third of pesticides used on food are suspected of being cancer agents in laboratory animals, another third may disrupt the human nervous system, and others may interfere with the endocrine systems. Residues exceeding MRLs are common, and persistent pesticides long-banned such as DDT (prohibited in the UK since 1984) are regularly detected. Because only a tiny minority of foods sampled – approximately 1 per cent – exceeds MRLs, conventional food is deemed safe to eat. The official annual report on pesticide monitoring, produced by the WPPR, states that the majority of foods have no detectable residues; while this is encouraging, it still means that pesticide traces, however minute, are detected in 30–40 per cent of the samples tested.

Testing for pesticides

Though the latest annual figures state that some 3,400 samples are taken and nearly 60,000 tests are currently undertaken, in addition to those carried out by industry, the amount of food tested is insignificant compared to that eaten. Sample sizes are small, and though basic food groups are constantly monitored, the range of foods tested is limited. Sampling tests do not cover all pesticides used, concentrating only on those in most frequent use or those most likely to be a problem. A graphic example can be found in the first Total Diet Survey (see p. 38), when an OP pesticide not found regularly turned up at levels calculated to be twice the ADI for infants.

MRLs are not set for every active ingredient or pesticide. Currently only about a third (117 out of 330) of active ingredients are covered, and this can and does affect monitoring results. For example, residues usually occur in most strawberries tested, but when the first analysis for the EU monitoring programme – which came into effect in 1996 – was done, residues had dropped fourfold. The EU surveys are directed at pesticides where MRLs have been set, while the UK surveys include a broader range and therefore more are detected. Further, apart from specific targeted examples – for instance, apples, bananas, peaches, pears, tomatoes, and imported lamb and Chinese rabbit – pesticide-monitoring on imported foods is even scantier, estimated at around one chemical analysis for every 6,500 tonnes. This means, effectively, that test results, whether negative or positive, can only be at best an indication of the real situation, and that their real purpose and value are regulatory.

It is now recognised that sampling techniques do not necessarily tell the whole picture. For example, residues that may be commonly measured in the skin or peel of a fruit can penetrate into the flesh. Pesticides can 'bind' to cereal crops in such a way that, until radio-tracer techniques recently became available, they have gone unnoticed. Indeed, improved sampling techniques are now showing that many pesticide residues may have formerly gone undetected. Moreover, the variability in residues is much greater than was previously thought, which means that *individual* samples of, say, carrots may have much higher levels of residues than found overall. This, according to the Ministry of Agriculture, 'may be the norm rather than the exception', and as a result, MRLs may need to be revised – which is little comfort for anyone who enjoys eating raw carrots. The same variability, ranging from twice to twenty-nine times greater than sample test levels, has just been found in apples, bananas, oranges, peaches, pears, nectarines and tomatoes. Potatoes, celery and kiwi fruit are next on the list to be investigated.

fact

£2 million is spent annually on detecting pesticide residues by the Working Party on Pesticide Residues alone. This is twice as much as the annual R&D budget for organic farming. £375,000 is also spent annually on monitoring pesticide usage.

Official advice

Official advice is based on the premise that pesticides are used and disposed of properly, always according to manufacturers' instructions. Unfortunately, misuse and pollution are rampant. The fact that most UK farmers are responsible people, actively trying to reduce pesticide use, is encouraging but of little consequence given that the food market is a global one. Reduction in the use of pesticides still means that 99 per cent of UK farmers are spraying a total of 23,000 tonnes, or about 1 billion gallons, in the UK annually. It also means that misuse occasionally continues to take place. The number of such incidents reported, published by the Health and Safety Executive (HSE), continues to rise: it was 250 in 1994/5. The 1995 WPPR annual report found no improvement in the use of non-approved pesticides on UK winter lettuce samples, 10 per cent of which were found either to have residues of non-approved pesticides or to be above MRLs; it also highlighted the use of non-approved chlormequat pesticide on UK pears. The 1996 report was much more encouraging, but found residues in over 90 per cent of samples, MRLs exceeded in some cases, and possible misuse of approved pesticides.

The daily dose

Exposure to pesticides is a constant drip process; it can occur through the skin, via inhalation, and through drinking water as well as through eating food. Generally, oral ingestion is the main route and results in the highest toxicity. To reassure people, the WPPR have just begun to calculate the average daily dose of pesticides received in the average diet, testing cooked as well as raw food, and to assess the risk factors involved for infants, schoolchildren and adults. This is known as the Total Diet Survey. Twenty different food groups have been analysed. Their results show that the average daily diet contains traces of thirty different pesticides, including OPs and OCs; DDT, for example, was found in eight food groups and lindane in five. In the vast majority of cases the levels ingested, calculated as risk levels, were below 10 per dent of the ADIs, and in some cases were less than 1 per cent. However, two OPs found in fruit scored too highly for comfort. One was found to be over 50 per cent and the other 140 per cent of their ADIs for adults; for infants this intake would exceed ADI by a factor of 1.8 and twofold.

The cocktail effect

When pesticides are developed, their effect on other pesticides is not generally taken into account or studied. Consequently, the cocktail effect of repeatedly ingesting infinitesimal amounts of different pesticides is not known. The official word from government advisers is that there is no danger to health. But many eminent scientists and doctors think otherwise, and studies, particularly from America, are now beginning to confirm their concerns. Two examples can illustrate this. A report published in the US journal *Science*, in June 1996, showed that combinations of two or three common pesticides, at low levels that might be found in the environment, are up to 1,600 times as powerful as the individual pesticides alone. More recently, researchers from New Orleans investigating the effects of pesticides and toxic chemicals – polychlorinated biphenyls (PCBs) – on the human hormone system have found that exposure to very tiny amounts of two chemicals at the same time can have an effect a thousand times greater than either chemical alone.

Can you wash pesticides off?

Washing removes a certain amount of some pesticides, but not all. Many surface-contact pesticides are designed to withstand rain, and tests show that anything between 75 and 93 per cent remains after washing. Peeling fruit, for instance, will remove more of a surface-contact pesticide than will washing. Systemic pesticides, on the other hand, enter the plant, remain within the flesh of the fruit, vegetable or grain and cannot be removed by washing or peeling. This is one of the probable reasons why residues are detected, for example, in shelled nuts or bananas.

fact

Over a hundred experimental studies have shown that widely used pesticides can alter and suppress normal human immune-system responses. This is now being confirmed by epidemiological studies. A new report from the World Resources Institute reaffirms these concerns and suggests that pesticides may worsen, and increase fatalities from, viral illnesses, particularly in children.

Products have now been introduced, such as Veggie Wash, which remove surface pesticide residues, including post-harvest treatments, microbial pathogens and other surface contaminants such as atmospheric pollutants, dust and dirt. A test performed by the Pesticides Trust found Veggie Wash effective in reducing the amounts of residues by around 40–90 per cent, depending on the pesticide. It can be bought at organic, wholefood and health food shops, and alternative supermarkets.

Do food-processing and cooking remove pesticides?

No one seems really sure. Cooking and food-processing are assumed to reduce residues, and indeed they do in some cases, but obviously much depends on the kind of pesticide concerned and its stability. For example, while the WPPR found none in processed tomato products, and amounts of some residues in potatoes were reduced when cooked, those in fruits used to make jams remained. Other examples in the book where pesticides – including OCs and OPs in some cases – have survived processing are breakfast cereals, biscuits, crisps and maize-based snacks, chocolate, dried pasta and bread. They have also been detected in infant meals. Although peeling will reduce residues, it also reduces fibre and nutrient levels.

The global perspective

The fact that the carrot you are eating may or may not have any detectable pesticide residues pales into insignificance compared to the worldwide use and misuse of pesticides. Nearly 5 billion lb of DDT have been used globally over the last fifty years, for example, and some 5–6 billion lb of pesticides are added to the world's environment every year. In the Third World, where there is inadequate information and training, and low literacy among many farm workers, misuse is rife. The Third World already uses many thousand of tonnes of pesticides, and is set to use double the present amount over the next ten years. It is seen as the major growth area for Western agrochemical companies, some of whom export pesticides banned in their own countries. Third World governments actively support increased pesticide use and offer subsidies to farmers and growers who use them. Older, more hazardous pesticides, or those whose patents have expired, can be produced cheaply in some countries. Rural communities have easy access to these dangerous substances. Often it is women and children who work in the fields who are the most exposed. Pesticides are commonly mixed by hand, used with no or inadequate protective clothing, and stored insecurely in gardens or homes.

The safe disposal of pesticides is minimally regulated; an estimated world total of over 100,000 tonnes of obsolete pesticides remains lying around waiting to be disposed of. The statistics in terms of human health are horrific: according to the World Health Organisation, an estimated three million cases of acute severe pesticide poisonings occur worldwide every year, including two hundred thousand fatalities.

The Pesticide File

Shopping for food and concern over pesticide residues in your food tend to overshadow the larger picture.

Pesticides and people

The Arctic has become the dumping-ground for pesticides used in tropical regions and for other toxic chemicals, because they are carried in the air and condense over the Arctic. As a result, the Innuit people suffer from the highest levels ever found of a group of polychlorinated biphenyl (PCBs) insecticides in their bodies. PCBs, banned in most industrialised countries, are suspected of causing cancer, suppressing fertility and damaging the immune system. Other Arctic peoples have seven times the amount of PCBs as people living in temperate parts of Canada. Innuit women also have some of the highest concentrations of OCs in their breast milk recorded in humans, while Greenlanders have more than seventy times as much of the OC hexachlorobenzene in their bodies. Polar bears, seals, fish and birds of prey are also heavily polluted.

Pesticides, resistance, and the treadmill

America provides a graphic illustration of the fact that, in the long term, pesticides are not as efficacious as they are presumed to be. In the last fifty years or so, insecticide use has increased tenfold, while crop losses from insect damage have almost doubled. Insecticides are used on three crops in particular: corn, cotton and apples. For corn, despite a thousandfold increase in insecticide use, it has been calculated that losses to insects have increased 400 per cent. Before the introduction of pesticides, there were three pests that affected cotton crops in Central America. With the advent of pesticides, applied eight times per season, three more major pests appeared. Pesticide applications were then increased to up to twenty-eight per season, eventually accounting for half of production costs. By the 1970s yields had begun to decline, there were now eight major pest species to contend with, and pesticide applications had risen to up to forty per season in some areas.

Pesticides and wildlife

By disrupting the food chain of various ecosystems, pesticides kill organisms not only directly, but indirectly too. Kill one pest and another species, who lives off that pest, dies. To take a simple example: before pesticides were introduced, 17 per cent of British flowering plants were found in cereal fields; now there are hardly any, and plants once thought of as troublesome weeds – corn buttercup, corn parsley – are now among the rarest in the country. The insects that live off those flowers have disappeared. Similarly, at least ten farmland bird species have declined by 50 per cent or more during the last twenty-five years, with the indirect effect of pesticides cited as a major cause. These include the tree sparrow (an 89 per cent decline), grey partridge (82 per cent), bullfinch (76 per cent), spotted flycatcher and song thrush (73 per cent), lapwing (62 per cent) and reed bunting (61 per cent). To halt the decline, the RSPB is pressing for major support for organic farming.

Pesticides and drinking-water

Pesticides in drinking-water supplies are a major concern, and it is clear that not all residues can be detected. In the UK, the major pesticides found are herbicides. OPs from sheep-dipping and from washing wool used in the textile industry are also common in the water of certain areas. The 1996 Drinking Water Inspectorate (DWI) annual report revealed twenty-three pesticides present above the EU standard of 0.1 microgram per litre; one, the OC heptachlor, banned in the UK since 1981, was present at levels four times above WHO guidelines. In another study on nitrates, pesticides and lead in water, for 1995/6, the DWI detected ten new pesticides above the EU standard, including OCs such as DDT and

NTAEs: new harvests, old problems

NTAEs, non-traditional agro-exports, is the term used for imported produce such as snow peas from Guatemala, asparagus from Peru, strawberries, peppers and tomatoes from Mexico, apples and pears from Chile, and exotic fruit such as mangoes, melons, passion fruit and pineapples from Latin America and the Caribbean. All, including the latest boom crops, flowers, are grown with heavy chemical inputs, including pesticides – even more, in some cases, than are applied to cotton, coffee and sugar cane. Ecuador's roses, for example, soak up three-quarters of production costs in insecticides and fungicides, Guatemalan snow peas over a third.

Pesticide-residue violations, through excessive application or spraying too close to harvest time, are a serious problem, especially in Guatemala and Mexico, leading to crops regularly being detained by US officials. Similar serious pesticide residues have been recorded for oriental vegetables grown in the Dominican Republic.

In Chile, where pesticide imports have more than doubled over the last ten years, and apples and pears are a major export business, the environmental and health damage caused by pesticides, including increasing numbers of children born with defects, is now a serious government concern.

Source Lori Ann Thrup, in *Growing Food Security.*

heptachlor. One-off accidents are also common. In 1996, a drum of lindane, dumped into a stream near Maidstone in Kent – described as an act of 'mindless vandalism' – caused Southern Water to close its drinking-water pumping station for a few days; the Dow Chemical Company was fined for a herbicide spill which polluted a Norfolk spring; and another herbicide applied to a farm pond in Devon made its way to the River Dart and to a local water-treatment works.

Water pollution is a major problem throughout Europe. In Germany, the Munich Water Company has decided that it is more cost-effective to pay farmers to go organic than to extract pesticide and fertiliser residues from drinking-water. As a result, nitrate residues have been reduced by one-third and the herbicide atrizine by four-fifths.

Pesticide Facts

- Ten companies now control over 80 per cent of the global agrochemical market, valued in 1995 at US$30 billion. Twenty-five per cent of sales are in developing countries, and this figure is increasing.
- Despite a tenfold increase in the use of chemical insecticides since the First World War, the loss of food and fibre crops to insects has risen from 7 to 13 per cent. At least 520 species of insects and mites, 150 plant diseases and 113 weeds have become resistant to pesticides meant to control them. An American study has shown that the European corn-borer moth lays eighteen times more eggs on sweetcorn plants grown in chemically farmed soils than on organic soils. Analysis revealed the mineral ratios to be responsible.
- In the agricultural sector worldwide, 14 per cent of all known occupational injuries and 10 per cent of all fatal injuries are caused by pesticides.
- Sixty active pesticide ingredients have been classified by recognised authorities as being carcinogenic to some degree. Eighteen pesticides have been identified as

disrupting hormonal balance. Oestrogen-mimicking chemicals, which include several pesticides, have been linked to falling sperm counts.

- Numerous studies show a higher incidence of cancers and related disorders in individuals occupationally exposed to pesticides. These include cancers of the lung and kidney, and testicular cancers and leukaemias.
- Organophosphates are the most widely used pesticides in the world.
- There are 330 active pesticide ingredients registered for use in the UK.
- A minimum of £2 million per year in the UK is spent on monitoring pesticide residues in food, twice the annual R&D budget for organic farming.
- It is estimated that one teaspoonful of concentrated pesticide could pollute the water supply of twenty thousand people for a day. A recent survey of drinking-water quality identified 298 UK water supplies contaminated with pesticides, with nearly a quarter exceeding the Maximum Admissible Concentration (MAC) of residues. Sixteen different active pesticide substances were detected.
- In the UK some vegetable crops may receive, on average, up to 9 pesticide sprays, soft fruit up to 10, and apples up to 24 treatments.

Sources *Pesticide Trust Review 1996*, *Pesticide News* (various), *Environment and Health News* (various), *The Environment Handbook*, 1997.

Pesticide Groups: The Basics

From the point of view of potential residues, pesticides fall into four main groups:

Contact pesticides are those that are sprayed on to the crop, remain on the surface and kill on contact.

Systemic pesticides are those that enter the plant or organism and remain in the tissues.

Persistent pesticides are those that are stable, do not biodegrade easily, and persist in the environment – and remain active – for anything from a few months to several years.

Non-persistent pesticides biodegrade and quickly become inactivated.

Persistent organic pollutants, collectively known as 'POPs', all break down very slowly and bioaccumulate in the tissues of living organisms; that is to say, they accumulate progressively, by being eaten, from plants to animals to humans, increasing in concentration as they advance up the food chain. They are found in all parts of the ecosystem – in the air, rain, ground water, sediments and soil, as well as in the plants and animals themselves; and, once released into the wider environment, POPs cannot be retrieved. They include major pesticides such as dioxins, dieldrin, PCBs, endosulfan, chlordane and DDT.

The two most important groups of pesticides that are regularly tested for residues are *organochlorines* (*OCs*) and *organophosphates* (*OPs*). Other important groups are *phenoxyacetic acids*, *carbamates*, *synthetic pyrethroids* and *EBDC fungicides*.

In the West, OCs have largely been replaced. OPs, carbamates such as carbaryl, aldicarb and pirimicarb, and synthetic pyrethroids such as cypermethrin and deltamethrin, are used extensively, the latter because they degrade relatively quickly and are generally not very toxic to birds and mammals. However, they are highly toxic to aquatic life, including fish, and to bees. EBDCs are a group of highly toxic fungicides extensively used worldwide. In fresh foods they are apparently unstable and residues are rarely detected. They can break down into ethylene thiourea which, if found present with the original EBDC, may increase when food is stored, cooked or processed. Both are described as 'toxicologically significant' and have been linked to animal tumours.

As far as residues in food are concerned, OCs and OPs are the most important and the ones that you see most often referred to in this book.

Organochlorines

OCs were the first pesticides to be developed, were used extensively during the 1940s–70s, and include most of the notoriously problematic ones such as DDT, and the 'drins' such as aldrin, dieldrin and endrin. They are highly persistent and volatile broadspectrum insectides, many of which, because of their persistence in the environment and their tendency to accumulate in food chains, in body fat, in plant oils and in the waxes on fruit skins, have now been banned in the West. They are ever with us, nonetheless: DDT has found its way to the remotest parts of the world, including Antarctica. They are found in human fat such as breast fat, and in breast milk, and appear to transfer freely across the placenta from mother to foetus. They have been linked to cancer and reproductive disorders; they kill wildlife and have been responsible for widespread reproductive failure in birds. Synthetic organochlorine compounds occur sparingly in nature. Vertebrates are not well adapted to dealing with them in large quantities, having little or no means of breaking them down. Once present in body fat, some may persist for a lifetime – DDE, which forms when DDT breaks down, for example, lasts almost as long as the average human life.

Many common pesticides other than OCs contain carbonchlorine bonds, but are not so persistent. For example, a quarter of the pesticides on the UK's approved list (118), including tecnazene used to prevent potatoes from sprouting, contain chlorine. Other pesticides, whose adverse effects are not so well known, are *presumed* 'safer' and more 'friendly'.

Lindane

Lindane is a special case. Though banned in many countries, it is the only remaining OC widely used in the UK as a domestic and agricultural insecticide, wood preservative and seed treatment, and to control headlice. In agriculture it is used on cereals, oil seed rape, sugar beet (a major ingredient in cattle feed); on a range of field vegetables such as brassicas and beans, and top and soft fruit; and it is also used in forestry, and on ornamental plants and turf. Highly volatile, when applied to field crops in particular, up to 90 per cent enters the atmosphere, later to be deposited by rain. It is found in increasing concentrations in the North Sea and is dangerous to fish. It features on the EU Black List of dangerous substances and on the PAN (Pesticide Action Network) 'dirty dozen' list of pesticides considered to be among the most dangerous in the world.

Though lindane degrades more quickly than other OCs, its breakdown products are more persistent and more dangerous. The manufacture of lindane produces highly toxic wastes, themselves used to make other OC compounds, referred to as the 'lindane chain of poison'. In Spain, every tonne of lindane has been shown to produce 5 tonnes of waste benzene hexachloride (BHC), an insecticide in its own right rejected as too toxic in twenty-eight countries.

Lindane is one of the most common pesticide residues detected in UK foods, particularly animal products. MRLs in milk have regularly been exceeded, and it has been reported in breast fat and breast milk worldwide. Infants and children are significantly more susceptible to its toxic effects. Other foods in which it has been detected include lettuce, chocolate, sweetcorn, eggs, meat, game, eels and potatoes.

Lindane is an endocrine disruptor, and is classed as a probable carcinogen. There is a significant body of evidence that suggests that where lindane is used extensively (such as on sugar beet in Lincolnshire) and where cattle are exposed to it, incidence of breast cancer is higher. Government authorities and scientists, describing it as a carcinogen that does not cause damage to DNA, state that traces of this type of carcinogen cannot affect human health; new research conducted in the USA questions this.

Lindane is known to penetrate the placenta barrier, and there is thought to be a link between lindane exposure and abnormal foetal development and spontaneous abortion. Other suspected

fact

The UK has the highest rate of death from breast cancer in the world. In Lincolnshire, the rate is 40 per cent higher than the national average. In Israel, since lindane has been banned, there has been a significant fall in the number of breast cancers, particularly among younger women; it is worth noting that dietary levels of lindane had been within the WHO ADIs before the ban.

effects include growth retardation, damage to the nervous system and liver, and immunosuppression. *Sources Dispatches*: *The Lindane Legacy*; Women's Environmental Network briefing paper; *Pesticide News*, fact sheet; *Chocolate Unwrapped*.

Organophosphates

OPs were developed to replace OCs, and are the most widely used group of insecticides in the world. In the UK, they account for around 60 per cent of the arable insecticide market. Anyone who has seen TV documentaries such as the 'World in Action' two-part series shown in Autumn 1997 cannot but have serious reservations about their safety. They are nerve poisons, developed originally as a by-product of nerve gases during the Second World War. When introduced they were declared perfectly safe for humans. Though less persistent than OCs, breaking down within a few months, they are acutely toxic to all vertebrates; they affect the central and peripheral nervous systems of humans, can cause irreversible damage and death, and are also toxic to aquatic life. Some have been found to damage DNA, while others – malathion, for example – break down when exposed to heat and air into more toxic compounds.

Organophosphates are described – and you will find this on the labels of domestic products containing them – as 'inhibiting cholinesterase activity'. What this means is that they inhibit the substance that helps nerve endings to transmit messages to each other. Without it, nerves can't work properly. The best-known organophosphates are those used in sheep-dips and during the Gulf War; dichlorvos, used in salmon-farming and in mushroom production; and those found in headlice treatments for children and in animals' flea collars. Another used regularly on UK produce, chlorpyrifos, has recently been criticised by the Environmental Protection Agency in America because of its adverse health effects. Over a hundred organophosphates exist, mainly insecticides, including contact, systemic and fumigant types, but there are also a number of related organophosphate herbicides and fungicides. In addition to their agricultural uses – they are applied to wheat, vegetables, top and soft fruit, for example – they are widely used in domestic and catering-industry pest control. While in agriculture their use is highly regulated and

Dear Doctor

Q I, like many parents, am alarmed by recent reports about dangerous levels of pesticides in our food. What, if anything, can we do to reduce any health risk?

A The health risks from eating food contaminated by pesticides are small and are more than outweighed by the benefits of eating five portions of fresh produce daily. That said, it makes sense to take steps to reduce any risk.

Use home-grown or organic produce where possible, wash all fruit and vegetables before cooking, and peel everything before eating.

– *Dr Mark Porter,* Radio Times, *Easter issue, 1997*

the dangers of too much exposure well known, this is not the case domestically, and I would strongly advise you not to use any products containing them in the home or garden.

OP residues in food are regularly detected. A large percentage of poisonings worldwide is due to occupational exposure to OPs. Other serious health effects due to OP exposure include psychiatric, nervous, cardiac, eye and chronic fatigue disorders similar to ME (myalgic encephalomyelitis). They have also been implicated in birth defects, though this is controversial, and in suicides. Recent research from Spain, for example, has shown that farmers using OPs are four times more likely to commit suicide. In England the suicide rate among farmers is two and a half times the national average. Psychiatrists and heart specialists have joined forces to persuade the government to ban OPs. All are on the Black List of harmful chemicals drawn up by the EU to protect aquatic environments. Little is known as yet about long-term neurological consequences from low-level repeated exposure.

Usage Worldwide, OPs and OCs are used on all arable crops: this includes fruit and vegetables, cereal crops and cotton.

In the UK, several OPs are used extensively. Those in regular use include:

- on fruit – fenitrothion, chlorpyrifos and pirimiphos-methyl
- on mushrooms – dichlorvos
- on potatoes – dimethoate and heptenophos
- on protected crops – heptenophos
- on outdoor vegetable crops – dimethoate, heptenophos, demeton-S-methyl and trizophos
- on wheat – dimethoate and chlorpyrifos

Lindane and endosulfan are the only two common OCs in general use. Lindane is used fairly widely on wheat, spring barley and sugar beet, on some apples and pears and on soft fruit such as strawberries and raspberries, in mushroom production and as a seed treatment. Endosulfan is mainly used on soft fruits.

Carbamates and synthetic pyrethroids are used widely on all crops; the use of synthetic pyrethroids is increasing, including in sheep-dips. For specific examples see pesticide usage and residue information in Appendix 1 on p. 325.

Genetic Engineering and GMOs

For the last fifty years we have been grappling with the effects of pesticides in our food; for the next fifty we will have genetically engineered foods to contend with too. As with pesticides, the fact that we eat them is just the tip of the iceberg. Their effects on animal and human health and the environment are completely unknown, and are likely to remain so for some time to come.

Genetic manipulation, genetic engineering, genetic modification and genetic biotechnology are different terms for the same process – namely, the extraction and insertion of genes from one species to another and from plants to animals, to create new types of crops and animals, and herbicide- and pest-resistant plants. These are usually described by the prefix GM (genetically modified), or GMO (genetically modified organism). Flavr Savr tomatoes, for example, contain fish genes to prolong shelf life, and Roundup soya beans contain genes from soil bacteria, cauliflower and petunias to make them herbicide-resistant. It is no accident that pesticides and genetically engineered food crops are often mentioned together, for they are often produced by the same chemical companies, who see biotechnology as the commercial opportunity of the future; by 1996, already over twenty thousand new GMO projects had been started, involving over six hundred companies in a market estimated at £330 million.

Flavr Savr tomatoes and Roundup soya beans have been developed by Monsanto chemical company, which also developed Bovine Somatotropin (BST), the genetically modified hormone used to stimulate milk production in dairy cows, currently banned in Europe for 'socio-economic' reasons until the year 2000. Polly, the cloned sheep, genetically altered to include human genes so as to produce a blood-clotting protein, is another of many instances of animals being used as 'bioreactors' to product pharmaceuticals in their blood or milk for human use, while the geep, a new animal bred from a goat and a sheep, offers the promise of a tough, woolly milker.

Reasonable concerns

Though genetic engineering, like Aladdin's cave, offers undreamed-of possibilities, it also generates many grave concerns. Genetic engineering is an experiment on a vast scale, with animals, human beings and the environment its guinea-pigs. Essentially a no-holds-barred, untested and imprecise technology which bears no resemblance to traditional breeding methods, it moves genes around at random to suit particular purposes. But genes are not discrete inanimate bits, nor do they work in isolation. They are fluid entities that interact with their environment, and just because a given gene has a particular effect in one organism does not mean it will have that effect in another.

There are many other implications. For example, GM plants bred to be pesticide-resistant are specific to a particular pesticide. They have to be grown in conjunction with that pesticide, which results in greater not less pesticide use, and estimates predict a threefold increase in herbicide use. Because they are living organisms and thus self-perpetuating, once in the environment, GMOs are here to stay. The repercussions of this are manifold. Natural species could be driven out, with GM plants becoming 'superweeds' and GM animals, such as salmon and carp, becoming 'superanimals' – a potentially disastrous outcome. There is also a real risk that GMOs will breed with native species, spreading GM genes to other species; this has already happened with radish, oil seed rape and potatoes.

Animal welfare is affected, too. Cloned sheep sometimes produce giant lambs up to twice the normal birth size, so that they have to be delivered by Caesarian, thereby causing their mothers unnatural stress and suffering. Health implications include the fact that GMOs are potential allergens and that the widespread use of antibiotic-resistant marker genes may render some antibiotics ineffective in the future.

Finally, there is the worry that genetic engineering could threaten one of the most important biological controls in existence. One particular bacterium, *Bacillus thuringiensis* (Bt), used to combat pests, has been the cornerstone of sustainable agriculture since the 1960s. Transgenic plants, with Bt in their genetic make-up, are now being approved; widespread use of these will lead to Bt-resistance in major pests and could destroy the effectiveness of Bt against some of agriculture's most intransigent enemies. At the time of writing, Austria and Luxembourg were considering suing the EU over its decision to lift its ban on Bt corn, and a legal petition has been filed against the Environmental Protection Agency in America for allowing the release of Bt crops.

The state of play

Market research shows that most consumers distrust genetic engineering and do not view the prospect of sci-fi plants and beasts with enthusiasm. Within the EU, either they have said no to GMOs, or they have indicated that they want the segregation and clear labelling of GM foods. Some member states have taken unilateral action to ban GM soya and maize or to insist on products being labelled, as have some of the biggest food manufacturers. Austria is holding firm in its ban. The UK government supports clear labelling but has taken no other action, the Food Safety minister, Jeff Rooker, merely stating: 'The use of genetics to produce better-quality food has tremendous advantages, but it needs to be regulated and labelled properly.'

At the moment, only a few foods such as soya beans, maize, oil seed rape and the Flavr Savr tomato have been released on to the world market, though GM enzymes are widely used in rennet to make vegetarian cheese. In the UK, GM sugar beet and oil seed rape are being trialled in Cambridgeshire and GM strawberries may be next. Many more GM foods are in the pipeline, including a wide range of vegetable crops. EU revision of rules on the release of GMOs into the environment is still being finalised, but does not bode well for consumers. On labelling, it has now been decided to have three sorts of labels for seeds, feeds and foods – namely, 'does contain GMOs', 'does not contain GMOs', or 'may contain GMOs'; the fear is that this will lead to ambiguity and to most foods being labelled as 'mays'.

Organic farming and genetic engineering

Organic farming is the only agricultural system to have rejected genetic engineering: it has declared unequivocally that genetically modified organisms have no place in organic farming systems. This covers the use of GMOs in crops, animals, food ingredients and processing aids, including enzymes such as genetically engineered rennet for cheese. Organic food is therefore the only food that is guaranteed to be free of GMOs, that offers no possibility of GMOs entering the food chain from animal feeds.

What's next on the menu?

A report in the *Guardian* in November 1997 highlighted what scientists say could soon be on our dinner plates with the aid of

> **fact**
>
> Monsanto predict that within a decade the majority of staple crops will be grown from GM seed; the area in the US used to cultivate GM crops increased from six million acres in 1996 to thirty million acres in 1997.

Ready for Roundup?

Genetically modified Roundup Ready Soya bean (RRS), developed by Monsanto and resistant to their own herbicide, Roundup (glyphosate), is a test case. The reason it is so significant is twofold. Soya is a major foodstuff, both as an important source of non-dairy protein for vegetarians and as a processing aid, with soya products found in over half of all processed foods and in some thirty thousand food products. Soya oil, soya flour and soya lecithin, for example, are used in bread, margarine, ice-cream, biscuits, chocolate, baby food, beer and other staple foods. Soya beans are also entering the food chain through being used extensively in animal feeds. This means that unless GM soya is segregated from conventional soya, it will be virtually impossible to avoid eating it. The same applies to maize and rape seed and their products, which are also universally used in processed foods. Already it's estimated that 40 per cent of all soya beans grown currently are GM soya beans. If legislation or clear labelling laws are not put in place to allow consumers to choose whether or not to eat GM soya, then many GM foods will follow in its wake.

genetic engineering. It includes low fat chips, fruits containing vaccines against diseases, super high protein rice that has genes from peas, pest-killing cauliflowers that have a snowdrop gene, and super fast-growing salmon.

what they say . . .

'I am worried by the complete commercialisation that is happening now in genetic engineering. It seems to me that we are at the beginning of a Gadarene rush irreversibly to transform the plants which constitute the staples of the human food chain within a few short decades. That food chain has always been taken for granted as part of the birthright of every person on this planet, and rightly: it has taken many millions of years to co-evolve with mammalian and other vertebrate species.

'Whenever a new technology emerges there is, by definition, very little evidence of its potentially harmful side-effects. It is invariably the unforeseen event which causes the most serious problem. When DDT and other bulk chemical pesticides were first introduced they were widely sold on the assurance that they were harmless to humans and fatal to insects. Who would have predicted their bioaccumulative chronic hormone-disrupting effects?

'History has a habit of repeating itself. Multinational conglomerates are moving away from bulk chemicals and heading instead into biotechnology, where there is still, as happened with pesticides, little evidence of the 'downside' and, as yet, relatively little regulation. The manufacturers of GM organisms are not in a position to give any reassurance on the long-term health implications of what they are doing. It is probably not our generation that will have to cope with any subsequent disasters, but our successors. However, there will be no chance of remedial action with GMOs that have gone wrong. We are told the risks are low, but it only has to happen once. Before Chernobyl it was always considered a "vanishingly small risk" that such a disaster could occur – until it did.

'Because genetic engineering tampers with life as we know it for evermore, it is imperative that everyone should feel some "ownership" of these issues, and that political decision-makers should learn from the historical evidence that we have of problems with pervasive technologies and lean towards scepticism about the claims of those who stand to profit directly from the gene revolution.' – *Dr Vyvyan Howard, President of the Royal Microscopical Society, Head of Research, Foetal and Infant Toxico-pathology Group, University of Liverpool. Abstracted from* Science in Parliament, *August 1997*

For more information on pesticide use, see Appendix 1, p. 325.

organic food and where to buy it

Where to Start

Given that potential residues concern most people, if you need to make choices – and most of us do – about what to buy, the pointers that follow may give you suggestions as to which basic popular foods to change to organic first. Fuller information can be found within the various sections. But remember that, while eating organic food will keep your intake of residues down to a minimum, organic food cannot claim to be pesticide-free. Also:

- When trying to decide, consider your own eating preferences and patterns. Wherever possible, make your organic priority those foods you eat a lot of.
- Include organic foods priced near to their conventional equivalents, or cheaper (see p. 29).
- Don't forget the foods you eat occasionally or consider as treats, such as chocolate, really good cream or butter, even cakes and biscuits. Judged per spoonful or slice, the extra cost is very little.
- Include bulk dried foods – brown rice, pasta, beans, sultanas and raisins. These store well and, again, the extra cost per serving is minimal.

● Finally, experiment. Sample different organic foods as and when you can. Biscuits, cornflakes, tinned tomatoes, passata, tortilla chips, crisps, tahini, mustard and stock cubes are all good bets.

Baby food An equally important question to ask is 'When to start?', and the answer to that is clear – from the earliest age. Babies and toddlers are particularly vulnerable to chemicals such as pesticides, so incorporate into their diet as much organic food, including fruit juices, as you can. For more on baby food, see p. 233.

Fresh produce Pesticide residues, however tiny, are undoubtedly present in most fresh produce. Crops that have exceeded the Maximum Residue Limits (MRLs) and/or that have caused most concern are carrots, cucumbers, lettuce, tomatoes and potatoes, and apples, citrus fruits (if you use the rind), grapes, peaches, pears and strawberries. So make all of these an organic priority. Also, sweetcorn, mushrooms and stored white cabbage, as well as any fresh organic produce priced attractively – that is, close to its non-organic equivalent. Plus vegetable juices, definitely, and fruit juices, especially organic apple juice, as and when you can.

Flour and breakfast cereals Pesticide residues in conventional wheat are a fact of life. Since most are present in the outer layers of the grain, white flour is less affected than wholewheat. Residues are also regularly detected in corn-based cereals. Make these, and organic wholewheat and brown breads, bran and bran products and wholewheat pasta a top priority. I would also add oats or oatmeal, and muesli and other corn-based products.

Baked goods The absence, in organic baked goods, of chemically hydrogenated fat, refined white sugar, preservatives and artificial flavourings is an added attraction. Start with wholemeal cakes and biscuits and flapjacks – and anything else that takes your fancy.

Other grains Any unrefined grain may contain pesticide residues; refined grains are far less likely to contain detectable amounts. It still makes sense, though, to make brown rice (which is good value) and any other whole grains your top priority. I would also add here any grains or seeds you buy for sprouting. Note, too, that products such as bulgur, as well as organic couscous and polenta, usually have more flavour.

Dairy produce Lindane (see p. 47) is the most worrying residue found in dairy products. Women and children are more vulnerable to any potential risks. To minimise this, it is a good idea to choose organic milk and yoghurt. If you eat a lot of cream, cheese or butter, switch to organic when you can.

Meat Given that meat is generally the most expensive item in the household budget, to prioritise it is difficult. Residues are not found in meat to anything like the same extent as in fresh produce. Organochlorine pesticide residues, particularly lindane, are detected in fat, especially beef, and antibiotic residues are sometimes found in pork and poultry. Residues in UK lamb are rarely detected, though DDT is commonly found in imported New Zealand lamb. With meat, animal welfare issues come to the fore. The only sensible advice can be to choose organic meat when you can, using the information in the chapter on meat (p. 179) to help you decide.

The wider picture

If you are concerned about how your food is produced with respect to human welfare, the health and conditions of workers, as well as heavy pesticide use and abuse, then consider all these factors in relation to tea, coffee, cocoa, chocolate, bananas, pineapples, sugar, rice and Third World, Asian and South American imported fruit and vegetables (and flowers). If you're thinking animal welfare, think hard about chicken, turkey, pork and veal. If it's the environment that particularly concerns you, it's

fact
People buy organic food for health reasons (46 per cent), to avoid chemicals and pesticides (41 per cent), and for its taste (40 per cent).

cereals, sheep (sheep-dipping), salmon-farming and GMOs that should be on your mind.

WATCHWORD: Price guides are given throughout the book and represent the recommended retail price range you can expect to pay for branded goods at the time of writing. They were compiled from regular shopping trips and wholesale catalogues and are intended as an aid and guide to pricing. Actual prices are bound to fluctuate, though, as a general rule, organic food prices are falling rather than rising. Because meat and fresh produce prices vary so much and are constantly changing, specific price guides have not been included for these.

what they say . . .

'I started to buy organic food, for environmental reasons, about ten years ago, though only the odd items such as bread and root vegetables since the only available source was our local health food shop. But a year ago I discovered the Better Food Company (p. 121) and the wonderful convenience of home delivery. Quite honestly, it's changed my eating habits dramatically.

'Now, all the food I buy is organic, for taste and health reasons as well as ethical and environmental ones. For the first time I really appreciate what I eat and have discovered the pleasure of cooking (previously a task I hated). I also admit to enjoying the whole shopping process, from ordering the food to receiving it – lovely muddy carrots, local green greens, eggs with taste and fruit free of pesticides. OK, so organic food is more expensive, but since I've stopped buying convenience food and eat out far less than I used to, I'm fairly certain I save money.'
– *Rosamund Kidman Cox, editor,* BBC Wildlife Magazine.

Supermarkets

Until recently, supermarkets were an insignificant part of the organic food sector. This is changing rapidly. As one supermarket executive put it, 'The organic market is ripe and ready for substantial development', so much so, in fact, that today four major supermarkets, Safeway, Sainsbury's, Tesco and Waitrose in the south, plus Booths supermarket chain in the north, stock some organic food. At the time of going to press Marks & Spencer are reconsidering their position and are expected to follow suit and Asda are retrialling organic fresh produce in their hypermarkets. All, too, are doing their best to develop the market further, for example through various initiatives with UK growers with Sainsbury's also the first supermarket to advertise organic food on television and in the press. There are bright new labels for organic produce and new lines gradually appearing on the shelves, and in time we can expect UK supermarkets to be a major source of organic food.

For the shopper, supermarkets offer convenience and ready access to organic food. Prices are becoming more attractive, and supplies more regular. Supermarkets currently offer a useful starting-point, especially for those who want to include just a few organic items in their shopping baskets each week.

Two important points to bear in mind are:

- Supermarkets currently sell a limited range of organic food, and sales of this represent a tiny amount of total sales – around 1–2 per cent. Moreover, they all sell approximately the same foods, and often the same brands. They are strongest in fresh produce and baby food, fair to good in dairy produce, patchy in bread and drinks, weakest in meat and – though this is already beginning to change – virtually non-existent in everything else.
- Availability varies considerably, with some branches having a few token items only. Stores in affluent areas and major cities, and large 'show-case' stores, contain more organic food than others.

What you can expect

- All produce is sourced through accredited suppliers and organisations. In addition, Sainsbury's and Waitrose operate their own independent monitoring. Fresh produce and meat usually carries the Soil Association symbol.
- Good organic buys in supermarkets are those items where supply, and therefore prices, are stable. These are also the ones most likely to be found in most stores most of the time. They include an increasingly wide selection of vegetables, such as mushrooms and potatoes, kiwi fruit and lemons, some dairy produce, and everyday breads and flour.
- Supermarkets adopt the same standards of quality control for organic as for conventional vegetables and fruit, though they allow some relaxation over the size and the cosmetic aspect of fresh produce.
- Supermarkets supply UK and imported organic produce. Because they endeavour to supply all year round, and need much larger quantities than other retailers, the level of fresh organic produce that is imported tends to be higher, currently around 75 per cent of all fresh organic produce.
- Organic goods may be grouped together, or found with conventional produce, or, occasionally, both, though the current trend for organic fresh produce to be grouped together – which offers organic shoppers greater convenience – is rapidly catching on.
- With the exception of Booths (see p. 65), as yet supermarkets do not stock locally produced organic food.
- Fresh produce is usually sold under their own label; dairy, meat and breads may be own-label or branded; shelf products are branded.
- Supermarkets offer limited information on organic food; on the shop floor, the level of expertise on the subject is minimal.

WATCHWORD: In addition to organic food, super-markets have their own brands of 'green', environmen-tally friendly produce – for example, 'Nature's Choice', 'Heritage', 'Farm Assured', 'Traditional', 'Naturally Reared' – and are also heavily committed to integrated crop-management schemes such as Leaf. Do not confuse these with organic food or associate them with organic methods of production. All use conventional methods of production and animal welfare.

NOTE: Tesco sell own-brand organic milk, beer and wine under the Nature's Choice label. Sainsbury's organic bread is also sold as Nature's Choice.

The big four

Safeway Nationwide, 380 stores, Safeway were the first super-market to start selling organic food, in 1981. Their commitment has been steady throughout, and they gained an early reputation for being the 'green' supermarket. They have an extensive range of fresh produce, including packs of assorted organic fruit and vegetables, as well as the biggest selection of organic wines, though they no longer sell organic meat. Organic milk, cheese and wines are available in all stores, fresh produce in most, and other shelf groceries in selected stores.

Sainsbury's Nationwide, 396 stores, Sainsbury's are one of the UK's leading supermarket chains and currently sell 25 per cent of the organic produce sold through supermarkets. They first started selling organic produce in 1985. They have expanded their range considerably. Their commitment has steadily increased, and they aim to become the leading supermarket for organic food. They are the only supermarket to have a full range of meat and are strong in fresh produce, baby food and dairy products. All of their stores sell some organic vegetables and fruit. In total, 150 lines are stocked of which 50 are available in over half their stores. New deli and dairy ranges are being planned. Their freephone Customer Careline 0800 636262 (Monday–Saturday) holds comprehensive computer data on organic produce and is splendid;

they will check which local stores sell organic produce, tell you what they stock, or where you can buy a particular product.

Tesco Nationwide, 530 stores, Tesco are the UK's largest supermarket chain. They first began selling organic food in a few selected stores in 1990. What began as an experiment in forty-five stores has continued, and currently organic produce can be found in over half their stores. Tesco have had a major impact due to their pricing policy, and in autumn 1996, they became the first supermarket to sell organic fresh produce at the same price as conventional produce: note that, though prices are lower, they correspond to premium, not standard, produce. Their range of fresh produce has increased. Milk and eggs can be found in most stores. Fresh and dairy produce, bread, and other lines – juices, rice and biscuits – can be found in larger stores. They do not sell organic meat.

Waitrose South-east England, 122 stores, Waitrose first started selling organic produce in 1983. Like Sainsbury's, their stake, range and commitment are steadily increasing. Unlike the other supermarkets they have not developed their own 'green label', preferring to offer organic food instead, and have publicly stated that they intend to sell only organic vegetables and fruit once supplies become available; their plans include a programme for helping organic growers improve their growing techniques to boost quality. Rather than out-of-town superstores, they have smaller ones, more of them in high streets, and respond actively to demands from local customers. All stores sell some organic produce, though the amount varies considerably – in total they list over 100 items and are strongest in fresh produce, dairy products and baby food; they are the first to sell organic ice-cream and trial organic sausages.

Others
The following supermarkets sell a token amount of organic food. This is what they stocked in 1997 (availability varies from store to store):

Asda Baby Organix baby food (15 lines), Yeo Valley yoghurts, Mornflake organic oats, Caledonian Brewery Golden Pale Ale, 2 organic wines. A limited range of fresh produce – carrots, mushrooms, onions, potatoes, tomatoes, apples and pears – are available in their thirteen hypermarkets, priced as near conventional produce as possible.

Co-op Baby Organix baby food, Yeo Valley yoghurts, fruit and vegetables in Scotland, 3 organic wines.

BOOTHS
'Traditionally better'

Booths is a family-owned supermarket chain, with twenty-four branches throughout Lancashire and Cumbria, that has been quietly selling organic food for several years. They do not yet sell organic baby food, but their shelf range is more extensive than that of major multiples; furthermore, they have a policy of selling locally produced organic food. Their commitment increased substantially in 1997, including securing more local home-grown organic produce for their customers. They stock over 100 items, including the full range of Rachel's Dairy products, most Village Bakery breads, cakes and biscuits, and Pencarreg, Tyn Grug and Tregaron organic cheeses. They also stock Doves Farm cornflakes, Mornflake oats, Meridian organic olive and pasta sauce, Whole Earth baked beans, Green & Black's chocolate, plus organic flour, vegetable juices, jams, peanut butter, tomato ketchup, margarine, honey, stock cubes, UHT milk, soya milk and Rice Dream drink, tea bags, and one organic beer, wine and cider. The latest addition is a range of La Terra E Il Cielo pastas and Graig Farm organic meat (p. 104). As with the major multiples, the range varies considerably from store to store.

How to Be a Supermarket Organic Sleuth

1 First, choose your supermarket. The availability of organic produce varies enormously from store to store within a chain. If you have the choice, check out other supermarket stores to see if their range is better.

2 Make a point of checking what organic produce is available every time you visit. The range available is often determined by each branch individually. If there is something you want that the store doesn't have, ask; as long as the chain stocks it, they will usually do their best to supply the item for you.

3 When comparing prices against non-organic items, double-check that you are comparing like with like; for example, check the prices per kilogram, or by weight of boxes.

4 Stock up on promotional offers.

5 Always make at least one organic purchase. This will help ensure that demand keeps rising and that supermarkets will keep stocking organic food.

Somerfield Some dairy.

NOTE: All supermarkets stress that things are changing fast, that they will respond to customer demand and are constantly reviewing the organic market. Watch this space.

Price guide

Supermarkets do not charge extra premiums for organic food, and the difference in price is a reflection of the extra money they have to pay to the suppliers. Wherever possible, all try to price organic food as near to conventional prices as possible. In reality, prices can fluctuate more than in other retail sectors, which means that sometimes their prices are much lower than those of small independent retailers, and sometimes higher. As a general guideline, though some items can cost more, expect to pay 10–25 per cent extra for most basic things.

> **NOTE:** Prices are becoming more attractive all the time. It is rare not to find at least one or two items that are the same price as the conventional equivalent, and sometimes cheaper. For examples, see p. 30.

Finally, and most importantly, don't presume automatically that the organic item is more expensive than the non-organic one, and double-check carefully that you are comparing like with like. To give a simple example, I once found bagged organic flat beans priced at £1.99 per lb, while the same variety of non-organic flat beans was priced at £1.19 a bag. Superficially it looked as if the organic beans cost 80p extra. In fact, the non-organic beans were £1.19 per 250g bag. A quick look at the price per kilogram revealed that the organic beans, at £4.39, were 37p cheaper than the conventional ones.

what they say . . .

'During the 1980s there was a profusion of labels and groups claiming to be organic, and relationships between organic organisations and supermarkets were poor or underdeveloped. This led to customers being confused as to what was organic, and criticism from the main growing sector that organic food could not be taken seriously.

'In the 1990s things have changed. All organic food must be approved by UKROFS via organisations such as the Soil Association. It is the Soil Association who have become the most respected guardian of organic food and today all multiples, including Waitrose, reflect that in the logo used and in customer

information. Other groups have either merged or become
significantly less important and there is an air of unity and
co-operation that was not apparent ten years ago.'
– *Alan Wilson, agronomist, Waitrose*

What they sell

This is what the major supermarkets stocking organic food had on
their shelves at the time of writing. The availability in any store at
any one time is more limited, depending on the season and availability, size and location of store, and which supermarket. Own
brands are available in selected lines, such as bread, milk, flour
and yoghurt.

Fresh produce: The range is steadily increasing – regular lines
commonly stocked are:

> *vegetables:* beans, broccoli, cabbage (green, red and white),
> carrots, cauliflower, celery, Chinese leaf, courgettes,
> cucumbers, garlic, leeks, lettuce, mushrooms, onions,
> parsley, peppers, potatoes, swedes, tomatoes, watercress

> *fruit:* apples, grapefruit, grapes, kiwi fruit, lemons, mangoes,
> oranges, peaches, pears, satsumas, strawberries

Safeway Stock further items, including Jerusalem artichokes,
celeriac, peas and various fresh beans, ready-shredded organic
coleslaw, greengages, blackcurrants and Scottish raspberries.

Dairy produce: Every supermarket sells organic milk (whole
and semi-skimmed) and yoghurt in all or most stores. Butter,
cream, crème fraîche and eggs are sold in selected stores. Cheese is
usually prepacked (Lye Cross Cheddar, Landsby Brie), with other
lines – for example, Pencarreg, Welsh Brie, Welsh Country
Cheddar – sold loose on selected deli counters.
Sainsbury's Sell Rachel's Dairy yoghurts and crème fraîche, and
Green & Black's chocolate ice-cream, Danish Grinzola cheese, in
selected stores. Sell organic butter in all stores.
Safeway Sell organic soya milk, but not cream.

Waitrose Sell own-brand organic vanilla ice-cream and organic soya and UHT milk in selected stores.
Tesco Sell virtually fat-free organic milk. Their organic cheese range has increased and includes Lye Cross Cheddar, goat's cheese and Gouda with nettles.

Baked goods: Bakery products are primarily limited to bread and rolls; as yet, apart from Booths, there are no organic cakes or other baked goods sold in supermarkets, except for Duchy Original and Doves Farm biscuits. White and wholemeal flour is available in most stores.
Safeway Sell Whole Earth and Doves Farm wholewheat organic bread, but available in very few stores; Duchy Original biscuits.
Sainsbury's Stock eight different breads, including Village Bakery rye breads and Cranks honey and sunflower bread; Doves Farm digestive biscuits, Doves Farm plain white flour and The Stamp Collection organic wheat-free flour.
Waitrose Have the widest selection of breads – twelve lines in total, including rolls, Village Bakery rye breads and Pane Toscano, and Duchy organic breads; Duchy Original biscuits and Doves Farm lemon and muesli cookies; also, self-raising flour.
Tesco Sell white and wholemeal organic sliced bread; Allinson's organic wholewheat flour, and Doves Farm strong white and wholemeal flour. At time of writing, they are planning to launch a range of organic biscuits.

Meat: Only two supermarkets, Sainsbury's and Waitrose, supply organic meat, and in selected stores only. The range of cuts is limited. All meat is prepacked. Sainsbury's are increasing the number of stores stocking meat.
Sainsbury's Sell ten different cuts of organic beef, eight cuts of organic lamb and P.J. Onions whole chickens. A full range of pork cuts has recently been introduced in a few stores, mainly in London. Beef is now available in over fifty stores.
Waitrose Sell Eastbrook Farm organic beef in fourteen stores; they are trialling organic sausages in selected stores.

Baby food: Organic baby food can be found in all or most supermarket stores; the range depends on the store.
Safeway, Sainsbury's, Tesco and Waitrose Baby Organix.

Sainsbury's Cow & Gate and Hipp.
Tesco Hipp.
Waitrose Cow & Gate; Hipp follow-on infant formula milk.

Breakfast cereals: Beginning to appear in selected stores.
Sainsbury's Whole Earth cornflakes and Swiss-style muesli; organic oats.
Safeway and Waitrose Mornflake oats.

Non-alcoholic drinks and juices: Tea-bags and ground coffee can be found in most or selected stores, depending on the chain. A very limited range of juices is stocked in selected stores.
Safeway Ridgeway organic tea-bags, Ashby's organic coffee. Eden bottled organic carrot and vegetable juice.
Sainsbury's Ridgeway organic tea-bags, Ashby's organic coffee; Grove Fresh Florida chilled organic orange juice.
Tesco Do not stock organic tea or coffee. Eden bottled organic carrot juice; Grove Fresh Florida chilled organic juice, 250ml and 1-litre cartons.
Waitrose Own-brand organic tea-bags and Percol coffee. Eden bottled carrot and vegetable juice and Grove Fresh Florida chilled organic orange juice, 1-litre cartons.

Alcoholic drinks: Organic beer, lager, cider and wine can be found in selected stores.
Safeway Have the best and widest selection of organic wines – over ten different kinds.
Sainsbury's Do not stock organic beer or lager, and stock one organic wine.
Tesco Do not sell organic lager or cider, and stock two organic wines.
Waitrose Stock one lager and cider and four organic wines.

Confectionery: Organic chocolate can be found in many stores.
Safeway, Sainsbury's, Waitrose Green & Black's chocolate.

Other: Very few other organic goods are sold, and in selected stores only.
Safeway Billington's sugar, Whole Earth baked beans, olive oil, honey, rice, dried herbs and spices.

Sainsbury's Billington's sugar, Country Harvest wholegrain rice, Meridian olive oil, Whole Earth peanut butter.
Tesco Country Harvest wholegrain rice.
Waitrose Billington's sugar, Whole Earth baked beans, olive oil, honey.

Source Compiled from information supplied by Safeway, Sainsbury's, Tesco and Waitrose.

Alternative Supermarkets: Shopping for a Better World

The mid-1990s heralded the start of a new shopping experience in the UK, when the first independent supermarkets dedicated primarily to organic food and sustainable consumerism entered the scene. Forget any notions of brown rice in sacks, hippy staff and heavy metal politics. Modelled on organic supermarkets in the USA, the modern alternative supermarket is slick, spacious, attractive, professionally run, innovative; it selects only high-quality goods, uses the latest technology and goes out of its way to offer every convenience. To step over the threshold is to taste the future.

What have alternative supermarkets to offer over conventional ones?
Alternative supermarkets look different – smaller, yet more spacious.

- They offer the best and largest range of organic/ethical produce it is possible to buy, including non-food items such as cleaning materials, pet food and books.
- Staff are generally more knowledgeable and more committed, and give better service and advice.
- Customer information is given a high priority: information about products is readily accessible and constantly updated. Alternative supermarkets offer a high level of customer involvement.

● They feel different – more friendly – and they aim to make shopping fun and stress-free.
● They hold events, regular tastings and presentations.

WATCHWORD: Alternative supermarkets sell not only organic produce, but also a wide range of conventional goods; everything they sell, though, must satisfy their own codes of ethical shopping. Like conventional supermarkets, they sell imported organic produce.

Price guide

Alternative supermarkets are keen to attract all shoppers, and price their goods as competitively as possible, Out of This World especially so. However, they do not have the buying power of major multiples – though this is beginning to change. Prices are generally similar to those in other organic shops. Special promotions and seasonal bargains are standard.

Planet Organic

Opened in 1996, in Westbourne Grove, London, near Bayswater tube station, and run by two Americans, Renée J. Elliott and Jonathan Dwek, Planet Organic is London's flagship alternative supermarket with, ultimately, several branches planned nationwide. In 1997 they were voted organic retailer of the year by *Daily Mail* readers.

They stock a huge range of organic foods and drinks, plus a wide range of health and cosmetic products, organic pet food, household cleaning materials, fresh (conventional) flowers and books. Their cheese counter and chilled foods sector are generally excellent; their Q Guild (see p. 187) organic butchery counter exemplary; their fresh fruit and vegetable aisle, second to none, though this also includes a small range of conventional produce. Another star feature is their juice bar – large cartons of delicious organic vegetable and fruit juices prepared to order, plus the latest juice craze, organic wheat grass; and organic coffee and teas. They also have a well stocked fresh fish counter. They have recently introduced organic sandwiches; organic herb plants will be next.

All their organic produce is certified; any non-organic produce is clearly labelled as such. Informed advice is always on hand. They do not stock any foods containing artificial additives or preservatives, hydrogenated fat or refined sugar, or foods containing GM ingredients, and offer organic wherever possible. They hold regular tastings and have regular promotional offers.

They can be found at 42 Westbourne Grove, London W2 tel: 0171 221 7171 Mon.–Sat. 9am–8pm, Sun. 11am–5pm. Local home delivery service available.

what they say . . .

> 'At Planet Organic you need not worry about the by-products of
> intensive farming or cheaply processed food filled with
> preservatives and artificial ingredients. We read the labels for these
> harmful by-products and will not stock them. The difference at
> Planet Organic is this: when other retailers ask, ' ' Will it sell?",
> we ask, ' ' Should we sell it?"' – *Jonathan Dwek, Planet Organic*

Out of This World

Described by the *Sunday Telegraph* as the most radical experiment in British retailing for one and a half centuries, and by the *Guardian* as Britain's most ethically sound supermarket chain, Out of This World is a modern ethical co-operative. The first three shops, in Bristol, Nottingham and Newcastle, were opened in 1996; their Cheltenham branch was opened in 1997. Three more are planned soon. Currently they have well over twenty thousand members who, as owners, participate in policy decisions and in running the business. To join, tel: 0191 272 1601.

The shops market themselves as neighbourhood grocery stores with a global dimension and stock a full range of fresh and processed foods and drinks, plus fair-traded items such as clothes; household cleaning materials and books. All products must meet their ethical standards and are selected for their contribution to healthy eating, community development, fair-trade, animal welfare or environmental sustainability.

Wherever possible, food products are sourced locally, which results in cost savings being passed on to customers. Their deli counters sell organic sandwiches, snacks and cakes. Unique to them is their computerised 'Worldly Wise' product information, which allows customers to see what is ethically good (and bad) about the products on sale. They sell only products guaranteed to be free from GM soya. Other innovations include a mail order catalogue, *The Natural Collection*, for clothes and household items, and a regular newsletter, *Shop News*, for each store.

Out of This World aim to sell organic produce as cheaply as they can; dried bulk basics, such as grains and pulses, are very good value. Where prices of organic produce match those of non-organic, only the organic item is stocked. For a list of these, see p. 31.

Their newest branch, in the centre of Cheltenham opposite Marks & Spencer, has a licensed organic café, sells freshly made organic sandwiches using the Authentic Bread Company's bread (p. 214), at the same prices as M&S's, home-made take-away meals and deli items using organic ingredients; it also features a wide range of fresh produce supplied by the Organic Marketing Company (p. 119). Stores are open Monday–Saturday.

You can find them at:
Bristol Clifton Down Shopping Centre, Whiteladies Road tel: 0117 946 6909 Mon.–Sat. 9am–6pm, late-night opening, Fri. until 8pm.
Cheltenham 6–8 Pitville Street tel: 01242 518300 Mon.–Sat. 8.30am–6pm, late-night opening, Thurs. until 8 pm.
Newcastle upon Tyne Gosforth Shopping Centre, High Street tel: 0191 213 0421 Mon.–Sat. 9am–6pm.
Nottingham Villa Street, Beeston tel: 0115 943 1311 Mon.–Sat. 9am–6pm, late-night opening, Thurs. and Fri. until 8pm.

what they say . . .

'We have no choice about being consumers, but we can make practical, ethical choices about where we shop and what we buy, and we can become part of the solution instead of adding to the problem.

'Out of This World sees the organic standard as the cutting edge of the movement towards food awareness. Our policy is to bring more organic produce into our range, to switch to organic-only ranges as soon as possible and to offer promotions when we can. We stock only organic fruit, vegetables, meat and meat products, pies etc., dairy products, herbs and spices, hot and cold deli items, sandwiches, dried fruit, nuts and grains, and have over five hundred certified products overall, of which about 40 per cent are fresh. All our produce is certified.

'We source fresh produce locally, whenever possible; up to half of our fresh organic produce can come from very local suppliers from August to January. At least half of our organic produce is the same price or less than the supermarkets' non-organic equivalents, as we do not have to prepack our range, as they are required to do, to prevent substitution. We also take size grade-outs of organic produce from wholesalers who are packing for supermarkets – we think that people have a much greater tolerance about the size of produce than supermarkets specify. We have permanent major display boards about organic food in the stores.'
– *Richard Adams, Out of This World*

Food Halls

Though Harrods does not, London's other two fine food halls, Harvey Nichols and Selfridges, stock a selected range of organic food, as does the Bluebird food complex on the King's Road. All are up-market, with prices to match. New lines are regularly being introduced, and promotions on organic food are becoming routine in-store events.

Bluebird, *350 King's Rd, Chelsea SW3* Terence Conran's not-to-be-missed food complex, comprising inside grocery store, bakery and deli, outdoor fruit and vegetable market, chef's shop and restaurant.

Extensive hand-picked selection of organic food with some staples sold loose, and including well known brands such as Rachel's Dairy yoghurt; Green & Black's ice-cream; Suma dried pulses, dried fruit, vegetable oils, canned soups and baked beans; Doves Farm cornflakes; Whole Earth peanut butter; Billington's sugar; Aspell's cider vinegar; Shipton Mill, Doves Farm and the full range of Maud Foster flours and muesli; De Rit basmati, wild and long-grain rice, waffles, langues de chat and baked beans; Eu Vita passata, and bio-dynamic pasta; Hipp baby foods; Eco baby apple rice; Kallo stock cubes and Bonsoy soya milk. They have a wide range of fresh fruit and vegetables supplied by the Organic Marketing Company, Hereford; eggs, dairy produce and cheeses, including Parmesan cut to order; a full range of fresh meat from Eastbrook Farm, P.J. Onions chickens, and Quiet Revolution fresh soups. Breads are made with organic flour. They also supply fresh herb plants from Jekka's Herb Farm, L'Estornell organic olive oil sold loose at £7.99 per 750ml, and Ecover washing and cleaning products.

Harvey Nichols, Knightsbridge SW1 A stone's throw from Harrods, Harvey Nichols has the smallest food hall but, fruit and vegetables apart, offers an impressive range of organic produce with over a hundred different items in total, including organic bean sprouts. Strongest in packaged and specialist foods, the range includes organic rice – brown, wild, Thai, red Carmargue and jasmine; flours; muesli; cornflakes; pasta and pasta sauces; Italian Gabro olive oil; snack foods; hummus; organic vegetable stock cubes; fruit spreads and honey; oatcakes, biscuits, cookies, waffles, crostini and Green & Black's organic chocolate. Their dairy range includes organic milk, eggs, butter, soft cheese, Rachel's Dairy yoghurts, The Elms Dairy goat's milk yoghurts and Rocombe Farm organic ice-cream and frozen yoghurts. They also sell organic Rice Dream drink. They have an excellent range of organic breads, Village Bakery cakes, and a small range of Eastbrook Farm meats – namely, organic leg of lamb, loin of pork, sirloin of beef and chickens – and Quiet Revolution fresh organic soups. At the time of writing they do not sell organic fruit or vegetables, or certified organic wines.

Selfridges, Oxford Street W1 Revamped and relaunched their organic food selection in summer 1997, and are steadily increasing their ever more impressive range of fresh, chilled and shelf groceries. Lines include breakfast cereals, spreads, salsas, tortilla chips, pasta sauces, pastas, tinned tomatoes and salad dressings; six olive oils; Martin Pitt eggs; Yeo Valley yoghurt; tofu; bean sprouts; De Rit honey cake, Doves Farm biscuits, waffles and rice cakes, and over 30 selected breads, cakes and biscuits from the Village Bakery. They sell selected prime cuts of Eastbrook Farm meat, including beef, veal, chicken, pork and lamb, ready-prepared stuffed organic joints, and pâtés, salamis, hams and other meats from Pure Organic Foods. They have a range of organic cheeses, prepacked and loose; Quite Revolution fresh soups; and eleven certified organic wines, plus cider and beer, soft drinks, Hambledon herb teas and hot chocolate. They do not sell organic fruit or vegetables. They offer organic beef in their Premier restaurant.

Shops

Ten years ago, shops selling organic food were few and far between. Today, hundreds of independent shops now stock organic food, and most counties boast at least one shop doing its best to sell as many organic goods as possible, selling fresh produce, including meat and dairy, bread, groceries, tea and coffee, drinks and wine and eco-friendly cleaning products. Some produce their own take-away organic meals, while others provide sandwiches and many offer home delivery. There are dedicated organic shops that sell only organic produce, and even a mobile shop, Midlands Organic Supplies (see p. 79). ' One-stop' shops, where you can buy everything, are tipped as the next major development. To find your nearest shop, consult the Soil Association's booklet, *Where To Buy Organic Food*.

Shops dedicated to organic food
These are the top of the pyramid, and they stock the widest range of organic produce possible. Many operate home delivery and/or box schemes (see p. 107), and sell produce from local organic

growers. All organic goods are clearly labelled and certified; the shops are run professionally, and owned by people who are committed to the organic philosophy.

Shops in this group may sell two to three hundred or more different organic lines. The best, such as Organic Health in Heanor, Derbyshire, and Infinity Foods, Brighton, have around five to seven hundred lines – as many or more than alternative supermarkets. Shops selling *only* organic food are Damhead Organically Grown Foods in Edinburgh, the Organic Store in London, Godshill Organics in Godshill, Isle of Wight, and the Organic Centre, Brighton. More are in the pipeline. For details, see p. 80.

Wholefood shops

Wholefood shops specialise in unrefined foods, but they have moved a long way from their original 'brown rice and sandals brigade' image, these days selling a wide variety of deli items and fresh foods also. Many cater for vegetarians and vegans, and most have always stocked some organic items. After shops specialising in organic food, they are usually the next-best place to stock up at. The best will offer between fifty and a hundred or more organic lines, and often offer discounts for bulk purchasing. *Wholefood co-operatives* are wholefood shops owned by their staff.

Health food shops

Despite their name, health food shops often sell as many and sometimes more health food supplements and herbal remedies and cosmetics as food items. Although they were generally indifferent to organic food in the past and slow to stock it, organic food is now a major growth area, though this does vary from shop to shop. They stock the same range as wholefood shops. The two major chains, Health and Diet Centres (south-east England) and Holland & Barrett, both stock some organic foods and are increasing their ranges.

NOTE: Wholefood and health food shops may or may not stock meat.

Delicatessens

Patchy. Some, like the splendid fine-food emporium, the Ramsbottom Victuallers in Ramsbottom, Lancashire (p. 83), are knowledgeable and dedicated to the organic philosophy and offer a wide choice, but others offer only a few token items. The better ones are beginning to stock more organic things – cheese and dairy products, breads, dried goods, olive oil, pasta, and so on.

Others

Everyone has an *Oxfam* near them, so it is useful to know that in addition to fair traded goods, they stock a small range of certified organic produce: namely, Zambian honey, Café Latino and instant Mexicafé coffee, Maya Gold chocolate bars, cashew nuts, dried apricots and sultanas. The range varies from shop to shop. All products are certified by the Soil Association; the honey, apricots and sultanas are excellent value. *Traidcraft* shops also sell own-label organic coffee beans, dried apricots and honey. Some conventional shops are beginning to stock a few popular items, such as dairy products and organic flour. Similarly with local multiples.

An organic mobile shop Midlands Organic Supplies, Wolverhampton tel: 01902 761803, mobile: 0468 625333 The UK's only organic mobile shop. Sells fresh meat and everything else except vegetables, at competitive prices. Operates on Saturdays at Garden Village garden centre on the A454, between Trescott and Shipley. Home delivery service rest of the week.
Organic farm shops Often sell an extensive range of organic products. See p. 85.
Food Halls See p. 75.
Markets See p. 89.

Price guide: As a rough rule of thumb, shops committed to organic food do their best to price competitively. Shops stocking the odd organic item do not, and sometimes put a higher mark-up on organic produce; exceptions are shops in rural areas serving as outlets for a local producer – for example, a supplier of organic eggs.

Also:

- Though, apart from seasonal differences, you can expect stable prices for most products, prices for organic foods tend to vary from one shop to the next. This is because overheads vary considerably, depending on the kind of shop, its location, and so on. A small shop in a region well serviced by organic producers such as Devon, Somerset and parts of Wales can source organic food easily; those in areas where organic suppliers are scarce must work harder and transport the food further.
- Small shops do not have the buying power of multiples, which means that they have to pay more for organic goods at wholesale. Also, they support small producers, wastage may be higher, and staff costs are considerable.

Star Performers: Organic Shops

Here is a brief selection of some of the best, that is, the most committed. Except where stated, all stock meat, dairy produce, fruit and vegetables, breads and other baked goods, dried foods, groceries, preserves, deli items, confectionery, wines, beers, juices and other beverages, herbs and spices and eco-friendly cleaning products.

Bumblebee, 30,32,33 Brecknock Road, London N7 tel: 0171 607 1936 Soil Association registered. A remarkable vegetarian whole-food enterprise, comprising three shops. Though not exclusively organic, it has one of the most extensive ranges of organic foods and drinks possible – wider than alternative supermarkets' – and an excellent choice of brands. Apart from meat and fish, there is nothing you cannot buy here. It stocks only organic fruit and vegetables, wines (60) and beers. Plus the full range of Rapunzel goods, 14 certified organic olive oils and 4 brands of organic baby foods; Celtic Baker's, Cranks, Neal's Yard, Village Bakery and Paul's breads; 15–20 organic cheeses, cut to order, and a full range of organic macrobiotic products and so on. They also operate a box scheme and publish a regular newsletter.

Other highly recommended shops in London offering an extensive range of organic foods include Wild Oats, 210 Westbourne Grove, W11, and the East–West Centre, 188 Old Street, EC1, which includes a macrobiotic restaurant, serving food made with 60–70 per cent organic foods.

Cook's Delight, *360–364 High Street, Berkhamsted, Herts.* tel: 01442 863584 Established in 1980 and certified by the Soil Association, a vegetarian organic shop, featuring a huge range of organic lines, including macrobiotic goods. They make their own frozen organic meals and also sell organic wines, cotton and ecological cleaning products. They have a box scheme and home delivery service.

Damhead Organically Grown Foods, *Lothianburn, Edinburgh* tel: 0131 445 5591 Demeter-registered. A 100 per cent organic farm shop which sells everything except wines and beers. All produce is certified. Fresh produce is sourced direct through local Scottish organic growers, supplemented by other UK and imported produce sourced from wholesalers. Local organic meat and Graig Farm meat; Loch Arthur dairy products and meat. Home delivery and extensive exclusively organic mail order catalogue.

Godshill Organics, *Yard Parlour, Newport Road, Godshill, Isle of Wight* tel: 01983 840723 Soil Association registered. A 100 per cent organic shop selling over five hundred lines, and the island's only organic smallholding, which grows an extensive range of vegetables and some soft and top fruit for sale in the shop, run by Ruth and Roy Illman. All lines are certified, except for bread baked by a local baker, but made with organic flour. They also operate a box scheme and home delivery service.

Infinity Foods, *25 North Road, Brighton, Sussex* tel: 01273 603563 Soil Association registered. One of the best traditional wholefood shops, established in 1971, now a co-operative, committed to organic foods; it also has a large wholesale company selling an extensive range of dried foods under the Infinity Foods label. Stocks over five hundred certified organic lines including fresh and dairy produce, and their own organic bread. No meat.

Infinity Foods are widely distributed throughout the south-east and London, and to many wholefood shops nationwide.

The Organic Centre, Telscombe Cliffs, Brighton, Sussex tel: 01273 585551 Soil Association registered. Britain's first 100 per cent organic shop, started in 1981, run by Pat and Bob Beaumont. They stock over seven hundred certified organic lines, including their own range of breads, have a home delivery service with drop-off points, provide discount bulk buying for families, and much more. They try to price as competitively as possible, and often have lines cheaper than conventional produce. Provide regular customers with food and health information and advice.

Organic Health, Marlpool, Heanor, Derbyshire tel: 01773 717718 A remarkable shop owned by Jackie Garfit, who has a certificate in organic agriculture and dedicates her life and considerable energy to providing her customers with organic food, sourced from local suppliers wherever possible, as cheaply as she can. Her organic shopping basket of basic foods costs less than the local supermarket's. A wide range of organic fresh food and grocery items is available, totalling around 750, plus an excellent mail order catalogue. She recently opened a farm shop at Perry Court bio-dynamic farm, Garlinge Green, near Canterbury, Kent. Both shops are registered with the Soil Association, and sell bio-dynamic produce.

The Organic Shop, The Square, Stow-on-the-Wold, Glos. tel: 01451 831004 A pioneering organic shop, opened in 1986, with over 80 per cent of its lines organic. They stock a full range of certified produce, including wines, dairy produce, breads, and excellent meat and vegetables. Also make their own soups, prepared meals, pasties, quiches, pies, cakes and flapjacks, using organic ingredients – all available from the take-away counter.

The Organic Store, 8 Staines Road, Twickenham, Middlesex tel: 0181 893 3310 Organic Farmers and Growers registered. Open 7 days a week. London's first 100 per cent 'one-stop' organic shop. They stock a full range of organic foods, wines, beers and other drinks from major organic suppliers; and a comprehensive range of fresh produce, competitively priced. The chilled section includes hummus made with organic chick-peas and organic pizzas, and quiches from Boulangerie Gaughier in Normandy. Excellent catalogue available. Home delivery service within ten-mile radius; local deliveries free. Business is booming.

The Ramsbottom Victualler, 16–18 Market Place, Ramsbottom, Bury, Lancs. tel: 01706 825070 Winner of the Best Food Shop Award, and an example of a fine food shop with a missionary zeal about quality and the benefits of organic food. They stock around 250 certified organic lines, a full range of seasonal vegetables, loose dried fruit, pulses, grains, olive oil and so on, and source from local suppliers wherever possible. Particularly knowledgeable about wines. Organic produce is used in their award-winning restaurant. They offer a regular newsletter, plus tastings and events.

Ryton Gardens Shop, Ryton Organic Gardens, Ryton-on-Dunsmore, Coventry tel: 01203 303517 Ryton Gardens is the centre for the UK's largest organic gardening association, the Henry Doubleday Research Association (HDRA), one of the foremost organisations promoting organic food and farming. Over 90 per cent of its products are organic, and the shop's policy is that where there is an organic equivalent to a conventional item they will stock it. Fruit, vegetables, bread, meat (from Eastbrook Farm and Graig Farm), dairy produce and wines are exclusively organic. All products are certified. They operate a box scheme, containing vegetables at similar prices to conventional ones in local supermarkets. Their award-winning restaurant specialises in organic food and serves fish supplied by Cornish Fish Direct (p. 207). Ryton Gardens bakery, due to open soon, will provide a restaurant and a shop with organic breads. Their other centre, Yalding Gardens, Yalding, Kent, also has a well stocked shop.

Also, three shops illustrating the diversity of shops selling organic produce in rural areas:

The Green Shop, *54 Bridge Street, Berwick-upon-Tweed, Northumberland* tel: 01289 330897 Sell only environmentally friendly, organic, fair-trade or local products. Their organic range includes over 120 items, Village Bakery breads and other baked goods, plus others using organic ingredients. Stock only organic fruit and vegetables. They also sell organic cotton clothes and bedlinen.

Greenlink Organic Foods, *9 Graham Road, Malvern, Hereford & Worcester* tel: 01684 576266 A friendly shop that claims to sell the widest range of organic produce in the county, including vegetables, fruit, Graig Farm meat, dairy produce, breads and wholefoods. They also stock eco-friendly cleaning products and toiletries. They operate a box scheme, and have a take-away counter and snack bar. Free local delivery service.

The Tree House, *2 Pier Road, Aberystwyth, Ceridigion* tel: 01970 615791 Soil Association registered. A small shop-cum-restaurant selling their own certified organic produce from their seven-acre market garden, organic fruit, meat from Graig Farm, Rachel's Dairy products, local and organic cheeses, Village Bakery breads, soya products, tea and coffee, jams and spreads. Ninety-five per cent of their stock is organic. Their restaurant uses organic ingredients where possible – around 80 per cent – including their own produce. The restaurant is vegetarian during the day; and open three nights a week, when organic meat is served. Provides a take-away service.

Also, see Star Performers: Organic Farm Shops, p. 86.

what they say . . .

'We have a God-given responsibility to look after this world. I welcome the chance to buy organic when it is available and buy locally when I can. We now have a regular supply of locally baked bread – organic bread, for instance – and when the supermarkets and local health food shop do stock organic items I buy them. If I am travelling near an organic farm I will buy meat or vegetables – whatever is on offer. I welcome initiatives like Out of This World, where local produce is sought out and companies are checked out . . . Roll on the day when there is such a shop near to where I live.'
– *Mrs S. Gibson, Salisbury*

'The level of service, information and friendly advice you receive from organic outlets makes shopping a pleasure rather than a chore. The fact that we are helping to support sustainable farming is simply a bonus.' – *Eddie and Gina Baines, Essex*

'Shopping organic involves a greater awareness and interest in what we consume. A piece of meat doesn't grow on the supermarket shelf pre-wrapped in three layers of Styrofoam and cellophane. Knowing that the carrot in your ratatouille comes from Cornwall and the blue broccoli from a farm just outside Canterbury adds value to the meal.' – *William and Gabriela Lana, Greenwich*

Farm Shops

Organic farm shops are springing up all over the country; most – over sixty – can be found in the Soil Association booklet, *Where to Buy Organic Food*, which includes bio-dynamic farms that sell produce under the Demeter label. All offer an opportunity not just to buy produce direct but to meet the producers, and see how organic fare is produced for yourself. They vary in sophistication from simple outlets to impressively well stocked shops. Several are exclusively organic. Note, too, that almost all are proper farm shops: that is to say, shops belonging to the farm rather than, as has often become the case, wholesale-type shops or stalls calling themselves farm shops selling bulk bought-in produce.

Remember:

- All organic farm shops sell produce from their own farm; many may also sell bought-in fresh organic produce.
- Many organic farm shops sell other products, such as bread, flour, dried goods, oils, drinks, wines, beers, jams and confectionery. Produce sold as 'organic' will be certified.
- Organic farm shops may also sell conventional wholefoods and other items.

- Some organic farm shops may specialise in only meat or only fresh produce.
- Farm shops are open all year; opening times vary, so telephone first to check.
- Farm shops must conform to the same health and safety, labelling and trading standards as all retail shops.

In addition to farm shops, many farms and smallholdings sell their organic produce direct. These are classified as 'farm-gate' outlets and are also listed in the Soil Association booklet, *Where to Buy Organic Food*. Prices are usually lower than those at a farm shop, but range and facilities are more limited. Phone first to check opening times and availability.

> **WATCHWORD:** Though reared or grown using organic methods, *not* everything produced on an organic farm is necessarily certified as organic; if this is the case, it will not be sold as organic. Some farm shops have a mixture of organic and high-animal-welfare, additive-free meat.

Price guide: Produce from the farm is generally excellent value. Fresh produce, in particular, can be 15–20 per cent cheaper than conventional greengrocers'; meat and dairy produce are also cheaper than in conventional shops. Bought-in produce varies, depending on the supply chain, for example, according to whether the farm shop buys direct from another producer, through whole-sale outlets or via intermediary sources. Discounts may be offered for bulk buying.

Star Performers: Organic Farm Shops

Phone ahead for opening hours.

Growing Concern, Home Farm, Nanpantan, Loughborough, *Leics.* tel: 01509 239228; open Thurs.–Sat. Organic Farmers and Growers registered. A dedicated family-run organic farm, specialising in high-quality meat from rare breeds, and the sole outlet for the traditional pure-blood, horned Hereford beef, said to be the best of all beef breeds for quality, and of which only 350 remain in the UK. They produce their own beef, lamb, pork (large blacks), ducks and Christmas poultry. The animals are sent to a small abattoir, then hung and butchered on the farm. Organic chickens are supplied by P.J. Onions. They offer excellent value – cheaper than supermarket prices in some instances. They also produce organic eggs, sold under the Cherry Tree Farm label. The farm shop sells a wide range of organic foods and staples, including locally grown Demeter-registered vegetables, home-baked goodies and meat dishes using organic ingredients; home-smoked bacon and hams, home-made sausages, cheese and dairy produce. Plus organic wines and other drinks.

Highfield Harvest, *Highfield farm, Topsham, Devon* tel: 01392 876388 open Tues.–Sat., Sun. am. Soil Association registered. An award-winning farm shop with a full range of organic produce, including over fifty varieties of their own vegetables, fruit, herbs and free-range eggs, Eastbrook Farm meats, Rachel's Dairy yoghurts, and an extensive selection of organic wholefoods and over fifty different wines and beers. They also stock more than twenty local farm cheeses. They operate a box scheme, supplying mainly home-grown produce; boxes come in two sizes, £5 and £8; they offer a home delivery service and publish a regular newsletter.

Marshford Organic Nursery, *Northam, Bideford, Devon* tel: 01237 477160 open Mon.–Sat. am Soil Association registered. A unique 100 per cent organic nursery, established in 1985, growing wonderful vegetables including salads, soft fruit, an extensive selection of herbs including basil and coriander, and cottage plants. The nursery includes a garden trail and herb garden. The farm shop stocks only organic produce, and sells an extensive range of meat, fresh and dairy produce, bread, cakes, dried and convenience foods, condiments, tea and coffee. It also offers first class seasonal vegetable boxes, at £8. Highly recommended.

The Old Dairy, *Hardwick Estate, Whitchurch-on-Thames, Pangbourne, near Reading, S. Oxon* tel: 0118 9842392 open Wed.–Sat. Soil Association registered. An award-winning farm shop offering an extensive range of organic foods, including their own meat, unpasteurised milk and cream, and vegetables and soft fruit grown by Iain Tolhurst (p. 117). They stock fresh and frozen meat, including home-made sausages, and an extensive selection of small-producer cheeses. Eighty-five to ninety per cent of the produce is organic, including fresh and dried herbs, wholefoods, flour, pulses and dried fruit, and wines, beers and ciders. All their meat is killed in a certified organic mobile abattoir.

Prospect Organic Growers' Farm Shop, *Prospect Cottage, Bartestree, Hereford* tel: 01432 851164 9 open Tues.–Fri., Sat. am Soil Association registered. Part of Green Growers' Co-operative, they sell an extensive range of home-grown vegetables and fruit including those grown in their twenty-five polytunnels, imported produce, and a wide range of organic wholefoods, dairy produce and Graig Farm meat. Over 90 per cent of foods sold here are organic. They also operate a box scheme, either standard boxes at £5 or £7.50, or customised orders.

Riverford Farm Shop, *Riverford, Staverton, Totnes, Devon* tel: 01803 762523 open Mon.– Sat., Sun. April–end Dec. A splendid family-run farm shop which makes all its own produce, using organic ingredients where possible, including a wide range of breads, pies, pâtés, smoked meats, frozen meals and preserves. They sell home-grown organic vegetables (p.117), organic and additive-free meat, game and poultry, home-reared pork, bacon, and hams, organic dairy products and selected groceries and organic wines and ciders.

Other farm shops selling exclusively organic produce include:
Claydon House Organic Gardens, *Middle Claydon, nr Winslow, Bucks.* tel: 01296 738061.
Flint Acres Farm, *Bury Gate, Pulborough, West Sussex* tel: 01798 831036.
Gold Hill Organic Farm, *Childe Okeford, Blandford, Dorset* tel: 01258 860293. Also have a stall in Castle Cary market Tuesday mornings.
Octavia's Organic Farm Shop, *Breakspear Farm, Old Horsham Road, Beare Green, Dorking, Surrey* tel: 01306 712376.

Scragoak Farm Shop, Brightling Road, Robertsbridge, East Sussex tel: 01424 838420. Another star performer.
Simply Organic, Sandylands, Market Weighton Road, Barlby, Selby, N. Yorks. tel: 01757 708540. Also stock fair trade foods and other goods.
Stoneybridge Organic Nursery and Farmshop, Tywardreath Par, Cornwall tel: 01726 813858.
Sunnyfields Organic Farm Shop, Marchwood, Southampton, Hants. tel: 01703 871408.

Also, see farmshops listed under mail order (pp. 97-107), box schemes (p. 120) and Old Plaw Hatch Farm (p. 168).

what they say . . .

> 'There have been times when I have found organic produce that is even cheaper than the non-organic produce in supermarkets. I buy from Brockfield Farm Organic Shop. They stock a comprehensive range of fruit and vegetables, dairy, meat, poultry and groceries, and even beer and wine. In fact, you can do most of your shopping in this one shop. I also enjoy the experience of shopping at the organic shop – it is so much more civilised than the supermarket. More like a village shop, with friendly and helpful service.' – *Lynda Jenkins, Bracknell, Berks.*

Brockfield Farm Organic Shop, Warfield, Bracknell, Berks. tel: 01344 882643 open Wed.–Sat. They sell only certified organic foods and foods containing organic ingredients, plus Eastbrook Farm and Graig Farm meats, as well as St Helena fish (p. 208).

Markets

Not much organic food is sold through traditional markets. *Organic market stalls* can sometimes be found in local markets – around twenty at the last count – usually selling local organic vegetables; or sometimes meat-producers have stalls selling their own produce at farm prices or thereabouts. Market stalls are a good idea for vegetables, especially, which are likely to have been picked fresh that morning. Occasionally, you find stalls such as that of Global Organics in Stroud market (Wednesdays and Fridays), which offer a very wide range of goods. Many are listed in the Soil Association's booklet, *Where to Buy Organic Food*.

In London, there are four *organic markets* where you can buy fruit and vegetables from producers direct, meat, dairy produce, breads and, depending on the market, other goods such as organic tofu, pickles and relishes, wines and other beverages. As with all markets, it pays to get there early, to get the best choice. Prices vary, but are lower than retail outlets; organic vegetables, for example, cost around the same price as conventional vegetables.

The London organic markets are:

Camden Green Organic Produce Market, *off Chalk Farm Road NW1* Open Sat. and Sun. 10am–6pm Fruit, vegetables, herbs, breads, cheese.

Greenwich Market, *off Stockwell Street SE10* Open Sat. 10am–4pm Fruit, vegetables, meat, breads, cheese.

Portobello Road Market, *Portobello Road W10* Open Thurs. 11am–6pm Fruit, vegetables, meat, breads, pickles and conserves.

Spitalfields Market, *Commercial Street E1* Open Fri. 11am–3pm, Sun. 9am–3pm Set up in 1992, this is London's largest organic market. Around a dozen stalls are housed inside a listed glass-covered Victorian building. Fruit, vegetables, meat, dairy produce, breads, cheese, tofu, tea and coffee, wines. Longwood Farm (p. 106) have a permanent shop for meat, open Friday and Sunday; and the shop next door, Unwin's Organic Provisions, open every day except Monday and Saturday, sell dairy produce, groceries and dried goods.

Farmers' markets

These have become a fixture in California and other parts of the USA, and offer an opportunity to buy direct from local farmers, growers and producers, who set up stalls to sell their goods. The first one in the UK started recently in Bath, organised by the Bath Environment Centre, and includes organic producers and those in the process of conversion from conventional to organic systems, selling fresh produce and meat. For details tel: 01225 460620.

WATCHWORD: An organic producer selling organic produce on a market stall will have his or her certification on display. A trader selling organic produce is unlikely to be registered; where products are not labelled, he or she must be able to provide proof of where the organic produce comes from, if asked; or you can check with the market manager.

Mail Order

Mail order is one of the best-developed sectors of the organic food market. The advantages are fourfold: it provides a greater variety of organic food; it offers the opportunity to buy direct from producers to whom you would not otherwise have access; it provides the ultimate in convenience shopping; and, in certain cases, it enables you to buy in bulk, which invariably works out cheaper. Standards are generally high. For many organic producers, mail order is the only or prime outlet for their goods – which means that they have to be good at it. The best, such as Eastbrook Farm Organic Meats, the Fresh Food Company, Graig Farm and Swaddles Green Farm, have developed considerable expertise and aim to give the highest-quality service, and can be said to have the leading edge in food mail order generally; while Longwood Farm and others can provide you with everything you will ever need – meat, dairy produce, vegetables, fruit, bread and groceries, and wine. The Soil Association's booklet, *Where to Buy Organic Food*, lists seventy-seven enterprises operating a mail order service. New and exciting developments have just come on stream, propelling organic mail order into the twenty-first century by enabling you to buy organic food on the Internet.

The variety of foods you can buy through mail order is much

larger than you would think: fresh and cured meat, cooked meat products, dairy produce, fresh fruit and vegetables, flours, bread and other baked goods, herbs and spices, wines and other drinks, tea and coffee and a whole range of dried, packaged, tinned and convenience foods. Latest hot news are organic chilli peppers and aubergines by post; and the ultimate in luxury, festive hampers and hand-made chocolates. Brief details of each group are set out in this section.

But first, a word of caution. There is a little more to mail order than simply ticking the boxes on the form. Unlike when sending off for clothes, where you can see a picture of what you're buying and you know it's easy to send an item back if you're not happy with it, shopping for fresh food by mail order can be more of a risk. But as with any kind of shopping, the more care you take, the better it will work out for you. So follow the simple guidelines under How to Be a Mail Order Sleuth (p. 94), and you will not be disappointed.

Also, as organic mail order specialists are the first to point out, although they make efforts to use, for example, recyclable plastics and non-PVC film where possible, mail order often inevitably entails the use of non-environmentally friendly packaging, and involves more food miles than supporting local shops. Purists, take note.

Points to remember:

- The same guarantees apply when buying organic food by mail order as from any other retail outlet. All producers and goods must be certified organic. All goods must be clearly labelled. Any company repackaging foods must be registered. If the company itself is not certified, anyone dealing with fresh food must be able to produce the relevant certification.
- Not everything may be available from the mail order list or catalogue at all times.
- There are two main types of delivery service. Perishables are delivered by an independent carrier within twenty-four hours, usually by a specified time and in special packaging to enable them to be kept chilled if necessary. Wines are also sent by independent carriers. Non-

perishables, including bulk purchases, are usually sent through the post and take from three to seven days, or occasionally longer.

● Promotional offers, discounts on bulk orders, bargain packs, free p&p for orders over a certain value – all these are part and parcel of mail order. Some companies make a separate charge for carriage costs, while others include it in the price of the goods.

● Mail order meat companies often have farm shops, retail outlets and their own delivery service to selected parts of the country; check to see.

How do I find out about mail order suppliers?

Food directories are the best source of organic food suppliers operating mail order. For a short list, see p. 363. Otherwise, consult the ads in magazines such as *Country Living*, the *BBC Vegetarian Good Food* and *Good Food Magazine*, the Soil Association's own journal *Living Earth*, and environmental magazines.

Is it cheaper? or more expensive?

People tend to have one of two views of mail order food: they think either that it is horrifically expensive or that it is very cheap. Neither is accurate. Pricing strategies vary, depending on the level of service, on whether or not the food is perishable, and on the type of producer. Prices also differ slightly from supplier to supplier on various items, but across the range they equal out.

Meat generally shows the greatest variation in price. It is certainly the most expensive food to mail, and prices will be slightly higher than the majority of retail outlets. Meat from small producers dealing with only their own meat is usually cheaper than that from larger specialist mail order companies, and can cost less than retail prices. Dairy products such as cheese are cheapest from the producers direct, who tend to charge farm shop prices plus carriage. Flour is very economical bought in bulk direct from the miller. Otherwise, expect to pay recommended retail prices plus carriage costs. Remember, too, that although you pay carriage costs, you save on petrol, parking and time.

How to Be a Mail Order Sleuth

Buying by mail order is straightforward. Suppliers are always keen to help and talk you through their products. In addition, bear these points in mind:

1 It's a good idea to shop around. The ranges of products, services and prices differ; this is especially so with meat. Where possible, begin by contacting a few suppliers so that you can compare and see which is likely to suit you best.

2 The 'feel-good' factor is important. Send for literature before placing an order; this will not only detail goods and prices but will give you a good idea of the people and how user-friendly they are likely to be.

3 Spend time on the phone talking to the supplier first; when buying meat, specify exactly what you want and discuss any special requirements.

4 Check how soon the order will be processed; delivery arrangements; substitutions – that is, whether you are willing for a similar item to be supplied if they haven't got exactly what you want; methods of payment; what happens if something goes wrong.

5 The clearer the order instructions, the better. Write out a detailed order on a separate sheet if there is not enough room on the order form, and keep a copy. If there is anything you definitely don't want, make this clear.

6 Get to know the supplier, or one particular person, and always ask for him or her by name. This way they get to know you and what you like, and you get to know them.

How does it work?

Service varies from the basic to the deluxe and from small producers with simple price lists where payment is usually by cheque, to specialist companies offering a broad range of goods and services, plus detailed literature, regular newsletters and recipe leaflets; the latter may also have fax, e-mail and internet facilities, and offer a premium service, including payment by credit card. But all operate the same way. You select what you want, telephone or fax the order, and it is then dispatched to you. Each company has its own terms and conditions – the small print – which you should read. Payment is usually on receipt of goods, but is sometimes requested with the order.

What happens if things go wrong?

They usually don't. Mail order works remarkably smoothly and most of the time goods arrive promptly, well packaged and in excellent condition. Occasionally there may be a minor mix-up in the order – usually due to a misunderstanding when the order was given.

If problems do arise, it's usually with the carrier. The answer is to act quickly:

- If for any reason the carrier has not delivered perishable goods by the time specified, ring up the supplier who can then chase the carrier.
- If goods arrive badly packed, inform the supplier, who can take it up with the carrier.
- If you're not satisfied in any way, inform the supplier. Most offer refunds or credit notes.
- Make sure you arrange delivery times when you know you will be at home, or ensure adequate alternative arrangements with a neighbour.

What and where to buy

The majority of mail order suppliers are organic meat producers, many of whom sell certain other fresh foods. Buying organic flour, cheese, juices and wines by mail order is also a well established practice. A few companies specialise in mail order of other kinds of food. The list below includes most major mail order specialists or suppliers, many of whom are described elsewhere in the book.

Meat: The most popular way to buy organic meat is through mail order. But it's a major purchase and the trickiest thing to buy, and it's well worth following a few guidelines and taking as much care as possible to ensure that you get exactly what you want. Standards of butchery, packaging, labelling and distribution are high.

Remember:

- Be cautious when buying meat from a supplier for the first time. Stick to tried-and-tested joints, favourite meats, good-value items. Be wary of diced meat.
- Unless you particularly want or need to, don't buy huge quantities or economy packs first, but select only what you know you will really like and will provide a good test of the supplier.
- Always discuss your order in detail. Check how long the meat has been hung and any other production and quality details important to you.
- Check that the meat is vacuum-packed. This is by far the best method of packaging, especially if you intend to freeze the meat. This is the norm except for whole poultry, which is difficult to vacuum-pack successfully.

For major suppliers, see Star Performers, p. 104. Other established meat-suppliers operating mail order services are:

Growing Concern, *Loughborough, Leics.* tel: 01509 237064/239228 The only supplier of rare-breed organic meat; see Farm Shops, p. 86.

Meat Matters, *Wantage, Oxon.* tel: 01235 762461 Operate a nationwide customised organic meat delivery service and a fruit and vegetable box scheme. Meat is sourced direct from Welsh farms through a Welsh butcher, who hangs and cuts the meat to order, as well as from Eastbrook Farm Organic Meats and Springfield Poultry. Other meat products include organic sausages, burgers and children's sausages, pâtés and pies. They also do veal, game in season, organic barbecue items in summer, organic turkey, geese, smoked wild Irish salmon and Crone's organic apple juice.

Naturally Yours, Witcham Toll, Ely, Cambs. tel: 01353 778723 E-mail orders @ naturally-yours.demon.co.uk. Website www. naturally-yours.demon.co.uk. Produce lamb, pork and chickens to Soil Association standards, plus additive-free beef. They also offer a range of home-made sausages, cooked meat dishes such as Hereford chicken, faggots, green chicken curry, spiced apricot lamb casserole, pâtés, vegetarian dishes and puddings such as rhubarb and orange crumble; also, organic barbecue, stir-fry packs, vegetable and mixed fruit packs. Note that not all items listed in their catalogue are certified organic; check to see. Free van delivery service extends over a wide area, including St Albans, Luton, Cambridgeshire, Rutland, Bury St Edmunds and Kings Langley.

Organic and Free-range Meats Ltd, Jamesfield Farm, Newburgh, Fife, Scotland tel: 01738 850498 E-mail 101566.2262 @ compuserve.com. Registered with the Scottish Organic Producers' Association. An organic farm since 1986, they produce organic beef, lamb, mutton and vegetables and free-range pork and poultry, sold through their farm shop and mail order next-day delivery service. Special requests catered for. Mail order also includes their own sausages and bacon, and haggis made for them by a local butcher; plus salmon and locally smoked wild salmon. The shop also sells a range of organic and ecologically sound staples.

Pure Meat Direct, Upper Stondon, Beds. tel: 01462 8515610 A specialist high-quality meat mail order company with a shop, B&M Seafoods, selling meat and fish, at 258 Kentish Town High Street, London NW5. Their organic beef, lamb and pork carry the Soil Association symbol. Other high-animal-welfare, additive-free meats include Eldon Wild Blue pork, poultry and free-range veal; game is also available. Stuffed meat specialities comprise a mixture of organic and additive-free meats, with organic stuffing ingredients.

West Country Organic Foods Ltd, Exeter, Devon tel: 01647 24724 Soil Association registered. A co-operative venture comprising various organic producers in the south-west. They supply, by mail order, beef, lamb, pork, poultry, dry-cured bacon, home-made sausages and meat pastry products. The meat is well hung to ensure good eating quality, and is also available in their retail shop, Packer & Son, High Street, Crediton, Devon. They can supply vegetables by request, with meat orders.

Also

***Welsh Haven Poultry**, Pembrokeshire* tel: 01437 781552 They supply chicken, ducks and geese. See p. 199.

General groceries: These include dried, tinned, packet and convenience foods, baby foods, staples, dairy produce, chilled products including vegetarian pâtés and spreads, drinks, herbs and spices, condiments, confectionery – in fact, everything from organic baked beans to blue corn tortillas and Japanese miso.

***Ceres Natural Foods**, Yeovil, Somerset* tel: 01935 428791 Their mail order wholefood/healthfood catalogue, which lists ingredients, contains a selected range of organic foods: dried fruit, seeds, nuts, pulses, rice, cereals, flours, sugar, pasta, dry ready meals, breads. Orders are accepted by post only, and require prepayment; no minimum order.

***Countryside Wholefoods Ltd**, London N13* tel: 0181 363 2933 They have two shops: 19 Forty Hill, Enfield, and 90 Aldermans Hill, Palmers Green. An extensive range of organic and conventional wholefood/health food products is available by mail order. Fresh and dairy produce, and other fragile items, are excluded. Their organic products are sold under the Devonshire Foods label, and are certified. Free delivery in London and surrounding areas.

***Damhead Organically Grown Foods**, Lothianbum, Edinburgh* tel: 0131 445 1490 See Star Performers, p. 81. An exclusively organic mail order service, they send orders by overnight courier, and include everything except meat and fresh fruit and vegetables. An excellent selection of baby foods and dairy produce. Non-food items include household goods and toiletries.

Longwood Farm, Suffolk tel: 01638 717120 See Star performers, p. 106. Can provide everything and has one of the best mail order lists for groceries.

Organic Health tel: 01773 717718 See Star Performers, p. 82. Mail order with a catalogue and personal service, from one of the country's leading certified organic food shops. Their list includes bread and cakes and wines. There is a small section of non-organic wholefood/health food, and non-food items too.

Also

Greencity Wholefoods, Glasgow tel: 0141 554 7633 A wholefood co-operative wholesaler with an extensive range of organic foods, they operate a bulk-buying delivery service for consumer groups at discount prices in Scotland, minimum order £100. They also offer a national mail order service to individual customers, minimum order around £25, goods priced at recommended retail price, p&p included.

Hampers Hampers, London N4 tel: 0181 800 8008. A luxury hamper gift service offering a variety of hampers priced from around £20 to £200, plus delivery, containing predominantly organic foods, wines and delectable hand-made Jeannette's Dutch chocolates (p. 281). Friendly, efficient service. Their hampers are also available through selected home delivery services, such as The Better Food Company (p. 121).

Take It from Here, Egham, Surrey freephone 0800 37064 A family company importing a select range of high-quality Italian foods personally sourced from small producers, including organic pasta sauces and dressings, La Selva tomato products and Roi olive oil, plus hand-produced jars of roasted organic aubergines and peppers in (non-certified) olive oil, also by La Selva.

Fruit and vegetables: These are available nationwide through two services. A few retail shops operating mail order offer fruit and vegetables; consult the Soil Association booklet, *Where to Buy Organic Food*. See also The Better Food Company and Sundrum Organics (p. 121) and Meat Matters (p. 96).

The Fresh Food Company, 326 Portobello Road, London W10 tel: 0181 969 0351 E-mail organic @ freshfood.co.uk.www.fresh-food.co.uk. Soil Association registered. Award-winning, deluxe (and therefore not cheap), nationwide, next-day home delivery service for fresh produce, Cornish fish and National Trust spring water. All produce is certified and cut to order, and comes from specified growers direct, either home-grown, primarily from Eastern County Organic Producers (ECOP), or imported. Produce can be bought as a mixed box, as separate modules including carrots, apples and oranges for juicing, or as individualised orders; 10 per cent discounts are given for two or more main boxes. They have recently expanded to include an extensive home delivery service covering south London, and are in the process of widening

Peppers by Post

A must for chilli and aubergine aficionados. A new mail order venture by chilli experts and growers Michael and Joy Michaud of Sea Spring Farm, West Bexington, Dorchester, Dorset tel: 01308 897892. The farm shortly receives its official Soil Association symbol in May 1998 – though they have always grown organically and pesticides have never been used. They supply an exciting range of home-grown fresh chilli peppers and aubergines unavailable anywhere else, grown in polytunnels, at £1.50 per pack, plus p&p, available July–November. Varieties of chilli include Poblano, Thai hot, Habanero, Hungarian Hot Wax and Yellow Cayenne. Selection depends on what's ripe and ready. Their mixed chilli bag includes new varieties under trial; a recipe leaflet is included with your order. They also produce tomatillos – a Mexican fruit known as the jam berry, which looks like a large pale-lime-green Cape gooseberry, with a flavour somewhere between this and cooked tomatoes and which is grown outside without pesticides, but not certified organic.

their range to a total fresh food service to include meat, poultry, game, Demeter-registered bacon, sausages, home-cooked meats, charcuterie, pies, quiches, a full range of dairy produce including Normandy organic butter, breads, apple juices, wines and beers. Friendly service; credit cards accepted; a regular newsletter, containing special offers and recipe ideas. They also supply Peakfresh preserving bags (p. 131).

Organics Direct, *London EC2* tel: 0171 729 2828 www.organics-direct.com. Soil Association registered. A new specialist mail order company, offering nationwide delivery of organic fruit and vegetable boxes supplied by the Organic Marketing Company, Hereford, and dairy and macrobiotic boxes. Other lines include baby food, Quiet Revolution fresh soups, wines, bread from the Authentic Bread Company, juicers, Christmas hampers, fresh herbs, oils and chutneys, and mineral water. Operate their own overnight delivery network and aim to price competitively.

Fish: see p. 205.

Dairy produce: Organic milk, cream, butter, eggs, ice-cream and cheese are all available by mail order. See Star Performers (p. 104); Rachel's Dairy (p. 165), Rocombe Ice-cream (p. 171), the Fresh Food Company and Organics Direct (above), Sundrum Organics and the Better Food Company (p. 121). For buying cheese by mail order, see p. 159.

Bread and other baked goods: See the Village Bakery (p. 218), Organic Health, Countryside Wholefoods, and Damhead Organically Grown Foods (pp. 98–99), Longwood Farm (p. 106), the Fresh Food Company and Organics Direct (above), the Better Food Company and Sundrum Organics (p. 121).

Flour, cereals: See Doves Farm, Shipton Mill, Little Salkeld and Pimhill (pp. 229–31), Organic Health, Countryside Wholefoods and Damhead Organically Grown Foods (pp. 98–99) and Longwood Farm (p. 106).

Herbs and spices: Hambledon Herbs see Star Performer, p. 252. Their comprehensive mail order catalogue includes organic herb teas, gift selections and flower essences. Also available from Organic Health, Countryside Wholefoods, Damhead Organically Grown Foods (pp. 98–99) and Longwood Farm (p. 106).

Olive oil: See p. 302.

Tea and coffee: *Tea & Coffee Plant* tel: 0171 221 8137 E-mail coffee @ pro-net.co.uk. Mail order catalogue includes organic Assam tea, loose and as tea-bags, and organic Colombian and Mexican coffees. Retail outlet at 170 Portobello Road, W11, and stall at Spitafield market. Also from Organic Health, Countryside Wholefoods, Damhead Organically Grown Foods (pp. 98–99) and Longwood Farm (p. 106); Hampstead Tea & Coffee (p. 259); Hambleden Herbs (green tea, p. 252).

Wines, beers, cider, spirits, juices: Available from wine merchants specialising in organic wines and other drinks and from specialist producers. Major ones are:

Avalon Vineyard, Glastonbury, Somerset tel: 01749 860393 Soil Association registered. An organic vineyard and fruit farm, producing organic wines, traditional cider and organic fruit wines – apple, red and white gooseberry, strawberry and tayberry – made from their own fruit. By mail order, available by the case, costs the price of ten bottles plus delivery charge. Also, direct sales from the farm shop – visitors welcome.

Chudleigh Vineyard, Chudleigh, near Torquay, Devon tel: 01626 853248 Soil Association registered. An acclaimed organic vineyard, producing its own award-winning wines. A selection of four white wines, dry to medium-dry, all one price, available by the case, £66.50 including delivery.

Dunkerton's Cider, Pembridge, near Leominster, Herefordshire tel: 01544 388653 Soil Association registered. An organic Herefordshire cider and perry producer, selling a range of blended and single-variety dry and sweet ciders, and dry to medium-sweet perry produced from traditional varieties of perry pears.

Minimum order 1 case, in litre bottles, from £36.50 including delivery. They also have a cider mill, a shop and their own restaurant, the Cider House Restaurant tel: 01544 388161.

The Organic Wine Co., PO Box 81, High Wycombe, Bucks. tel: 01494 446557 Specialist mail order organic wine merchant, supplying 150 organic wines plus beers, cider and brandy. Also, Il Casale Tuscan olive oil and oak-aged wine vinegar, gold- and silver-award Mas de Gourgonnier Provençal olive oil, grape and apricot juices, UK apple juice and French tomato juice. Mail order catalogue and newsletter available.

Sedlescombe Vineyard, near Robertsbridge, East Sussex tel: 01580 830715 Soil Association registered. Supply organic wines, cider and juices. Mail order catalogue available.

Vinceremos Wines and Spirits Ltd, Bramley, Leeds tel: 0113 257 7545 E-mail Vinceremos @ AOL.COM. Specialist organic wine merchant, selling a full range, plus beers, ciders, spirits and juices. Mail order catalogue available. Also run the HDRA Organic Wine Club.

Vintage Roots Ltd, Farley Farms – Bridge Farm, Arborfield, Berks. tel: 0118 976 1999 Specialist organic wine merchant, stocking over 250 wines, plus beers, ciders, spirits and juices. Mail order catalogue available. Exclusive supplier of Broughton Pastures organic mead and ginger wine.

Why Buy Organic Wine?

Wine production is highly intensive. It is estimated, for example, that vineyards account for only 10 per cent of arable land but over three-quarters of herbicides and nearly half of all pesticides used (for pesticide usage on UK vines, see p. 339). A recent three-year study of French farmers has concluded that there is a significant link between bladder cancer and pesticide exposure in vineyards. Residues are frequently detected. The last time wine was tested, in 1993, half of imported red and white wine samples and three out of five samples of English wine contained fungicide residues. In addition, a cocktail of chemicals is used to make cheap wine, and chemicals such as sulphur are used to preserve it – if you get a headache from wine, high levels of sulphur are the likely reason. Organic grapes are grown without the use of artificial fertilisers or synthetic pesticides, though Bordeaux mixture, a copper compound used for many generations to protect against mildew, is permitted. Vine varieties are selected for disease-resistance and character rather than for high yields, crops are grown between the vines to provide fertility, and vine prunings are returned to the land. Like all fine winemakers, organic winemakers produce their wines with a minimum of added permitted chemical treatments and low levels of sulphur, and do not use animal fining agents. Yields are smaller, which means better-quality wine; conventional makers of good wines are increasingly adopting the policy of not using artificial fertilisers precisely because the best way to improve quality is to reduce yields.

There are over three hundred organic wines available, and the range is steadily increasing. The majority are made by small family growers. Over half are French; look for the words *vin biologique* on the label. Many of the best winemakers have always used organic methods of agriculture, though are not certified; many more are turning to organic methods, especially bio-dynamic cultivation techniques which, they believe, produce finer wines. Wine experts comment on the purity of organic wines, finding that they typically have a fresher taste, express the grape variety and *terroir* better, and do not give you a headache. They cost around 5–10 per cent more, less for wines over £5.

Star Performers: Mail Order

Four of the best:

Graig Farm, Dolau, Llandrindod, Wells, Powys tel: 01597 851655/ 07000 E-mail sales @ graigfarm.co.uk. www.graigfarm.co.uk. Soil Association registered. An award-winning company specialising in organic and additive-free meat produced to highest welfare standards; poultry-producer, exclusive supplier of St Helena fish, and supporter of the fair-trade scheme. They sell a full range of organic meat, ham and bacon, meat products, including cooked meats, pâtés, biltong (spiced dried meat) and dairy produce, all produced locally. Another first from them is organic ostrich meat, which eats like beef but is lower in fat and cholesterol than poultry. They produce hand-made pies with mainly organic ingredients, such as mutton and ale, and chicken with apricot and tarragon, as well as ready-made convenience meals such as St Helena bake (fish pie), Welsh mutton bake and pizza. Dairy products comprise organic milk, butter, cream and a few cheeses. Additive-free meats include chicken, duck, quail, goose, guinea-fowl, wild boar. They also stock local wild venison and rabbit and are the only supplier of organic mutton. My favourite chicken-producer – their chicken livers and home-made faggots are excellent value.

Other lines include organic peanut butter, herbs, spices, and spice pastes from Zimbabwe, organic teas from the Seychelles, plus tropical dried fruit, tomatoes and mushrooms from Uganda, local wildflower honey and Pimhill cakes. Friendly, efficient sales staff; special requests catered for; credit cards accepted; detailed literature supplied on request; regular newsletter; gift service. Produce also available direct from the farm shop. They operate an extensive home delivery service and have over thirty retail outlets. Nationwide deliveries free for orders over £40. Now stock wines.

***Eastbrook Farm Organic Meats**, Bishopstone, near Swindon, Wilts*. tel: 01793 790 462/460 E-mail eastbrookfarm @ compuserve.com. Soil Association registered. One of the country's best-known award-winning organic meat-producers. Their mail order service comprises their own beef, lamb, veal, pork, offal, award-winning dry-cured bacon, ham and gammon, eight different kinds of sausage, including their award-winning spicy lamb merguez, P.J. Onions organic chickens and organic cheeses. Veal is becoming a speciality; calves are mothered by nurse cows, given their own new specially designed housing, are fed on warm milk, and graze outside in summer and are fed hay or silage at other times; they are killed at six months and hung for twelve days. The company offers a full range of prepared cuts including beef olives, stuffed noisettes of lamb and pork; a children's range; barbecue boxes in summer, including smoked chicken. They also buy in meat from other farms, sell free-range and organic chickens including their latest addition, rare-breed organic table chickens, and free-range ducks. Friendly, efficient sales service; special requests catered for; credit cards accepted; a regular (humorous) newsletter, containing special offers and recipe ideas, is included with the order. They hold regular open days, run Eastbrook Farm Club for kids, 'The Piglets', and have a retail shop, 50 High Street, Shrivenham, Oxon. tel: 01793 782211. Local delivery service.

Longwood Farm, *Tuddenham St Mary, Bury St Edmunds, Suffolk* tel: 01638 717120 Soil Association registered. A remarkable venture which includes a farm shop, two permanent shops in Spitalfields Market, London (see p. 90), plus stalls at Portobello Green and Greenwich markets, London. They have one of the most comprehensive mail order lists for dairy and non-dairy produce and groceries, featuring over five hundred lines, plus a large selection of fresh produce and bread. They have recently acquired a drinks licence. Produce and sell all their own meat, sausages, cured and cooked meats and poultry, including Christmas geese and turkeys, from the farm shop and through mail order. Their meat is well hung and cut to order. Friendly efficient service; special requests catered for; separate mail order list for groceries; a regular newsletter.

Swaddles Green Farm, *Hare Lane, Buckland St Mary, Chard, Somerset* tel: 01460 234387 E-mail organic @ swaddles.co.uk. Website http://www.swaddles.co.uk. Soil Association and Organic Farmers and Growers registered. Described by the *Sunday Telegraph* as 'gastronomes who produce the kind of food people go to France for', this is another award-winning meat-supplier that produces an impressive range of home-made organic everyday and special-occasion ready meals (meat and non-meat), excellent organic charcuterie, pâtés and pies, soups and desserts, all made on the premises. The meat is raised on their own farm and on neighbouring farms, to their own specifications, to ensure highest eating quality; for example, all beef is from traditional beef breeds, has proper conformation of fat and is hung for three weeks. All meat is cut to order. They offer a full range of beef, veal, lamb, pork, chicken and delicious duck; offal; bacon and hams; barbecue and picnic packs; sausages and burgers; children's burgers and sausages; chorizo, saucisson d'Arles, spiced beef, rillettes, cooked glazed hams, veal, chicken and duck galantine, and so on – plus thirteen different pies and ready-to-eat pizza. They also sell organic chicken bones for stock (a bargain), organic marinades, stocks, eggs, butter, Cheddar, chutneys and relishes, organic beer, wine and cider. They now operate a grocery round including freshly harvested produce, freshly baked bread and fresh farm milk bottled the same day. Friendly, efficient service and advice; special requests catered for; credit cards accepted; excellent literature, including recipes. Extensive free home delivery service to London, Surrey and Middlesex.

Also, something slightly different:

Higher Hacknell Farm, Burrington, Umberleigh, Devon tel: 01769 560909 An award-winning organic farm – awards include the Lorraine Award for conservation – that has developed its own mail order fresh-meat box system to supply their pedigree suckler, richly flavoured South Devon beef and lamb direct to customers at exceptionally affordable prices: only £6 per kilo for beef and £5.95 per kilo for lamb, plus a standard £5 charge for nationwide delivery. The meat is well hung, professionally butchered and vacuum-packed. Customers receive a mixed box containing (all cuts are included) 10–12 kilos of beef or 8–10 kilos of lamb, which is easily manageable for a family with a large freezer. The boxes are available approximately every three weeks. Individual cuts are also available, priced accordingly. Free local deliveries. The farm produces a regular newsletter, and organises farm walks; it has been managed organically since 1988 and has never had a case of BSE. They also grow and sell potatoes. Their meat can be enjoyed at the nearby country hotel, Northcote Manor, which uses mainly organic food.

Box Schemes

Box schemes have revolutionised the buying of organic vegetables and have been a phenomenal success. Demand far exceeds supply and, as with any rapidly developing sector, standards vary. The best enterprises are excellent, enabling consumers to enjoy a weekly box or bag of some of the freshest and healthiest locally produced seasonal vegetables it is possible to eat, purchased direct from the grower at highly competitive prices, and with a flavour that can be out of this world. Such schemes are also the most environmentally friendly and sustainable way to buy vegetables, while forging that valuable link with the land that modern lifestyles have lost. Many intermediary schemes also exist, involving growers who buy in supplementary produce or middle men who buy produce from a number of sources. Some retail outlets also offer box schemes and home delivery services offer vegetable and sometimes fruit boxes as well.

All box schemes offer the opportunity to buy a mixed box of vegetables that vary from week to week. But though they share common characteristics and aims, the schemes vary in the scope and kind of services they offer. So it is well worth checking those available in your area, to see which is likely to suit you best. Broadly speaking, they divide into two groups: traditional producer-operated box schemes where the grower produces and dispatches the vegetables, and company-operated box schemes run by private individuals, who buy in produce.

It is as well to be aware that standards do vary. And eating in season has its high and low points, too. While summer boxes are universally a delight, most winter boxes inevitably major on roots and greens. A friend who is a well known food writer living in London, committed to his weekly box scheme – though, like most people, liable to get fed up with swede – asked me to say: 'Stay with it.' In other words, in order to flourish, box schemes, like any business, need support throughout the year.

Producer-owned schemes

Rural, predominantly seasonal, box schemes run by the growers themselves who, in the main, operate within a radius of twenty miles or less and for part of the year only, from early summer onwards. Each week the grower harvests whatever crops are in season, makes up the bags or boxes and then takes them to central delivery points for customers to collect. Crops are harvested, bagged and ready for collection generally within 24–36 hours. The grower determines what goes into the box – the customer does not find out what the week's box will contain until it arrives. To offer more choice, some growers also buy in a few extras such as mush-rooms, lemons or avocados as optional extras.

Company-operated schemes

Generally but not exclusively urban schemes, catering for the ever-growing demand for box schemes in towns and cities, and operating all year round. The best companies buy direct from selected growers or well known wholesale companies dealing exclusively with organic produce. Others may use some 'grade-out' produce – that is, produce that does not meet the cosmetic standards required by large retailers. They operate from a central depot where bought-in produce is immediately bagged and boxed and delivered to the customer's home rather than to a central pick-up point. Some have an arrangement whereby the produce is bagged for them, on the spot, by the grower. The age of the produce depends on the supply chain: for example, whether it has been bought direct from a farm or via whole-salers.

> NOTE: Buying in produce means that company-oper-ated box schemes have more flexibility, and are able to offer their customers more conventional choice. Increasingly they offer self-selection. It is also means, however, that some produce is imported (thus more food miles) and that selections will contain out-of-season vegetables.

- Many box schemes, especially if the grower has a farm shop, or if the scheme operates from a retail outlet, offer additional goods including meat, dairy produce, bread, groceries and eco-friendly cleaners. Some produce regular newsletters and recipe leaflets too.
- Some box schemes offer more flexibility than others: for example, some will take into account customers' likes and dislikes.
- Many box schemes, rural and urban, offer home delivery; some make a delivery charge, some deliver free.
- A growing number of box schemes now also include fruit; a few company-operated schemes offer separate

fruit boxes. Most fruit is bought-in.
- If, for any reason, the customer is dissatisfied with a particular produce, a refund or substitution is usually offered.
- Customers acting as pick-up points or co-ordinators receive a discount or a free box.

What will the box contain?

Depending on the season and size, boxes contain six to twelve or more different vegetables. Basics – potatoes, roots, onions – will always be included. You can also expect at least one green vegetable and seasonal salad stuff, plus unusual vegetables, mushrooms and seasonal treats such as strawberries and asparagus, if grown. These real-life examples of summer and autumn boxes are from Northwood Vegetable Boxes in Devon (p. 116).

20 August
bunched carrots
coriander
courgettes
cucumbers
French beans
green peppers
potatoes
ruby chard
snap peas
spring onions
Lollo Rosso and Green Salad Bowl lettuce

15 October
beetroot
carrots
cauliflower or calabrese
coriander
courgettes
fennel
onions
parsnips
potatoes

salad bag: rocket and Red Salad Bowl lettuce, endive,
   radicchio, marigold and nasturtium flowers
sweetcorn
tomatoes

- Traditional box schemes are likely to contain more
  variety overall and more unusual vegetables, though will
  contain less variety at certain times of the year.
- Box scheme growers produce a diverse range of crops,
  from traditional stalwarts such as potatoes to fancy
  salad crops, strawberries, herbs, and unusual vegetables
  like Swiss chard and Chinese lettuce. Traditional
  varieties and varieties renowned for their flavour are
  often preferred so that, ironically, though the customer
  may have very little say in what goes into the box, the
  choice can be better than that found in retail outlets.
- Box scheme growers take great pride in their vegetables,
  and quality control is important. But though
  presentation matters, cosmetic 'finesse' and fancy
  packaging are less important. So expect healthy, fresh
  vegetables of excellent quality in their natural state –
  that is, as harvested. This means they will be unwashed,
  and presented with a minimum of trimming. Salad stuff
  will be packed separately, but most vegetables will be
  loose. You should expect imperfections in size, blemishes
  and the occasional insect. But you should not expect old,
  badly damaged, or severely wilted produce.
- The range and type of vegetables grown are governed by
  what grows best for each grower. This means that every
  box scheme grower's portfolio will be slightly different,
  varying according to which part of the country the crops
  are grown in.

fact

Crops grown with heavy inputs of fertilisers are more
prone to disease, so need more pesticide sprays.

Handling and Storing

Freshly harvested growers' produce is just like your own home-grown produce, and should be treated in exactly the same way. Unlike conventional produce, it has rarely had its field heat removed, nor has it spent time in high-tech storage or been packaged or sprayed to improve its shelf life. It comes to you in its prime as nature intended, and to enjoy it at its best you must treat it differently:

1 Unpack your box as soon as you get home – don't leave it to wilt or hang around in the garage.

2 Sort the vegetables into categories: roots, salad stuff, green veg and the rest.

3 Inspect for insects, baby worms and the like, and remove.

4 Pick out any yellowing or damaged leaves, paying particular attention to salad leaves and crops such as spinach and Chinese vegetables. Wrap immediately in thick plastic bags or Peakfresh bags (p. 131), and store in the fridge.

5 Keep roots in brown paper bags in the salad drawer or somewhere cool; it's easier to wash these while the dirt is still moist, though they will keep better unwashed.

6 Eat fresh!

● Company-operated box schemes that buy in offer standard retail produce including seasonal, out-of-season and imported produce – which includes 'exotics' such as avocados, kiwi fruit and lemons. Standards of freshness vary.

Price guide: Prices depend on the type of scheme and the size of the box, and are fixed for the year, irrespective of what the box contains. They start from as little as £3 and go up to £15–£20, with £7–£10 the average price you can expect to pay. In London, you may pay more.

Producer-owned box schemes may be up to 30–40 per cent cheaper than retail prices. Most growers offer a choice of box sizes, and many offer optional seasonal items at a small extra charge as well as bulk buying of surpluses.

Company-operated box schemes usually, though not always, charge slightly less than retail prices. Most offer a choice of box size. Those that offer self-selection have printed price lists.

Are box schemes for me?

Box schemes of one sort or another now supply an estimated fifty thousand households nationwide, including celebrities such as Ruby Wax and Julian Clary and pop stars. Many become enthusiastic devotees. Research has shown that those who join a producer-operated box scheme don't just rediscover how good vegetables are and how much flavour they have – they rediscover also the joy of eating in season. Knowing the producer adds a human dimension that a supermarket never can. People find that they eat and cook more vegetables, and that their children eat more too. Many are surprised to discover that the lack of choice is not a drawback but a bonus – there is an excitement in what this week will bring, and you find yourself cooking vegetables that you may not usually cook, such as beetroot or Swiss chard. Many of those who join company-operated box schemes also speak enthusiastically of the flavour of the vegetables and the convenience they offer.

However, getting the best out of a box scheme is a two-way process, and requires a change of attitude in the customer too. A box scheme does not offer you a year-round supply of anything you want, and, as already mentioned, the produce is not cosmetically perfect. Delivery in cities can be erratic. If your vegetable consumption is very low, or you don't relish the thought of eating parsnips (or swede), however fresh, every week for two months, are wedded to your weekly supermarket shop, or don't particularly value the less tangible benefits they offer, box schemes are probably not for you.

Still busting for organic vegetables? Try a customised home delivery service instead (p. 120).

How do I join?

Box schemes are available nationwide; southern counties have the most, with twelve to thirty-plus outlets, and far northern counties the least. London is very well serviced and most major cities and towns boast several outlets. This means that though traditional rural producer-owned box schemes still number less than a hundred, there will be a box scheme of some sort in your area, and most people will have a choice. The Soil Association booklet, *Where to Buy Organic Food*, contains a full list, tel: 0117 9290661. Alternatively, consult *The Organic Directory*. Box schemes are also advertised locally, generally through health food and wholefood shops selling organic produce, or via leaflet distribution.

- There is no subscription or conditions attached, nor do you need to commit yourself to any fixed period of time, though some company-operated box schemes may ask for a week's cancellation notice. Unless the scheme operates a door-to-door delivery, you may be asked to join the rota for pick-up and delivery points.

NOTE: Some box schemes are better than others. Boxes of drab and tired-out vegetables, with far too many potatoes, do happen. If so, don't continue with that particular scheme – try to find a better one.

fact
Non-organically grown vegetables may contain up to 20 per cent more water than equivalent organically grown vegetables.

Box-Scheme Checklist

Personal recommendation from someone you know who uses a box scheme is always the best starting-point. Remember that standards do vary, so phone around first. Don't be afraid to ask questions, seek advice or discuss any teething problems. The aim is to find which of the available schemes suits you best. Most have literature they will send to prospective participants.

1 Ask about the range of vegetables grown, other goods and/or services provided, whether customer likes and dislikes are taken into account, complaints procedures and, of course, delivery arrangements. Ask what happens if you are out at work all day, and if necessary arrange to have the box delivered to a neighbour; or give specific instructions about a safe, cool place where the box can be left, or inquire whether the operator can help with special packaging to protect the produce better.

2 Check price(s). Ask what a typical box contains in summer and in winter.

3 Check credentials. Is the box scheme registered? If not, what guarantees do they provide that produce is genuinely organic? If buying from a company-operated box scheme, ask where they source their supplies.

Star Performers: Box Scheme Operators

There are many excellent box schemes. The following five, producer-owned, are examples of what you can expect from the best.

Growing with Nature, *Bradshaw Lane Nursery, Pilling, Lancs.* tel: 01253 790046 Soil Association registered. An award-winning, dedicated husband-and-wife team. They grow over thirty-five crops, freshly harvested and delivered to the door or via agents throughout Lancashire, the South Lakes and as far as Settle, North Yorks. Now linked with three other local growers whose produce they market, enabling an all-year-round service. They offer a 'grower's choice' traditional box scheme, featuring approximately 10–14 seasonal vegetables and salads for £7.50 or £10, and a 'customer's choice' individualised list. Mushrooms, avocados, citrus, kiwi fruit, cheese, and truly free-range, additive-free eggs are also included. They hold regular open days, produce an informative leaflet and a periodic newsletter.

Crops include potatoes, onions, leeks, roots, cabbages, kale, sprouts, broccoli, celery, courgettes, squashes, tomatoes, cucumber, peas and beans, salad crops and herbs.

Unusual crops include kohlrabi, chard, Jerusalem artichokes, mixed salad leaves in spring and summer, and stir-fry greens in winter.

Merricks Farm, *Langport, Somerset* tel: 01458 252901 Soil Association registered and winners of the 1997 Organic Food Award for box schemes. Traditional seasonal box scheme servicing about 150 households locally. Grow over a hundred different varieties of vegetables and salad plants, plus soft fruit and herbs. They offer four standard boxes, priced £4–£10, or a customised order list. Operate end May to end February. They also sell their own pork raised from rare breed crosses and stock organic beef, lamb and eggs for sale at the farm.

Crops include: asparagus, aubergines, celeriac, Jerusalem artichokes, peppers, ten different varieties of potatoes, garlic, red and white onions and shallots, cabbages, courgettes, spinach, peas and beans, broccoli, kale, winter squashes, strawberries, raspberries and black and redcurrants.

Unusual crops include: sugar snap peas, chillies, heritage tomatoes, oriental vegetables, ruby chard, mooli radishes and banana peppers.

Northwood Vegetables Boxes, *Northwood Farm, Christow, Exeter, Devon* tel: 01647 252915 Soil Association registered. One of the original pioneering box schemes, the epitome of local food for local people, this enterprise has provided inspiration and a role model for countless others. Set up in 1991 by Tim and Jan Deane, who grow over sixty varieties of vegetables and salads, and operate from July to March. Freshly harvested, the produce is mainly delivered within a three-mile radius supplying 130 families. The emphasis is on high quality and standards in every respect, including presentation. They buy in some maincrop potatoes and onions, or produce needed to replace crop failures, but otherwise all produce is their own. Boxes contain 8–12 different seasonal items, in three sizes, at £6–£9. Customer likes, dislikes and special requests are catered for. They have a regular newsletter and hold an annual open day.

Crops include potatoes, roots, leeks, snap peas, brassicas, celery, cherry and beefsteak tomatoes, salad crops, peppers, aubergines, fennel, sweetcorn, squash; and herbs – basil, coriander, parsley, chervil and mitsuba.

Unusual crops include winter chicories, celtuce, mixed oriental greens including mitsuna and komatsuna, Hamburg parsley, winter radish, hungry-gap kale and romanesco.

Riverford Farm near Buckfastleigh, Devon tel: 01803 762720 Soil Association registered. One of the largest organic growers in the south-west, this is part of the same family concern as the Riverford Farm shop (p. 88), but run independently. A vegetable gourmet's delight, they grow over eighty crops, from basic staples (including the largest, juiciest carrots in the world!) to fresh herbs, globe artichokes, fennel, courgette flowers, aubergines and winter squashes, picked fresh, and often sold at half supermarket retail prices. They operate a year-round service, supplementing home-grown produce with bought-in organic produce during late March–May. Boxes contain 8–15 seasonal items and are available in three sizes, at £5–£7.50. Organic eggs also available. An excellent leaflet, a booklet including cooking hints, and a regular newsletter are provided free. Farm walks are held every month during April–October. Produce also available at the farm shop.

Tolhurst Organic Produce, West Lodge, Hardwick Estate, Whitchurch-on-Thames, Pangbourne, near Reading, S. Oxon. tel: 01734 843428 Soil Association registered. A classic, traditional box scheme run by one of the most experienced organic growers in the country, Iain Tolhurst. Save for mushrooms, no produce is bought in. They grow fifty-four crops, including (superb) strawberries, raspberries, melons and grapes in a large walled garden, plus further field crops. They operate ten and a half months of the year. Offer small, medium and large boxes, containing 5 or 6, 7 or 8 and 10 or 11 different seasonal vegetables and salads, at £3.50, £4.50 and £6.50 respectively. Supply an extras list for seasonal bulk items such as potatoes, carrots and onions, and for specialities such as pink fir potatoes and soft fruit, at prices guaranteed to be competitive with supermarkets. Produce also sold (at retail prices) through The Old Dairy, Hardwick Estate, Pangbourne (p. 87).

Crops include potatoes (4 varieties), onions, leeks, roots, swede, summer turnips, cabbages (5 varieties), cauliflowers, sprouts, broccoli, leaf beet, spring cabbage, peas and beans, courgettes, spinach, salad plants, celery, tomatoes, peppers, aubergines.

Unusual crops include celeriac, fennel, winter squash (5 varieties), Chinese vegetables, winter radish, garlic, scorzonera, salsify, red lettuce, rocket and ruby chard.

Company-operated box schemes: a few examples

Limited Resources, *Hulme, Manchester* tel: 0161 226 4777 An award-winning urban box scheme supplying local outlets in central and south Manchester, and a member of Organic 2000. They supply home-grown and imported produce all year round, including bread, eggs, milk and environmentally friendly cleaning products, available as singles', standard or 'grower's choice', at £5, £6.50/£7.50 and £9.50, or as customised orders. Most produce comes from the Organic Marketing Company, Hereford. They are committed to reducing food miles, and 90 per cent of deliveries are made by bicycle and trailer.

Organic Connections, *Wisbech, Cambs.* tel: 01945 773374 Soil Association registered. A family business with their own organic farm offering a modern box scheme serving postal areas PE and

CB, covering a wide area including Cambridgeshire, Lincolnshire, Norfolk and Essex. They specialise in produce from local growers, and offer standard boxes and add-on modules including pasta and salad boxes, bread and dairy produce and their own organic apples and apple juice. Produce is individually wrapped. They publish a regular newsletter.

The Organic Marketing Company, near Ledbury, Hereford tel: 01531 640819 A major wholesaler and distributor who supply local home-grown and imported organic produce (around 50 per cent of each) to eighty box schemes throughout the country. Ring them and they will try to put you in touch with the nearest box scheme or mail order supplier. They also supply the Authentic Bread Company breads (p. 214).

Organic Roundabout, Hockley, Birmingham tel: 0121 515 3524 Soil Association registered. One of the country's best-known and largest company-operated box schemes, supplying over two thousand households in the Midlands, recently expanded to London and Brighton. They work with growers direct, and supply home-grown and imported produce all year round via the Organic Marketing Company. They aim to provide a selection of 40–50 fruits and vegetables every week, available as a standard box at £6.50 or as customised orders. In 1997, in conjunction with others, they launched Organic 2000, a campaign to supply fresh organic produce direct from the fields to as many households as possible by the end of the century.

London: London is well serviced for box schemes and specialist organic home-delivery services, which may incorporate vegetable boxes. Each offers a slightly different service; most offer a range of foods. Ring for details. London box schemes include:

The Beacon, Kingston tel: 0181 547 0507 Free delivery in Kingston and Surbiton.
Farm-a-Round, SE23 tel: 0181 291 3650 The largest, sourced primarily from growers direct.
The Fresh Food Company, W10 tel: 0181 969 0351 Nationwide delivery. See Mail Order, p. 100.
Green Adventure, SE5 tel: 0171 277 2529 A buying club where

Little Ash Eco-farm

A remarkable experimental farm situated near Oakhampton in Devon tel: 01647 231394 that practises a radical completely self-sustaining ecological farming system. The farm buys nothing in and sells only what it produces. Available direct from the farm, their produce includes fruit and vegetables, home-milled wheat and triticale ancient wheat flour, oats, ewe's milk and cheese, lamb, mutton, beef, goat and poultry as well as wool and mare's milk. Calves are never taken from their mothers, even in the case of dairy cows, and live in family groups. They sell their produce locally only, and have recently begun to offer seasonal fruit and vegetable boxes, delivered locally, usually by horse.

members help pack and deliver. Delivery in SE postal area, by bicycle.

Inner City Organics, *SW9* tel: 0171 733 4899 Home delivery to South London, Mon. and Fri. and a market stall in Brixton market, Mon., Thurs. and Sat.

Just Organics, *N1* tel: 0171 704 2566 Serve Camden, Islington and east London.

Organics Direct, *EC2* tel: 0171 729 2828 Nationwide delivery. See Mail Order, p. 101.

Spring Green, *NW6* tel: 0181 208 0855 E-mail springgreen @ dial.pipex.com Deliveries throughout London.

Also, see Bumblebee Wholefood shop and the Organic Store, pp. 80 and 82.

Home delivery services

These offer a bridge between box schemes and retail shops, as well as the convenience of having organic produce delivered to your door. Many exist. Most offer meat, dairy, and vegetable boxes as well as customised orders, and all offer other groceries as well. Three typical examples are:

The Better Food Company, *Barrow Gurney, near Bristol* 01275 474545 Soil Association registered. A comprehensive organic and fine food home delivery service run by Philip and Geraldine Haughton. It includes fruit and vegetables supplied by the Organic Marketing Company, Hereford; meat from Welsh suppliers; dairy produce; wines; an extensive range of groceries, including pastas, oils and vinegars; and Heritage fish and game. They produce an excellent catalogue and newsletter. Overnight home delivery within a thirty-mile radius of Bristol; nationwide deliveries also, including Christmas hampers and fruit and vegetable boxes. They also supply Rocinantes restaurant in Bristol, run by Barney Haughton, which promotes organic food and use organic ingredients wherever possible.

Green Cuisine, *Cardiff* tel: 01222 498721 Organic Farmers & Growers registered. A husband and wife team, Andrew and Marcia Robinson, who provide the largest range of organic produce available in Cardiff, including an extensive range of fresh meat from Black Mountain Foods (p. 203), cut to order, fresh produce, dairy products, groceries and tea and coffee. All goods are certified.

Sundrum Organics, *Mauchline, Ayrshire* tel: 01290 426770 E-mail: sales @ sundrum.force9.co.uk. Soil Association registered. A vegetarian box scheme and home delivery service that have recently won the Organic Food Award for their deluxe organic muesli. Extensive catalogue includes fresh organic ginger, sprouted seeds, delicatessen products, dairy, Engine House breads and tofu products, wines, beers and household products. Offer vegetable and fruit boxes, priced £6 and £10, or customised orders. Local produce used where possible. Evening deliveries within Scotland, free for boxes or orders more than £35. National delivery and discounts schemes available.

For a further list of box schemes and home delivery services, see Appendix 2, p. 351.

what they say . . .

'We find the textures and tastes of organic foods more like the foods from our pasts. The spinach is more like celery at the stalk, and just as juicy.' – *Mrs Carol Sykes, Mirfield, West Yorkshire*

'Greatly disturbed when I became aware of the pesticides used on edible crops, I placed an order to have delivered weekly a box of organic vegetables, and occasionally to have included fruit and groceries when required. Good value? I am delighted with the superior taste of all the items and, in particular, feel they have contributed to the well-being of my husband, who has been ill for nearly three years. As for me, their excellent results in my body have assisted me in caring for him. He is seventy-nine and I am eighty-one years old. So, I feel the extra cost of buying organically is of little importance.' – *Alice Donaldson, Grimsby*

'I find an excitement in handling, cooking and eating vegetables straight from the fields, which goes beyond freshness and flavour. We are what we eat, and it is important to feel a connection and trust in our food that are denied by modern farming and retailing.' – *Guy Watson, Riverford Organic Vegetables*

vegetables and fruit

Organic produce is better for your health and infinitely better for the environment – two powerful reasons for buying organic vegetables and fruit when you can. Buying organic means that you no longer need to worry about whether you should peel your carrots or apples – now the official advice – or whether you should eat the skins of potatoes. Research shows that people enjoy eating organic produce more, and countless numbers enthuse about its flavour.

Fresh produce is one of the most important foods for health, if not *the* most important. Concern over pesticide residues and nitrate levels resulting from modern farming practices, together with concern about how fruit and vegetables are grown, has never been greater – the now familiar scares about carrots underpinning how serious the problem is. Progress is slow. For example, the EU recently set lower levels for the maximum amounts of nitrates permitted in vegetables. Some UK-grown lettuce and spinach exceed the new levels, but instead of trying to find ways of resolving this, the Ministry of Agriculture, Fisheries and Food has

---

fact

In 1995, the Ministry of Agriculture issued a health warning about UK carrots after residues of five toxic chemicals including OPs, up to twenty-five times higher than expected, were found. In March 1996, after OPs exceeding the recommended maximum residue limits (MRLs) were found in a test sample of apples and peaches, government health officials advised the peeling of fruit to be eaten by children as a 'sensible additional precaution'.

---

negotiated an exemption – which means that these vegetables can continue to be sold in the UK though they cannot be exported, while imported lettuce and spinach will have to comply with the new levels.

Fresh produce is also a major force in the world economy: the rise in pesticide use globally, and the development of genetically engineered crops, are two of the most serious environmental and health issues facing the twenty-first century. Buying organic vegetables and fruit is the single most important contribution you can make to minimise these.

Range and price – and how easy is it to buy?

Sales of organic fresh produce have soared, and there is now a real choice for every shopper. The phenomenal growth in box schemes (p. 107) has widened that availability further. Though the quantity of organic produce is tiny compared to non-organic, the means of obtaining it are more varied and creative. You cannot buy conventional fresh produce by mail order, but you *can* buy organic in this way. Convenient home-delivery services are much more widespread than in the conventional sector. And only the organic sector offers you the opportunity of subscription farming, whereby you pay an annual subscription to an organic farm which grows your organic produce for you. Four major supermarkets now stock it, which means access to some organic produce for everyone. With a few noble exceptions, the only sector that has been slow to respond is independent greengrocers.

A few points:

● The rise in consumer demand – an increase of 50–60 per cent every year for the last three years – has fuelled the increase in choice and availability. Appearance and presentation have also improved substantially, such that shabby-looking organic vegetables are rapidly becoming a thing of the past. As retailers gain more commitment to, and expertise in handling, organic produce, this will improve further. Organic frozen vegetables – broccoli, carrots, peas and sweetcorn – have now come on stream, with others due to be added.

- As demand and supply rise, prices are becoming more competitive daily. Common organic vegetables like onions, potatoes and mushrooms are *not* expensive. Shop around, and you will find regular bargains and promotions, too, on a wide range of other fresh organic produce, such as avocados, kiwi fruit and lemons. For more, see p. 29.
- The amount of organic produce grown in the UK compared to conventional produce is tiny, and currently about 75 per cent is imported. Supermarkets, which rely mainly on imported goods, are now encouraging their UK growers to convert to organic production, so the situation will change. But it will require the same kind of substantive political change as elsewhere in Europe before any really significant improvement can be made. Meanwhile, one of the best ways of buying home-grown organic produce is through box schemes and local outlets. For a select list, see p. 351.

WATCHWORD: Various green-label schemes such as 'Leaf' purport to grow crops in environmentally friendly ways by using integrated crop-management (ICM) schemes. Though a very positive step, with the objective of substantially reducing the use of pesticides, ICM is not organic farming, but best-practice chemical farming. The same range of artificial fertilisers and pesticides is used, but used less and in more controlled ways. Though such schemes encourage greater use of biological controls, there are no provisions or recommendations for building up soil health or the organic quality of the soil, and protocols are intended as general guidelines only.

Looks versus health

This is a hotly debated issue, one in which consumers can help enormously. Briefly:

- Organic vegetables and fruit are not, and never can be, cosmetically perfect clones. The only way to achieve this on a commercial scale is to grow them with an armoury of chemicals – it appears that as many as 80 per cent of pesticides applied to vegetables and fruit are used for appearance purposes. But improvements in organic growing techniques are constantly being made and, already, up to 70–80 per cent of crops look as magnificent as they taste.
- The drive for uniformity and a blemish-free appearance has been set by retailers and consumers alike, and this has resulted in more healthy organic produce being rejected than need be. Extensive use of biological controls means that the occasional friendly insect may turn up in organic vegetables, but this should not be a cause for concern.
- Beauty is more than skin-deep, and freshness and health are what matter most. Organic produce in its prime has an extra depth of colour, sheen, bloom, smell and vitality. These are the things to look for when buying organic produce, rather than a certain size or shape, or uniformity.

Nutritional superiority

It's well known that organic produce generally has lower nitrate levels and contains less water, and can have higher vitamin C levels. Tests carried out by Camden Food and Drink Association have shown that in addition to vitamin C, organic fruit and vegetables contain more essential nutrients, with organic potatoes containing a quarter more zinc, and organic tomatoes a quarter more vitamin A, than the chemically grown varieties.

Other differences relating to health have also been found which, though not conclusive, highlight potentially important benefits. For example, a study on the effect of the 'green revolution' in South Asia, where crops are now grown with extensive use of chemicals, published in *Nature* recently, found that intensively grown crops were nutritionally deficient, particularly in iron and zinc, and that the IQ of children who had consumed a diet largely based on these crops had dropped by ten points.

But perhaps the most potentially controversial studies of all are those relating to sperm counts. Several have shown that the sperm counts of Western males have dropped dramatically over the last fifty years. The most recent, from Finland, showed that only 27 per cent of men who died in 1991 had produced sperm in normal amounts, compared to 56 per cent who died in 1981. Pesticides that act as endocrine-disruptors, many of which are used in fruit and vegetable production, are among the possible causal factors cited. By contrast, Danish research has shown that the sperm counts of organic farmers and growers were 50 per cent higher than average. At the same time, significant increases in testicular cancer have also been recorded in Western countries, and the number of couples who are unable to conceive, living in countries where such low sperm counts have been recorded, is also rising. Further work is being carried out to see if this is conclusive. In late 1997 a team of some 1,800 American scientists, reviewing over sixty studies, has confirmed that the decline in sperm counts is real – at a rate of 1½ per cent a year for American males and about twice that for European males – and its research has strengthened the view that chemical pollutants are to blame. Watch this space.

Flavour

Organic produce is allowed to grow at its own pace, without chemical feeds or artificial nitrates (which increase uptake of water). Because of this, is usually tastes better. To give a simple example, organic carrots spend around three weeks longer in the soil than conventional carrots, take up water at a slower rate and develop a higher fibre content, all of which contribute to extra flavour.

fact

Vegetables grown conventionally have lower mineral contents now than in the 1940s, when artificial fertilisers and pesticides were not in common use. Comparing published tables, there was almost 50 per cent more magnesium and well over a third more iron in basic vegetables in 1939 than in 1991. Potatoes had 58 per cent more potassium, 55 per cent more calcium, 43 per cent more magnesium, 85 per cent more iron and 9 per cent more phosphorus.

But extra flavour cannot be guaranteed. The flavour of any vegetable or fruit is a complex combination of many factors, including the variety, where it is grown, how fresh it is and the skill of the grower. The flavour of a crop also varies from season to season, and this variation is more apparent in organically grown crops precisely because they are grown naturally. In addition, organic crops are grown over a wider range of soils than non-organic crops, which are grown in highly specialised ways, including soil types, some of which are not as suitable as others for a particular crop. This, too, has a bearing on flavour.

- The best organic produce has not only a better flavour, but also a sweetness that conventional produce never has.
- The need to supply fresh organic produce all year round has a bearing on the flavour – produce is likely to be better flavoured at certain times of the year. Shoppers can help by giving supermarkets and retailers feedback.
- Freshly harvested vegetables grown locally and sold through box schemes are usually uniformly excellent in flavour.
- Imported and larger-scale commercially grown organic produce is variable; it can be excellent, but can also be no better in flavour in some cases than conventional produce.
- Flavour variations show up more in some crops – tomatoes, carrots, potatoes and certain lettuce types – than in others. Organic green celery is superb.
- Organic apples and pears, the two most commonly available fruit in supermarkets, are usually imported and are better at certain times of the year than at others. Organic oranges generally have a superb flavour.

How well does organic produce keep?

In many cases, as studies confirm, organic produce keeps better, because it is inherently healthier. It is grown in healthier soils, has not been forced and has a lower water content. All the same, too few people experience the luxury of spanking fresh organic produce. In practice, the keeping quality depends on the kind of crop, and how it has fared post-harvest: that is, the amount of care

How to Buy

The best approach to buying organic produce is to be an opportunist. Rather like when buying fish, the golden rule is to buy what looks best on the day.

1 Snap up local produce when you can.

2 Take advantage of seasonal produce and special offers.

3 Don't worry about minor cosmetic blemishes, irregular sizing, minor bruises or the occasional insect. Do worry about any slugs and caterpillars – remove them immediately as they will continue to eat their way through the leaves and make a mess of your vegetable. Avoid badly bruised fruit.

4 Store properly.

5 Eat fresh.

that has been taken to ensure freshness from the moment of picking until it is sold by the wholesaler or retailer, and the degree of technology employed in storage – storage of conventional produce, sold in millions of tonnes, is a high-tech business, aided in the case of many fruits, for example, by post-harvest pesticides. In this respect, it has to be said that retailers bear part of the responsibility: some still seem to think that being organic is enough to sell the produce, and do not put sufficient effort into keeping it in good condition. Turnover is also slower, which means that on average most organic produce stays on the shelves longer.

- As long as they are stored correctly – that is, in cool conditions and with leafy crops kept in bags to retain their turgidity – freshly harvested organic vegetables have as good a shelf life as conventional vegetables. The same goes for soft fruit.

Where to Buy

Organic produce is widely available – though where you live will affect how hard you need to look for it.

1 Major cities and towns throughout the country are amply served, as is any part of the country where there are clusters of organic growers, such as Devon and part of Wales. The north is more patchy, though things are improving steadily.

2 The kind of outlet you buy organic produce from is important. Here freshness and how many links there are in the distribution chain after the produce has been harvested are the key.

3 If you want the freshest vegetables, buying direct from the farm or through a traditional box scheme is best. Check out local market stalls, too. If you want convenience, a supermarket or shop specialising in organic foods is best.

4 Seek out shops or supermarkets with a wide selection and a good turnover.

5 If you don't have a local shop or supermarket that stocks organic food, check out box schemes, home delivery or mail order.

- Organic maincrop potatoes are not sprayed with post-harvest chemicals such as tecnazene. Once out of cold storage, they do not keep as well as potatoes that are.
- Organic citrus fruits are not sprayed with fungicides or, usually, edible wax; their shelf life is much shorter. Organic lemons should be stored in the fridge and used within two or three weeks. Don't ask me why, but organic grapefruit keep longer.

TIP: To extract maximum juice, warm organic lemons first.

Remember, fresh produce is not meant to last. Though you can slow down the staling process, the sooner it is eaten, the better. For more notes on storing, see p. 112.

Peakfresh preserving bags: These roomy green plastic bags, made in Australia and organically certified, are designed to keep produce fresher and crisper, claim to preserve vitamin C, and can be washed and re-used for up to two months. They are impregnated with oya stone, a pulverised mineral from Japan that absorbs the ethylene gas given off by ripening fruit and vegetables and that accelerates ageing; it also has an anti-fogging treatment to inhibit bacterial growth and allow the passage of gases from the inside of the bag to the outside. My own trials on home-grown produce are encouraging, though some moisture does collect on the inside of the bag and it's worth wiping this out with kitchen paper. It's also important to make sure the produce is cold before putting it into the bag. Full instructions are included. Available in packs of ten from Planet Organic, other good retailers and the Fresh Food Company tel: 0181 969 0351.

Finally, don't buy bruised, dried-up or mouldy vegetables or fruit just because they're organic. And if they deteriorate too quickly, return them to the shop.

Fresh Produce Facts

- Worldwide, there are up to twice as many pesticides used on fruit and vegetables than on any other major crops.
- It takes around five hundred years to accumulate an inch of top soil. Soil erosion due to intensive agriculture is now a serious problem, costing an estimated £24–£51 million per year.
- An organic grower aims to have at least one million worms per acre. Fertile soils should have more than twelve worms in a spadeful.

● It can be done . . . In 1990, Cuba adopted organic agriculture as part of its official policy. By 1996 it had become self-sufficient in basic fruit and vegetables, all grown organically. Pesticide use and nitrate fertilisers have been reduced dramatically, and 80 per cent of pest control is now based on biological means. Sweden, also, has reduced the amount of pesticides used since 1986 by 75 per cent, and banned thirty-seven pesticides for health or environmental reasons.

what they say . . .

'I started my career in the conventional world some fifteen years ago now, and have always hated spraying crops. I was, however, always told that without sprays one would get total crop failures. Three years ago I became involved with experimental growing in an organic system. I was amazed – no sprays, and clean crops. One day a crop of cabbages had a cloud of aphids descend upon them, then two days later the crop was clean. This really made me look in the organic direction.

'In the conventional world chemical after chemical is 'banged on'. A crop such as lettuce may have been sprayed ten or more times, the last spray the day before harvest. This for me is rather scary; how many chemicals must we consume from eating conventional vegetables each week?

'The organic market is increasing rapidly but demand still outstrips supply. As soon as you think you have planned enough volume, the goal-posts have moved again. I am very confident this will continue to be the case, and any growers looking to convert can do so knowing there is a good and growing market for organic produce.' – *Paul Burgess, Production Manager, the Organic Marketing Company*

Vegetables

The more organic fresh produce you buy, the more you will enjoy and appreciate its flavour and the peace of mind it brings.

Because pesticides of one kind or another, be they soil fumigants, herbicides, insecticides, fungicides or post-harvest treatments, are used extensively, it is difficult to pick out with any certainty produce that is most or least affected, though you may like to note that compared to most other vegetables, squashes receive far fewer treatments, and residues are not generally detected. Official statistics pick out the worst offenders, though different countries' surveys highlight different ones, and tests by no means cover all potential residues. On a reassuring note, the amount of pesticide residues is tiny and the safety margins employed very large. For more information on pesticide usage and residues, see Appendix 1, p. 325.

The following list, drawn up with the help of Josa Young, who runs a box scheme, describes a selection of vegetables you may like to start with, and also gives a few extra tips on storing and using them. Other organic vegetables you will find, particularly in box schemes or organic shops where fresh produce is a speciality, are peas, turnips, beetroot, celeriac, asparagus, spinach, spinach beet, spring onions, sweetcorn, peppers, fennel, aubergines, curly kale, Chinese leaf, radish and a wide range of exotic salad leaves.

Josa Young's daily dozen

Beans A truly seasonal group of vegetables, starting with broad beans, then French beans and runner beans, UK organic beans are available throughout the summer. Imported Heleda flat beans, which are similar to runner beans, are available in spring and autumn. To enjoy them at their best, eat them as soon after you buy them as possible. Sizes of individual beans vary. Flavour differences are more detectable in some beans than in others; broad bean varieties such as Aquadulce or Claudia can be sublime, runner beans are sweeter, but French beans taste the same as the commercial variety. Freshness and youth are the key. A good tip for older beans is to chop them and stew them in olive oil with onions and tomatoes and serve at room temperature. A cheap gadget called the Krisk bean-stringer deals with runner beans quickly.

Broccoli A more intense, sweet flavour when very fresh – otherwise, a similar flavour to the conventional version. Firm, deep-blue-green heads are the ones to look for. The key variety is Marathon, in season from July to October. Winter-sprouting broccoli, available from late winter through spring, is a treat; trim away the leaves, and use them as greens.

Brussels sprouts An excellent flavour, richer, and more delicious than your average sprout, which can seem lack-lustre and have a bitter edge by comparison. In box schemes, and sometimes shops as well, they come attached to their stalks – a good idea, as they keep better this way. The flavour of any Brussels sprout deteriorates quite quickly, so eat as soon as you can. The stalks will invariably present you with sprouts of varying sizes, and they may need more trimming. Sprout tops are excellent; use like cabbage.

Cabbage Generally sweeter than the conventional kind, and can be truly delicious. It stores well, wrapped, in the fridge. All kinds are available, at different times of the year, from summer onwards. They may harbour insects in the outer leaves, so inspect first, and remove. All conventional brassicas may be sprayed several times.

Carrots Organic carrots are a number one priority, especially for children. The flavour is usually noticeably better than that of the conventional kind, partly because they contain less water. Their flavour is also dependent on the kind of soil they are grown in. Available all year, key varieties bred for sweetness include Nirobi, Boston and Nandor. Keep them dry and in the dark, though they are pretty robust, anyway. Unwashed carrots keep better than washed ones. Choose organic parsnips, too.

Cauliflower Available all year except mid-summer. The intense flavour is usually a revelation. Standard varieties are Linas and Nomad. Look for a firm, creamy head. Check the leaves for insects. They will keep in the salad drawer for three or four days, though the colour will dull. A good idea is to break off the individual florets from the outside first, leaving the rest intact for another meal.

Celery A top priority. Residues are found in almost all conventional celery, and multiple residues are common. Organic celery is greener, the greener the better – so snap really green ones up as they have a superb flavour. Outside stems are coarse, but excellent in soups and stir-fries, as are the aromatic leaves.

Cucumbers An excellent flavour, though the organic ones have thicker skins and sometimes come in weird and interesting shapes. Several varieties are available, such as Danima mini-cucumbers and Flamingo long ones. They are available from spring to autumn, though supplies may be sporadic. Make sure they are firm all the way along. Store in the salad drawer of the fridge, but don't let them get too cold as this spoils them.

Lettuce Best in its natural season, spring to autumn. If you want winter lettuce, choose organic. Residues are found in three-quarters of conventional ones. Flavours vary, depending on the season and whether home-grown or imported. Key varieties include Little Gem, Red Salad Bowl and Red Oak Leaf. There is likely to be more waste – untreated lettuces are vulnerable – so inspect for insects, trim off any damaged leaves, wrap and store in the bottom of the fridge and eat soon. To crisp up a floppy lettuce – surprisingly – douse in warm water for a few minutes, then dry carefully.

Mushrooms Good value, and an excellent flavour. To find out what *isn't* done to organic mushrooms, see p. 139.

Onions Good value, and often stronger-flavoured. British ones are available from autumn through winter. Key varieties are Goldito and Dorado. And the organic ones are untreated, so keep them dry and well ventilated to prevent moulding. They sprout faster than conventional ones; snip the sprouts like chives and use for soups and stir-fries. The same applies to organic garlic. Organic leeks may need careful washing; use the green parts for soups and stocks. A good idea for storing leeks is to clean them up, then put them in the salad drawer of the fridge.

Potatoes Another top organic priority, especially maincrop, in which residues are commonly detected in conventional ones, particularly in the skins; stored potatoes sprayed with tecnazene fungicide do not have to be declared as treated, so there is no way of knowing if they have been sprayed. Everyone, including many chefs, agrees that the flavour of organic potatoes is superior. Not expensive, and available all or most of the year, but best in autumn/early winter for maincrop. Varieties include Nicola, Désirée and Santé; traditional box schemes often feature rare and interesting varieties, too. Remove them from their plastic bags, store them in brown paper bags in the dark, and keep them cool. New potatoes are best eaten as soon as you get them, but can be put in the fridge to prevent sprouting, if you like. Organic main-crop potatoes are not treated after harvesting, so are more suscep-tible to moulding or greening. Unwashed potatoes keep better than washed ones.

Squashes Organic courgettes are available from summer to early autumn, and usually have a better flavour. Fresh ones have unbe-lievably glossy skins and feel hard. Various varieties of winter squashes are available from autumn onwards and have the virtue of storing supremely well if left whole, improving in flavour with time, the flesh becoming sweeter and harder as they shed moisture. Orange-fleshed kinds – Crown Prince, Turk's Turban – are best. You need a sharp, heavy knife to slice them; peeling is easier once they've been cooked. Wonderful for soups, baked, roast or puréed.

Swede Cheap, durable and with an excellent flavour.

Swiss chard A favourite with box-scheme growers, as it's easy to cultivate and can be grown for much of the year. One of my favourite greens, it has large, strikingly handsome, dark-green, crinkly leaves with a broad white or red midrib. The young leaves are as tender and delicate as spinach, while the older leaves are more resilient and have a stronger flavour. Think of them as spinach that can be used like cabbage – shredded and stir-fried, for example, or included in pâtés. The midribs are usually cooked separately, and served in a cream, cheese or tomato sauce, or can be egg-and-breadcrumbed and fried. Store well-wrapped in the fridge, cutting off the stems first if the leaves are too large.

Tomatoes Best in their natural season, summer to early autumn. Often but not always better flavoured, thought the *best* organic are much better than the conventional. Out-of-season tomatoes are never as good as the ones grown in summer. If not completely ripe, leave them for a few days at room temperature, to ripen. UK crop available May to October. Key varieties include Evita cherry tomatoes, Shirley and Gardener's Delight. Often more fragile than the conventional sort, so can get squashed easily. Try keeping smaller ones in egg boxes, stalk down, or in the egg rack of the fridge, but take them out well before eating to allow the flavour to develop at room temperature. Pesticide residues are detected in up to half of conventional ones.

Price guide: Though prices are coming down dramatically (see p. 31), organic vegetables and fruit are more expensive to produce, are in far shorter supply and therefore cost more. Wastage due to cosmetic imperfections is also higher. Currently organic vegetables cost anything from 0 to 30 per cent more. The price differential for organic fruit is wider, anything from 0 to 50 per cent, or even higher for exotic fruits. But there are occasions when organic produce on promotion will be cheaper than the conventional line – the ultimate bargain.

Where to buy: The best place to buy spanking-fresh produce is undoubtedly from the grower direct, either via a box scheme or from the farm gate. Fresh produce constitutes the major part of supermarket organic food, though range and availability depend on the store and on location. Alternative supermarkets, dedicated organic and farm shops offer a very good selection, and are usually strong on local seasonal produce. The selection in whole-food/health food shops varies; some are excellent, but some have limited supplies and range. Many operate a home delivery service. Though there are exceptions, greengrocers still do not generally stock organic fresh produce. If none of these outlets are available to you, or if you want the convenience of not having to shop at all, mail order could be your answer. For details, see p. 99.

Frozen vegetables Sold under the Whole Earth label, these are available in cheerful 450g packs, in shops specialising in organic food. Broccoli, carrots, peas and sweetcorn are currently available.

Organic chillies and aubergines Have arrived! Available by mail order from Sea Spring Farm, Dorchester tel: 01308 897892. See p. 100.

Organic mushrooms

Organic mushrooms are an excellent buy, and available most of the time. Brown-caps, which are a lower-yielding crop but much better value for the customer, and with a better flavour – more like that of a field mushroom – contain less water, so cook better and last longer. The main brand, Chesswood Produce, is widely available. Fresh organic shitake mushrooms and extra-large open-capped white mushrooms were introduced in 1997. More varieties are expected soon.

Gourmet Mushrooms UK A new company, registered with Organic Farmers and Growers, producing new and flavoursome varieties of exotic mushrooms which are sold primarily to top chefs and have already received rave reviews. The mushrooms are cultivated wild varieties that grow in clusters. There are two new oyster mushrooms, Sonoma Brown with a sweet flavour and firm texture and Colchester Blue with a more peppery flavour, and a dark-chestnut-brown button mushroom called Albarelle 'Little Caesar', with a nutty flavour and crisp texture. Also available in selected London stores such as Fortnum & Mason, Planet Organic, House of Albert Roux, Antonio Carluccio's and in the Japanese supermarket, Yaohan Plaza, at 399 Edgware Road, Colindale.

> **TIP:** Mushrooms need plenty of air to store well. Never keep any kind of mushrooms wrapped in clingfilm or plastic. Take off the clingfilm immediately, place a piece of kitchen paper in the bottom of the box to soak up any moisture, and keep the mushrooms uncovered in the bottom of the fridge; or put them in a brown paper bag. They will then keep for up to 5–7 days.

Growing organic mushrooms Organic mushrooms are grown naturally, and pest control is achieved by using air-filters and by biological means. The following substances and practices are all prohibited under Soil Association regulations:

- Chemical pesticides, whether in the compost, sprayed on the crop or as a fog.
- Chlorinated water for disease control.
- Formaldehyde for sterilisation.
- Fumigation by methyl bromide.
- Bleaching.
- Post-harvest treatment of composts with fungicides.

Organic watercress Organic watercress, packed with flavour, certified by Organic Farmer's & Growers, is grown in the traditional way at Hill Deverill, near Warminster, Wilts. (tel: 01985 840260) by John Hurd who has been growing watercress for forty years and uses the classic late flowering variety, rather than the newer varieties which are sown repeatedly and mechanically cropped when very young. No chemicals are used. The watercress grows naturally and from March to early December is cut by hand. Available from the packing sheds direct or the nearby Deverills Trout Farm. Widely sold through box schemes, home delivery services and some specialist organic shops throughout the country, as well as from Planet Organic, Waitrose and selected Sainsbury stores. Snap up a bunch when you can.

what they say . . .

'The difference between when we first started selling organic produce twenty-two years ago and today is dramatic. Organic growers are infinitely more skilled, quality-orientated and professional, and very aware of modern consumer needs. The future looks very bright. I can hardly think, for example, of anything that is not available organically at most times, with the exception of some exotics and some ethnic products. Shoppers can expect more loose organic produce, more variety, better consistency, increasingly more attractive prices and regular promotions. The biggest challenge is to increase our home-based organic vegetable and fruit production. A staggering two-thirds of the organic crops we import could be organically grown here. Conventional growers are responding to consumer interest and are converting, but this will take time.

'As a responsible producer and marketeer, we have to create real choice and the infrastructure to deliver that choice. We don't know how many BSEs are waiting in the wings – OPs in carrots, fungicidal cocktails sprayed on to fruit, genetically modified crops – who knows? We have to create the opportunity for consumers to have an alternative when they need somewhere safe to flee. Only organic food offers that safe haven. It is our responsibility to ensure everyone has the right to buy it.'
– *Peter Segger, OBE, Managing Director, Organic Farm Foods*

'In the next few years many more of our vegetables will be grown organically, but the task of changing over is a colossal one, and changes cannot be made overnight. As shoppers, all we can do is support the change and accept the unusual shapes and slight blemishes of organic produce. Frankly, I think it makes shopping more interesting. Come on, do we really want six absolutely identical, perfectly round tomatoes?' – *Nigel Slater, food writer*

'Organic produce tastes better and must be beneficially better without the pesticides. I never mind if the vegetables have been attacked by insects etc. If they still eat them, I know it is safe for humans.' – *Helen Hibben, Kent*

'Scientific evidence is gradually revealing that chemicals are detrimental to our health . . . I try, wherever possible, to limit my and my family's exposure to such chemicals, and this includes the consumption of organic food . . . Fruits and vegetables may not be uniform or cosmetically pretty, but it is reassuring to know that the skin is safe to eat, that the risks of pesticides and fertilisers do not outweigh the advantages of consuming natural vitamins and proteins, and we find that they actually taste better. Prices are more expensive, but becoming lower as competition increases, and I believe I cannot put a price on my family's health.'
– *Jacqueline Page, Thame, Oxfordshire*

'The taste of organic lettuces is so superior to the non-organic variety that it almost defies description.'
– *Ian Plummer, Slough, Berks.*

Fruit

Fruit poses a particular dilemma. Everyone is being encouraged to eat as much of it as possible for their health, yet fruit crops are sprayed repeatedly with pesticides – over 130 are licensed for use on apples, for example, and up to 50 of these are actually used. We are told to eat the skins for fibre and because the highest levels of vitamins are found just beneath the skins, but at the same time we are advised to peel them as a precaution against pesticide residues. In addition, the amount of commercially home-produced organic fruit is minimal, which means, ironically, sacrificing local fruit in order to eat organic. To give you some idea: though there are over 240 UK organic symbol holders growing fruit, currently only eleven growers are registered with the Soil Association exclusively for fruit, and these account for 30 per cent of organic fruit production in the UK. Furthermore, only four acres of one of our most popular fruits, strawberries, are under organic cultivation. As a result, almost all our most popular top fruit – apples, pears and plums – as well as soft fruit, is imported, and you are much more likely to be able to buy organic apples from Argentina and organic strawberries from Spain than from Kent.

It is technically difficult in our climate to produce perfectly formed organic fruit, especially top (orchard) fruit, and, as one grower explained, most consumers and retailers alike are so attached to cosmetically perfect fruit that they are willing to eat organophosphates for the privilege. Also, organic yields are lower. UK government aid for organic conversion is minimal compared to the rest of Europe – one-tenth, one-ninth and just over one-fifth of what is given in Holland, France and Spain, respectively, for orchard fruits, for example – and, until recently, there was simply insufficient demand to make the sums work for anyone thinking of changing over. Demand is now increasing fast, and more growers are converting, so we may hope that the picture will not look so bleak in the future.

Imported versus home-grown

Given that pesticide use is even more extensive in some major fruit-exporting countries such as South America than in the UK, buying organic imported fruit when you can, especially apples, pears and strawberries, makes sense. Whereas everyone can buy imported organic fruit easily, anyone who can buy home-grown organic fruit is very lucky. Think of it as the ultimate treat.

Quality and flavour

Although organic fruit is never uniform and top fruit rarely blemish-free, without exception the flavour of all the organic fruit I have eaten is better – in some cases, much better – than much conventional fruit. A good case in point is imported Granny Smith and Golden Delicious apples – one bite and you immediately taste the difference. It's the same with organic peaches. Organic oranges for juicing are tangier and much fruitier, and UK organic strawberries can be superb. Grapes are more variable. Imported organic apples and pears are generally good-quality; here, the main fault is bruising. I also find the skins of most imported apples quite thick and tough. UK top fruit tend to be smaller and more variable in size, and are less blemish-free.

Because they are not treated with fungicides, organic soft fruit should be eaten as soon as possible. Although they haven't got waxed, shiny skins I find that organic apples (and pears) keep well – apples for up to two weeks and pears for three to ten days, depending on ripeness.

Points to remember:

- Though organic pear varieties are quite well represented, apple varieties are severely limited. Though there are gaps a fair amount of imported fruit is available all year round. Quality does vary with the season.
- There are currently over a hundred Soil Association registered growers who grow some fruit that they are likely to sell at the farm gate or locally; a few, also, such as *Garlands Farm Shop, Upper Basildon, Berks.*, tel: 01491 671556, offer pick-your-own. Registered organic farm shops are a good bet for local seasonal fruit, and box-scheme growers often grow some soft fruit or have a few apple trees. Shops specialising in organic food will always stock local fruit when they can. The best guide

for local sources of fruit is the Soil Association's booklet, *Where to Buy Organic Food.*

● The main varieties of home-grown fruit that you will find are apples, pears, plums, strawberries, raspberries and other berries and currants. Whichever you buy, it will be seasonal. Don't expect organic English apples in May, or English strawberries at Christmas!

WATCHWORD: A wide range of conventional fruits, including citrus, apples, peaches and melons, are often *waxed.* Waxes may contain shellacs, paraffin, palm oil, synthetic resins and in some countries a range of fungicides such as benomyl and diphenyl to prevent fruit from moulding. Organic fruit is not waxed and is not treated with fungicides.

Bananas Organic bananas are in very short supply and therefore expensive, though things are just beginning to improve. Their thick skins do not give complete protection from pesticide residues: the developing fruit is wrapped in plastic bags infused with pesticides, massive amounts of which are used. The production of bananas is a major environmental concern, as are the working conditions of farmers and plantation workers – see the Banana Story below. For this reason, try to buy the occasional organic banana, or fair traded bananas, when you can.

The banana story
Bananas are the fifth most important food commodity in world trade, controlled mainly by a few transnational companies including Geest and Del Monte. They are the most popular fruit in the UK, where consumption has doubled in the last ten years to around 10 kilos of bananas per person per year, and are cheap and available all year round. Consumer preference is for spotless, yellow fruit, of uniform shape and taste. Around 90 per cent are produced from one variety, the Cavendish, which gives high yields but requires large inputs of artificial fertilisers and pesticides.

In Costa Rica, the one banana-producing country where reliable information exists, the average annual use of pesticides on banana plantations is as high as 44kg/hectare, compared to 2.7kg/hectare for most crops in industrialised countries. Many of the pesticides used on bananas are restricted in use or banned in their country of origin, and 30 per cent are classified as 'extremely hazardous' or 'highly hazardous' by the WHO. Insecticides are used, as well as fungicides and herbicides, and nematicides to destroy soil organisms.

Fungicides account for three-quarters of the pesticides used. Most are aerially sprayed, and an estimated 90 per cent is lost to drift, washed off by rain or applied to surrounding soil. They are also used in packing plants. Herbicides such as paraquat and nematicides (the most toxic pesticides used) are applied by hand, directly on to the plants from backpack sprayers carried by workers. Blue plastic bags, impregnated with insecticides, cover each bunch of bananas; the bags are left scattered around, find their way into watercourses and do not rot down easily. The result is that pesticide poisonings are three times higher in the banana regions than in other parts of the country. Many workers are given short-term contracts only for dangerous jobs; instruction on how to use pesticides safely remains inadequate; protective clothing is not always available, and is not fully protective anyway.

The environmental impact is devastating: severe pollution of watercourses – killing fish – and of the coastline, where at least 90 per cent of coral reefs are dead; the highest rate of deforestation in the world; soil erosion on hillsides, and the wholesale loss of the biodiversity of flora and fauna.

Source   The Banana Link

Strawberries and methyl bromide

Methyl bromide is a highly toxic soil fumigant, herbicide and fungicide, used to combat soil-borne diseases, insects and weed seeds in field crops and in glasshouse crops such as lettuce, tomatoes, celery and cucumber. It is used against insects in mushroom compost and against grain storage pests. It can be used to fumigate nuts, dried fruit, herbs and spices, as well as the containers, machinery and processing facilities (fabric treatments). It is lethal to both targeted and non-targeted organisms, and dangerous to wild birds, animals and bees. It has been classified as a class 1 ozone-depleter, many more times damaging than chlorofluorocarbons (CFCs), and studies show that between 50 and 90 per cent of methyl bromide used as a fumigant is emitted into the atmosphere. Because of this, it is due to be phased out of use by 2010; UK strawberry-growers and fumigant companies are lobbying against this.

Its prime use in the UK is on field strawberries, including pick-your-own, and it is estimated to account for three-quarters of methyl bromide usage on outdoor crops; it is used most in Kent. It does not leave harmful residues on the fruit, though it is highly toxic when inhaled, can cause death and is mutagenic to bacteria and plants. It was phased out in the Netherlands by 1992, and all strawberries grown in Germany, the Netherlands, Sweden, Switzerland and Denmark are already produced without methyl bromide.

Source   *The Food Magazine, June 1997, The Pesticides Trust*

For more information on pesticides in fruit, see Appendix 1, p. 334.

what they say . . .

'I have been employed for over thirty years now as a farm secretary, my time being split between a cereal grower, the largest producer in Europe of tomatoes, and, at the moment, a top fruit and soft fruit grower. It is only when you actually see the number of sprays used – apples and pears are subjected to sprays at least three times per week during their growing season – that you begin to understand that nothing is spared in the line of quantity. I am afraid that, though taste is beginning to be mentioned now and again, it is quantity only that is seen as essential.

'I feel that organic producers have never had encouragement from any government, and when you see how long they have to be spray-free, you can understand why the price has to be high. They should, to my mind, be given the same status for grants that all our other farmers have, and then maybe we would be able to have a real competitive choice in our food.

'I am sure the majority of people do not realise that for years tomatoes have been grown in rockwool (the same material used in our house walls) in glasshouses, and only grow through it when pumped full of fertiliser and nutrients. They look beautiful but, never having seen soil or the outside, it is no wonder that they are completely tasteless.' – *Mrs M. Cheesman, Kent*

dairy produce

The fundamental difference between organic and conventional dairy produce lies in how the milk is produced and in the fact that organic dairy enterprises are predominantly, though not exclusively, small-scale, and make no compromises to quality. Thus organic dairy produce – milk, butter, yoghurt, cream and cheese – offers as yet unrivalled purity and generally a better, cleaner, richer flavour. Milk, especially, is an important part of many people's diet. Persistent OC residues, particularly lindane, are a fact of life; drinking organic milk especially, and choosing organic dairy produce when you can, is the best way to minimise the effects of this – and a particularly wise precaution, it seems to me, for pregnant women, infants and children.

Organic Milk

Organic milk in particular is a major success story, to the extent that organic producers could already sell twice what they produce, and already 10 per cent of organic milk consumed or processed is being imported from Holland. Available everywhere (but not yet, alas, through milkmen), together with yoghurt, it's the most popular organic item sold in supermarkets. Fresh milk is available as whole, semi-skimmed or homogenised; a small amount of green-top (unpasteurised) milk can still be bought, though only direct from producers. Long-life and powdered organic milk is also available.

How organic milk is produced

Organic milk comes from cows that graze on organic pastures and are fed hay or silage. Feed, medication, welfare considerations and husbandry practices are all designed to ensure the maximum health of the cow and therefore of the milk:

Feed Only feedstuffs natural to herbivores are allowed. All animal feedstuffs – meat, fishmeal and bonemeal – are banned; in conventional systems, only mammalian protein is banned. At least 60 per cent of feed must come from forage. Most (85 per cent) of feed must be organic, the remainder from strictly controlled permitted feedstuffs. Feedstuff containing genetically modified organisms (GMOs) is forbidden, as are growth-promoting substances.

Medication Prophylactic and routine use of antibiotics – as, for example, in 'dry-cow' therapy used in herds to treat mastitis – and other medicines is prohibited. Instead, alternatives such as homeopathic remedies are preferred. Antibiotics must be and always are used where necessary, but the period before the milk can be sold is two to three times longer than that allowed in conventional herds and is a minimum of fourteen days.

Welfare Organic cows cannot be kept permanently tethered or permanently inside. Stocking densities are normally at least 25 per cent lower than on conventional farms. Organic calves must be weaned for a minimum of nine weeks, and are not allowed to be sold through livestock markets at less than one month old, as opposed to seven days old with conventional herds. Organic calves are never sold for veal export.

For pesticide residues in milk, see Appendix 1, p. 343.

fact | McDonald's restaurant chain in Sweden have been using certified organic milk in all their restaurants since December 1996.

The flavour of organic milk and cream

The flavour of organic milk and cream varies. This is because the flavour of any milk and cream depends on the lushness and complexity of the pastures, on the fat content, on the breed of the cow, on whether the milk is from a single herd or from several, and on whether or not it has been pasteurised. What is noticeable is its sweet, clean flavour.

Generally:

- Because all organic milk and cream are produced to the highest standards from animals grazing on organic pastures, it all has a good flavour.
- Standard organic milk, collected from various sources, pasteurised and cartoned in the same way as conventional milk, loses any flavour nuances it may have had. Semi-skimmed pasteurised organic milk, unless bought direct from a small producer-retailer, tastes the same as good-quality conventional semi-skimmed milk.
- The best organic milk, such as that of green-top producers like Julian Rose of Hardwick Estate near Reading, is sublime, and has a sweetness and delicacy never found in standard commercial milk, which invariably has a flat, 'dead' flavour, often with chemical undertones.
- Unlike the standard pinta or tub of cream, the colour of organic milk and cream also varies with the season and the cows' diet, ranging from pale white in winter to deep yellow in spring and summer, when the cows are feeding on fresh grass; this, too, comes through in the taste.
- The higher the fat content of a dairy product, the greater the difference between what it *can* taste like and what it often *does* taste like. Organic cream, which mainly comes from small producers, is a revelation to those who haven't tasted it before, and is uniformly excellent; here the richness depends on the breed of the cow, Jersey or Guernsey being the most delectable in this respect. As one head chef said to me, 'It looks better and tastes better, my customers love it, it's superb to cook with, never splits when I'm making sauces and is so rich that I

need to use only half the amount – which actually makes it cheaper than ordinary cream.'

Major brands of organic milk are:

Evernat Organic milk powder.
The Farmers' Dairy Co. The major independent company, selling milk under two brand names – this one and Hergest Court Farm.
Hergest Court Farm Milk comes from farms in Hereford, and is the major semi-skimmed brand. The Farmers' Dairy Co.'s excellent thick double cream is also sold under this label.
Manor Farm Their milk comes from farms in Dorset and West Sussex and is the major whole-milk brand.
Meadows Farms Semi-skimmed milk from Devon.
Molkerei Weissenhorn and Bio-H Organic long-life milk, whole- and low-fat.
Skane Swedish organic semi-skimmed UHT milk.

> NOTE: Much of the organic milk found in supermarkets is sold under their own labels, and is supplied either by Malthouse Dairies or the Organic Milk Co-operative.

Buying and storing: For choice, buy full-fat organic milk, which has the richest flavour and the highest nutritional value. Organic pasteurised milk has the same storage life as conventional milk.

- For maximum enjoyment, always buy the freshest milk you can and consume it quickly. Organic milk bought direct from the producer is the freshest you can get.
- Store in the coldest part of the refrigerator. Fresh milk will keep four or five days.
- Spoon off the cream from full-fat milk in bottles or plastic containers to enrich soups, sauces, dips and dressings.
- Homogenised milk may be frozen.

Price guide: Organic milk costs around 10–12p more than standard supermarket milk, 4–5p more than delivered milk and only 2–3p more than premium milks such as Channel Islands or breakfast milk. Bio-dynamic milk is slightly more expensive. Prices do vary from outlet to outlet, so it's worth shopping around if you buy a lot of milk. Expect to pay around 35–41p per pint, or up to 10p per pint less if you buy from the producer direct.

Organic cream is a luscious luxury product that you can't really compare with mass-produced cream. Most organic double

Green-top: the Crème de la Crème

Pasteurisation denatures milk, reducing its nutritional value and its flavour components. In addition, it kills the beneficial bacteria which protect milk from foreign bacteria so that, contrary to popular mythology, fresh unpasteurised milk and cream are likely to keep fresher longer and store better than the commercial pasteurised equivalents. Unpasteurised cream can be sold through shops; unpasteurised milk cannot, except from producer-retailers who have their own retail outlet.

Almost all organic green-top milk is sold to cheesemakers, making organic green-top milk and cream the rarest dairy products in the country – rarer than truffles. Organic green-top is without doubt the finest milk and cream you can buy; don't miss the chance to try some if you get the opportunity. Two suppliers who have local milk rounds and farm shops are Old Plaw Hatch Farm, East Grinstead tel: 01342 810857, and Hardwick Estate, The Old Dairy Farm Shop, Reading tel: 0118 9842392. Domini Quality Foods (p. 152) is another green-top producer. Note that official advice is that infants, pregnant women and elderly or infirm people should not drink green-top milk and cream.

Domini Quality Foods

A gem. One of the longest-established organic farms and one of the first to hold the Soil Association symbol in 1972, the Capon family's Village Farm, Diss, Norfolk tel: 01359 221 240/333 produces unpasteurised milk, cream and farmhouse butter from their Jersey herd that grazes on two-hundred-year-old pastures. They also produce their own milk-fed pork (which makes proper crackling), bacon and gammon, lamb, Aberdeen Angus beef, poultry, eggs, wheat and wholemeal flour. Livestock are fed home-grown grain, are never hurried, and live as natural a life as possible. The farm is very small and sells its produce by prior telephone appointment only. The meat is well hung and usually sold frozen. Prices are exceptionally reasonable.

Their milk, cream and butter are now available through Pure Organic Foods Ltd (p. 203). Because green-top milk cannot be sold through shops, each customer must sign a form which is kept by the farm, who supply Pure Organic Foods, who then supply the shop with that customer's order.

cream retails for around £1.50–£1.75 per glorious 250ml tub – that is, about twice that of standard cream, but three or four times the quality. Supermarket organic double cream is cheaper, at around 90p–£1.20 per 250ml. The superb Farmers' Dairy Co. double cream sells for around £1.20 per 250ml.

Where to buy: Organic cow's milk is one of the most widely available organic foods. Safeway, Sainsbury's, Tesco and Waitrose stores all stock it at similar prices; other multiples also stock organic milk. Sainsbury's and Waitrose sell organic cream in selected outlets. Waitrose sell Skane UHT milk in selected stores. Alternative supermarkets all stock organic milk and cream. Organic/wholefood shops and some health food shops sell organic milk and sometimes organic cream. In London, Selfridges and Harvey Nichols food halls and Bluebird sell both. Neal's Yard in Covent Garden sell organic milk.

Direct from the producer There are several small producers of organic milk who sell their milk direct. Consult the Soil Association booklet, *Where to Buy Organic Food*. See also Caerfai Farm, p. 160, Old Plaw Hatch Farm and Court Farm, p. 168.

Others Some box schemes and many home delivery services supply organic milk and cream.

Mail order:

Organic milk and cream can be ordered direct from Graig's and Swaddles Green Farms (p. 104 and 106). The Fresh Food Company (p.100) offer unpasteurised organic Jersey milk and cream. Longwood Farm (p.106) sell organic cow's and goat's milk and cream and Rachel's Dairy buttermilk.

Organic cream and crème fraîche Organic cream and crème fraîche are luscious stuff! The two best double creams generally available, thick and moreish, are Rachel's Dairy and the Farmers' Dairy Co. Delicious crème fraîche is produced by Rachel's Dairy and Yeo Valley; the latter is half-fat. See also p. 168.

Organic buttermilk Produced by Rachel's Dairy, see p. 165.

Organic clotted cream Produced by Rachel's Dairy, see p. 165.

Organic quark Produced by Old Plaw Hatch Farm, see p. 168.

what they say . . .

'I strive to give my cows best-quality organic food, comfortable quarters and a stress-free life, in return for longevity, good health and milk-production efficiency. The calves suckle for four months to build up their immunity to illness. Conventional medicines are used in rare cases of acute suffering, or to save a life. I prefer the use of alternative treatments and complementary medicine. My Ayrshire cows have taught me much and I enjoy being their student!' – *Nick Rebbeck, organic dairy farmer*

'I always used to be a firm believer in tradition, i.e. in having milk delivered by a milkman. However, when I wanted organic milk, he was unable to provide it, forcing me to buy milk at Tesco. I had got used to skimmed milk and didn't notice the watery taste and consistency until I tried organic. Not only did it have a fuller flavour, it was creamier, and I felt as if I could have got it from the farm that morning. I've felt more vitality since drinking and eating organic products – whether it's partly in the mind, I don't know, but I feel great!' – *Mrs T. Bonser, Kent*

'A pint of organic full-cream milk from the supermarket (Farmers' Dairy) tastes like delicious Jersey milk and is cheaper than ordinary full-cream milk purchased at a local corner shop, where 46p is the norm.' – *T. Riglan, Harrow, Middlesex*

Organic Butter

Organic butter is a treat. The flavour, particularly that of yellow butters, is better than many commercial brands, which taste flat and uninteresting by comparison. Unlike most commercial brands, organic butter is made in small quantities from fresh milk from known sources. In Britain, it is made by hand on a very small scale and in one or two small commercial dairies. Excellent Danish organic butter is readily available. Organic French butter is due to arrive soon, as well as more brands.

For pesticide residues in butter, see Appendix 1, p. 343.

Hand-made farmhouse butter
This is a luxury food and therefore expensive. Produced and churned in the traditional way, it is not pasteurised and varies slightly with the seasons. The two main producers are Rachel's Dairy and The Elms Dairy (pp.165–67), each widely distributed. Other organic butters are made locally by small producers and sold at the farm gate, through farm shops or local stores; two such are Radford Mill Farm, Somerset, and The Barn, Cornwall (see p.

168). Domini Quality Foods, near Diss, Norfolk, also produce hand-made salted and unsalted organic butter from Jersey cows.

These are the *major brands* of commercial butters:

Cornflower organic butter Produced by a small organic co-operative dairy in Grinsted, northern Denmark, using milk from their own farms. Pale colour, typical Danish butter flavour, available both salted and unsalted, certified by the Soil Association. They also produce *Thise Mejen* unsalted Danish butter, sold under their Grinsted Dairy label.

Harmonie butter Made by the manufacturers of Lurpak, an excellent organic sweet-cream Danish butter available in selected Tesco and Waitrose stores. Good value.

Hergest Court Farm organic farmhouse butter (Farmers' Dairy Co.) A small dairy in Hereford, which uses traditional methods and local organic milk supplies, certified by the Soil Association. A slightly salted, pale-golden-yellow butter with a rich, creamy flavour easy to become addicted to.

Lye Cross Salted organic butter, available in selected outlets.

Yeo Valley organic butter Due soon.

Buying and storing: Hand-made farmhouse butter is a different product from commercially made butter. Gloriously sweet and creamy when freshly made, it does not keep well and should be bought as fresh as possible and eaten within two weeks. For this reason, check the date stamp and only buy when very fresh. Commercially made organic butter is made from pasteurised milk and has the same shelf life as conventional butter.

- Always store butter in the fridge well wrapped in greaseproof paper; this protects it from absorbing other flavours that might be around.
- The best way to store hand-made organic butter is to cut it into conveniently sized small blocks, wrap well in greaseproof paper and keep in a box in the freezer. If

you use small quantities, do the same with other organic butters.

Price guide: Hand-made organic butter can cost three or four times more than cheap butters but is about the same price as up-market French butters; expect to pay around £2.20–£2.50 per 225g. Commercial organic butters vary, depending on the outlet; the best advice here is to shop around. Expect to pay anything from £1.20 to £2 per 225g. Organic butter from supermarkets, usually the cheapest places to buy it, can cost 30 per cent less than at other retail outlets.

Where to buy: Most major supermarkets now stock organic butter in selected stores: Safeway and Sainsbury's sell Cornflower, Waitrose and Tesco sell Harmonie and the northern chain, Booths, sell Rachel's Dairy butter. Alternative supermarkets and specialist organic/wholefood shops all stock organic butter.

Others Organic farm shops, some box schemes and most home delivery services.

Mail order: Hergest Court Farm farmhouse butter (Farmers' Dairy) is available from Graig Farm, Damhead Organically Grown Foods, the Fresh Food Company, Longwood Farm (Rachel's Dairy) and Organics Direct. See Mail Order, pp. 98–106, for telephone numbers.

Organic Cheese

Organic cheese uses milk from animals grazing on organic pastures, and raised organically on farms or holdings, without routine antibiotics, using extensive methods of husbandry. Cheesemakers who have switched from conventional to organic milk remark on the difference it has made to the flavour of their cheese. No artificial flavourings, additives or synthetic colourings are included, and in the UK only vegetarian rennet (non-GM) is used, so all UK cheeses are suitable for vegetarians. If no organic equivalent is available, up to 3 per cent of non-organic ingredients such as garlic, herbs and spices is permitted.

Organic cheeses are gaining more recognition, and several are now exhibited at cheese shows. Many are made by individual cheesemakers who use milk from their own animals, or buy accredited organic milk from known producers. The remainder are made in small and medium-sized dairies, including the rising number of imported organic cheeses coming on to the shelves. Cow's milk cheeses account for about one half, goat's and ewe's milk the other. About half are unpasteurised. The cheeses range from conventional hard ones such as Cheddar, Gouda and Edam, organic Brie and organic blue-veined cheeses, to smoked goat's cheese and cheeses flavoured with herbs, garlic and spices such as caraway seeds. Some imported cheeses use animal rennets, so if you're a vegetarian you may want to check first. Sadly, apart from Rapunzel feta, most organic feta is too hard, and a pale imitation of the real thing. A better bet is organic parmigiano cut to order, described by the head chef of Bluebird in London as 'brilliant'. Prepacked organic cheese is readily available; organic cheese (Pencarreg minis) is served in British Rail dining cars.

For Pesticide residues in cheese, see Appendix 1, p. 343.

Buying and storing: The same rules apply as to any high-quality cheeses. When buying loose cheese, look for one that is in good condition; avoid dried-up, sweaty or obviously unloved cheese; ask to have it cut on the spot rather than taking a piece that has been prepacked; always taste first, and seek advice if you need it.

Any high-quality cheese must be stored at the correct temperature; this varies with the individual cheese, but is usually around maturing temperature, 10–14°C/50–60°F. Whenever possible, check with your cheesemonger. A cool larder, or failing that, a plastic box in the salad drawer of the fridge is acceptable. It must also be wrapped well; waxed paper is by far the best – plastic film is not a good idea and will make the cheese go sweaty in time. Neal's Yard Dairy recommend storing cheese wrapped in greaseproof paper in a cardboard box, to create the right humidity. Allow cheese to come to room temperature before eating.

- The softer the cheese, the fresher it must be and the shorter the shelf life.
- If buying a whole cheese, ask how long it has been matured for, when it will reach its peak and the best way to store it.
- Soft curd cheeses are best bought prepacked.
- Once cut, use hard cheese within seven days; soft cheese such as Brie or soft goat's cheese within three to five days, curd cheeses and crème fraîche as soon as possible.

Price guide: Organic cheeses are all high-quality, predominantly farmhouse cheeses. Those already made in relatively large quantities such as Lye Cross Cheddar and Brie and stocked by supermarkets represent excellent value and cost very little more than conventional equivalents – 5–10 per cent at most, and in some cases less – with Lye Cross Cheddar approximately the same price. Organic farmhouse cheeses are in the same price range as other high-quality cheeses, around £9–£15 per kg (£4.50–£7.50 per lb). Look out for promotional offers in shops and specialist cheese stores.

Where to buy: Supermarkets are a good place to start; they all offer approximately the same cheeses, competitively priced. At the time of writing, Safeway sell Lye Cross organic Cheddar, grated organic Cheddar and Pencarreg; Sainsbury's sell organic West Country farmhouse Cheddar and Welsh organic Brie; Tesco have the widest range – Brie, Cheddar, blue cheese and soft goat's cheese – though only in a few stores; Waitrose sell Lye Cross organic Cheddar and Landsby Brie. Otherwise, cheese is an expensive purchase and you need to be sure you're getting it in good condition. Specialist cheese shops, which usually sell some organic cheeses, are the best place for this; failing that, shops that are cheese enthusiasts. Alternative supermarkets, organic/wholefood and some health food shops all stock organic cheeses. Finally, the cheapest and one of the nicest ways to buy cheese is direct from the producer at the farm gate.

Others Organic farm shops, home delivery services, or direct from the producer.

Mail order: Cheese specialists who offer mail order cheese are Neal's Yard Dairy, London; the Cheese Shop, Chester; and Iain Mellis, Edinburgh (see below). Organic mail order companies offering cheese include Damhead Organically Grown Foods, the Fresh Food Company, Longwood Farm, Organics Direct and specialist meat mail order companies such as Graig Farm, Meat Matters and Swaddles Green Farm. For telephone numbers, see pp. 96–107.

Star Performers:
Specialist Cheese Shops

The following shops, three of the best of their kind in the country, offer a mail order service, specialise in British farmhouse cheeses, including farmhouse organic ones, lovingly looked after, matured in their own cellars and sold in prime condition.

The Cheese Shop, Chester tel: 01244 346240 Stocks over a hundred British cheeses, is particularly strong on Welsh ones, and has a large range of organic farm-made cheeses comprising Staffordshire, Penbryn, Llangloffan, Pencarreg, cow's milk cheeses, Cornish herb, garlic and peppercorn full-fat soft cow's milk cheese, and Acorn organic ewe's milk cheese, available plain or saffron-coated (Lady Llanover). Mail order service available: the cheese is cut and dispatched to order, then sent in chilled packaging to reach customers within 24 hours.

Iain Mellis, Edinburgh and Glasgow tel: 0131 226 6215 Scotland's premier cheese merchant, with shops in Edinburgh and Glasgow. They stock 70–80 farm-made cheeses. Their organic cheeses include Loch Arthur, Staffordshire and Orla Irish sheep's milk cheese. They also sell organic olive oil from Spain, oatcakes, Loch Arthur organic yoghurt and Rachel's Dairy products.

Neal's Yard Dairy, Covent Garden, London WC2 tel: 0171 379 7646 A mecca for anyone who loves real cheese. Their organic cheeses include Llangloffan and Loch Arthur cow's milk cheese, St

Tola goat's milk cheese and Orla Irish sheep's milk cheese. They publish a comprehensive catalogue and advisory leaflet, *Taking Care of Your Cheese*, and run an excellent mail order service: the cheese is freshly cut to order, wrapped well and packed in a cardboard box (for keeping it in at home), and arrives next day. Their mail order list also includes organic red wine vinegar, French preserves, Dijon mustard and L'Estornell Spanish organic olive oil.

Also Ramsbottom Victuallers tel: 01706 825070 A keen cheese enthusiast. See p. 83.

Popular British organic cheeses

Look out for these British organic cheeses – some well known, some new:

Caerfai Cheeses A new farmhouse cheesemaker, at Caerfai Farm, St Davids, Haverfordwest, Dyfed, making unpasteurised Cheddar, Caerphilly, and Caerphilly with leeks and garlic. Soil Association registered. The farm also sells green-top milk and has camping and holiday cottages. Cheeses available from the farm, or nationwide at selected outlets; or by mail order, and can be vacuum-packaged tel: 01437 720 548.

Franjoy An unpasteurised medium-mature farmhouse Cheddar, made from Jersey milk by Franjoy Dairy in West Wales. Widely available. Retail price around £7.50–£8.50 per kg.

Llangloffan Farmhouse A delectable, rich unpasteurised Cheshire-style cheese, made with a mixture of Jersey and Brown Swiss cow's milk on Llangloffan farm near Haverfordwest, Dyfed. The cheese is made only when the cows are outside, feeding on fresh pasture. Available plain, flavoured with chives and garlic and as red Cheshire. Sold at the farm shop, which also stocks other Welsh cheeses and Rachel's Dairy products. Widely available. Price at farm, around £7.20–£7.60 per kg. Run a mail order service for all the cheeses they stock, minimum order 1.5kg tel: 01348 891241.

Loch Arthur A range of delicious unpasteurised bio-dynamic hard and soft cheeses produced by the Loch Arthur Creamery in

Beeswing, Dumfries (see also p. 168), from milk from their own Ayrshire cows. The range includes an award-winning traditional Cheddar, available plain or with herbs or caraway seeds, a twelve-month-aged Cheddar, a small soft cheese called *Crannog*, available plain, herbed or with green peppercorns, a semi-soft rind-washed cheese called *Criffel* and a smooth, creamy, pasteurised fresh curd cheese. All carry the Demeter symbol. The cheeses can be bought at the creamery and through mail order. Widely distributed throughout Scotland, including Iain Mellis' cheese shop (p. 159), London, which stocks Loch Arthur Cheddar. Prices from creamery direct range from £7.70 to £8.80kg for both hard and soft cheeses. For mail order details, including gift mixed-cheese platters and baskets tel: 01387 760296.

Lye Cross Pasteurised mature Cheddar, produced in Somerset by Alvis Brothers Ltd at Lye Cross farm near Bristol. Probably Britain's best-known organic cheese, it is available loose or prepacked and has a rich, toothsome flavour; excellent value, and widely distributed nationwide. Carries the Soil Association symbol. Expect to pay £7.50–£9 per kg, depending on the outlet. Find it also at supermarkets: Sainsbury's, in the south-west stores; Safeway, 120 stores; Tesco, 300 stores; Waitrose, all stores.

Lye Cross organic cheese A new range of Lye Cross speciality unpasteurised cheeses, flavoured with chives, mixed herbs, wild garlic, apple mint or oak smoked.

Malthouse Cottage Farm Cheeses, Ashington, Pulborough A range of goat's milk cheeses including a soft herbed and a hard, white-moulded, blue-veined cheese made on the farm. Carries the Soil Association symbol. Available mainly in London in whole-food and specialist shops.

Penbryn Britain's only organic Gouda, made at Ty Hen farm, Penbryn, Dyfed. Unpasteurised, moist, mild and sweet when young, ripening to a firm, dry, full-flavoured cheese. Carries the Soil Association symbol. Sold at the farm for around £5.50 per kg tel: 01239 810347. Widely available throughout Wales, and elsewhere through specialist cheese, organic and wholefood shops. Retail price £7–£8.50 per kg.

Pencarreg Britain's best-known organic Brie-style cheese made in Lampeter from pasteurised milk, with a mild flavour ripening to a soft, rich creaminess. Also available prepacked as segments and minis. Pencarreg Blue is a mild, soft blue-veined version. Carries the Soil Association symbol. Widely distributed. Pencarreg minis are available on British Rail. Expect to pay £7.50–£9 per kg for plain and £9.50–£10.50 per kg for Pencarreg Blue. At supermarkets: Booths (north of England), Pencarreg and Pencarreg Blue minis; Sainsbury's, Pencarreg minis, selected stores; Safeway, Pencarreg, Welsh stores; Tesco, Pencarreg and Pencarreg Blue, selected stores; Waitrose, Pencarreg, Monmouth store.

Staffordshire Organic A popular, good-value, unpasteurised Cheddar-style cheese made at New House Farm, Acton, in Staffordshire using local organic milk. Available as cloth-bound truckles or in vacuum-packed portions direct from the farm, both plain and flavoured with fresh herbs, dried herbs or wild garlic. Widely available through specialist cheese, organic and wholefood shops. For sale at their own farm shop, which also sells their meat and a wide range of organic foods. Price around £5–£5.50 per kg direct from the farm, or £7.50–£9 per kg from retail outlets. Mail orders by request tel: 01782 680366.

Whittington Made by Malvern Cheesewrights, this is a new organic cloth-bound Gloucester-style cheese made from Ayrshire cow's milk and matured for six months. Widely available, including at major multiples. Retail price around £9 per kg.

Yan Tan Tethera sheep's milk cheese: see p. 169.

See also Ashdown Foresters cheese, pp. 167–8.

Popular Irish cheeses
Desmond and Gabriel Cheddar, St Tola goat's milk log cheese from County Clare, and Orla sheep's milk peccorino-style cheese from County Cork.

Imported cheeses

Many organic cheeses are made throughout Europe, and some of them are beginning to be imported. With one or two exceptions, you will not find these cheeses in supermarkets or in most shops selling cheese. Look for them in organic shops, alternative super-markets and cheese specialists.

A few examples are:

Cornflower A range of Danish cheeses produced by the Grinsted organic dairy. The range includes Cornflower Brie; two mild, creamy Danish blue cheeses, Danish Blue and Grinzola; a Brie-style sliceable cheese, White Cornflower; St Paulin, Samsoe, Havarti, cow's milk feta; a plain cream cheese and a cream cheese flavoured with freshly crushed organic garlic. Prices around £4.50–£6.00 per 500g, depending on the cheese. Selected lines available in some Sainsbury's stores.

Hedwigshof A hard Gouda-type goat's cheese from Holland, available plain or flavoured with herbs and paprika, nettle and onion, and basil and garlic. Carries the ECO symbol. Retails at around £18 per kg.

Landsby Brie A rich, golden, creamy Danish pasteurised Brie, made by Tholsrup, Denmark's largest family-owned cheesemaking company. Comes in prepacked segments also. Available at Waitrose. Price around £10 per kg, or £1.49 per 150g pack.

Parmigiano Reggiano Genuine organic parmigiano reggiano is beginning to make its appearance and is available, for example, cut to order from Bluebird and Planet Organic in London and selected outlets elsewhere. It is generally superb, with a rich, sweet, complex flavour – as good as the parmigiano you will taste in Parma itself. Prices range from around £24 to £34 per kg. One to look out for is made by the Santa Rita co-operative, comprising thirteen small family-run organic farms situated in the hills near Pompeano and Selva in Modena. Its dairy has been making cheese organically since the early 1990s, and is certified by the AIAB (Associazione Italiana per l'Agricoltura Biologica).

Rapunzel A range of prepacked cheeses: Emmenthal; feta; cream cheese (Philadelphia-style), plain and with herbs; and grated Parmesan.

Others Swedish Farms organic cow's cheese; French mountain cheese (Comté); Emmenthal (Bavaria); Edam and Gouda, plain, herb and garlic. A new range of traditional high-quality cheeses from Allgau in Germany includes Rigatino, Montana and Bergkase, an unpasteurised typical mountain cheese made with Demeter milk; some of their cheeses use animal rennet. German organic cow's milk mozzarella is available under the Mozza brand.

Organic Yoghurt

The most popular organic food you can buy, available everywhere, and with sales increasing over 300 per cent in the last couple of years. For anyone new to organic food, yoghurt is the perfect thing to start with. Healthy, convenient, delicious and not expensive, unlike many other yoghurts it contains only real ingredients, no refined white sugar (organic yoghurts tend to add less sugar, anyway), and is completely free from artificial flavourings and additives. Stop press news is that frozen organic yoghurt has just arrived – and is wonderful.

There are two main types, commercially made and individual producer-made:

Commercially made Made primarily from organic cow's milk in the same smooth, thick style as conventional yoghurts, and can be used in exactly the same way. Available plain and flavoured, wholefat and low-fat. See Star Performers opposite.

Individual producer-made Mainly made from the producers' own organic cow's, goat's, or sheep's milk; mostly natural yoghurt, but a few producers make a small amount of fruit yoghurt. More like home-made yoghurt – with a creamy crust if made from whole milk, for example, or with a slightly thinner, grainier texture that yoghurt buffs appreciate and that is best for eating rather than cooking with. Like hand-made cheese, yoghurt may also show seasonal variations. For examples, see p. 167.

> **WATCHWORD:** Organic yoghurt contains 95 per cent or more certified ingredients. Only organic milk, milk powder, cream and fruit can be used. Non-organic ingredients may include added pectin or starch in fruit yoghurts. Yoghurt made by small producers is usually 100 per cent organic.

Star Performers: Yogurt

Rachel's Dairy Soil Association registered. An award-winning Welsh dairy, the first to produce an organic Greek-style cow's milk yoghurt and the only one to produce a low-fat natural yoghurt that does not contain milk powder and is made from fresh milk only. They make wholemilk and low-fat natural; 'really delicious', creamy wholemilk fruit (strawberry, raspberry, peach, apricot, Garden Fruits and Forest Fruits); and low-fat fruit yoghurts (strawberry, raspberry and apricot). A proportion of Guernsey milk is used in all their yoghurts. The fruit ones contain whole pieces, cooked first to a jam with cane sugar; no pectin or starch is used, giving the yoghurts a clean aftertaste. Recently introduced, a sugar-free fruit yoghurt, available at Sainsbury's. For their other products, see pp. 153–4.

Yeo Valley Soil Association registered. The major award-winning UK brand, which now commands a 1 per cent share of the market for all yoghurt – a first ever for an organic dairy product. It has recently opened a new organic dairy, Cannington Creamery, near Bridgwater, Somerset. They produce wholemilk and low-fat natural and fruit yoghurts (apple and blueberry, banana, strawberry, blackcurrant) and delicious half-fat crème fraîche. Their fruit yoghurts are made with fruit purées sweetened with organic apple juice and thickened with a little pectin or starch. The new dairy plans to produce a full range of dairy products. Look out for Yeo Valley organic cream, Greek-style yoghurt, butter and cheese.

Also Sainsbury's own-brand organic yoghurt, made by Rachel's Dairy; and Tesco own-brand and Baby Organix yoghurts, both made for them by Yeo Valley.

Rocombe Farm frozen organic fruit yoghurt The latest addition of the Devonshire ice-cream makers, made to their usual high standards and unbelievably good. Plain, which tastes almost as rich as ice-cream, blackcurrant, raspberry and strawberry flavours are available, with more planned. For details on Rocombe Farm, see p. 171.

Stonyfield Farm frozen yoghurt Not to my taste but virtually fat-free American flavoured organic yoghurts made from organic skimmed milk and cane sugar, available in 473ml tubs in vanilla, vanilla fudge swirl, chocolate, raspberry and decaffeinated coffee. Registered with Quality Assurance International in America and the Soil Association in the UK. Note that American organic standards differ and these yoghurts contain permitted stabilisers, emulsifiers, natural colourings and other ingredients such as rice syrup and whey protein. For more information about the company, see Stonyfield ice-creams, p. 170.

Baby Organix yoghurt See p. 234.

The Elms Dairy Organic Soya milk yoghurt, see opposite.

Buying and storing: Organic yoghurt is exactly the same as conventional yoghurt in these respects. Unopened, plain yoghurt stores very well in the fridge for two to three weeks, but changes in flavour, becoming more acidic with time and gradually thickening. Fruit yoghurts should be eaten as soon as possible.

Price guide: Commercially produced cow's milk organic yoghurts are approximately the same price as equivalent – that is, premium – conventional brands, currently around 99p per 500ml tub. Fruit yoghurts are only around 5–10p extra. The major organic UK brands all sell for roughly the same price. Look out for promotional offers in supermarkets. Yoghurt made by small producers is usually more expensive. In all cases, large tubs are more economical. Stonyfields frozen yoghurts are around £3.20 per large tub.

> **PRICEWISE:** Supermarkets and chain grocery stores sell organic yoghurt competitively; mark-ups are higher in independent shops and small outlets, and vary considerably.

Where to buy: Rachel's Dairy and Yeo Valley are available nationwide in major multiples, small grocery chains such as Spa, Leo's and Mace, organic/wholefood/health food shops, and some delis. Small producers sell primarily through local outlets, including farm shops. Planet Organic in London sells The Elms Dairy and other small-producer yoghurts.

Mail order: Damhead Organically Grown Foods, Longwood Farm and Organics Direct supply Rachel's Dairy yoghurt. For telephone numbers, see pp. 98–101. Rocombe Farm (p. 171) operate their own mail order service, including their frozen yoghurts.

Small-scale yoghurt and dairy producers

The Elms Dairy The Elms Dairy, at West Compton near Shepton Mallet, Somerset tel: 01749 890371 produce excellent organic goat's and sheep's milk yoghurt and goat's milk cream from their own herds, organic cow's milk and soya milk yoghurt, and organic milk, cream and delicate-flavoured, unsalted hand-churned butter; plus a small amount of sugar-free organic fruit yoghurt – the fruit is home-grown. All produce is pasteurised and made on the farm, and carries the UKROFS and Organic Farmers' and Growers' symbol. Outlets are concentrated in the south-west and a few shops in London, including Planet Organic.

Duddleswell Dairy A small family-run dairy at Putlands Farm, Duddleswell, Uckfield in East Sussex tel: 01825 712647 producing a range of sheep's milk and organic cow's milk dairy produce. The organic range is certified by the Soil Association, is sold under the Putlands Farm label and includes creamy, thick-set, low-fat bio-yoghurt made with Guernsey milk from which the butterfat has been removed; low-fat fromage frais-based soft cheese, plain, and garlic and herb; pasteurised organic Guernsey cream; small quantities of Guernsey unsalted butter, and the superb and delectably rich Ashdown Foresters hard cow's milk cheese. All their products are excellent; the low-fat products do not taste low-fat. Their products can be bought from the farm direct, are widely distributed throughout the South, and their hard cheeses are available by mail order.

Old Plaw Hatch Farm Voted by *Harpers & Queen* magazine as the best farm shop in the country, Old Plaw Hatch Farm at Sharpthorne, East Grinstead tel: 01342 810652 is a bio-dynamic farm under the ownership of a charitable trust and specialising in dairy produce – green-top milk, unpasteurised cream, ice-cream, yoghurt, quark, Cheddar-type cheese, and vegetables. They sell single, whipping and double cream (so thick it's more like quadruple cream), plain full- and low-fat yoghurt, and pure 100 per cent organic fruit yoghurts made with UK-produced organic fruit, mainly their own, and organic sugar. Their dairy produce is sold through the farm shop, throughout the south-east in small outlets, and in London. They are now in partnership with another nearby bio-dynamic farm, Tablehurst Farm, selling beef, lamb and pork. All products carry the Demeter symbol.

Also

The Barn, *Leswidden, St Just, Penzance, Cornwall* tel: 01736 787953 Currently in conversion, awaiting the Soil Association symbol (due shortly). Home produce – organic plain yoghurt, Cornish vanilla ice-cream, butter and cheese; vegetables, pork, bacon and ham – sold from the farm gate.

Court Farm, *Winford, Somerset* tel: 01275 472335 Soil Association registered. Yoghurt – plain organic yoghurt and fruit yoghurts made with organic milk; plus unpasteurised milk and cream; pork and beef. For sale at the farm and locally.

Loch Arthur Creamery, *Beeswing, Dumfries* tel: 01387 760296 Their produce carries the Demeter symbol. Full- and low-fat plain yoghurt, curd cheese, soft cheese and Cheddar-type cheese, sold on the premises. Wide distribution in Scotland. For more information on their cheeses, including mail order, see p. 160.

Radford Mill Farm, *Timsbury, Somerset* tel: 01761 472549 Soil Association registered. Home produce includes organic plain and fruit yoghurts, soft cheese; vegetables, turkeys, eggs, herbs; lamb, beef and pork to order. They operate a home delivery and box scheme, and have a stall in Glastonbury market on Tuesdays.

Yan Tan Tethera, *Llugwy Farm, near Llandrindod Wells, Powys* tel: 01547 550641 OF & G registered. Produce Greek-style sheep's milk yoghurt and sheep's milk cheese, for sale from the farm and locally. Hoping to start mail order. Phone for details.

Organic Ice-cream

Organic ice-cream is unlike most ice-cream you have ever tasted. Made from organic cream, milk, sugar and fruit, it contains minimum added ingredients and no artificial flavourings or additives. This means that it tastes superb: rich, clean and delectable. Nor do you pay for expensive advertising campaigns – which makes it even better value.

Comparing organic and non-organic ice-creams, there are two other important things to note:

- The vast majority of conventional ice-creams are made with a range of artificial emulsifiers and stabilisers. Their function is to enable maximum air to be incorporated and to develop a creamy feel in products which do not necessarily contain any cream. The only stabilisers allowed in organic ice-cream are guar, xanthan and locust bean gums, the only emulsifier, lecithin; all are natural products.
- Ice-cream is sold by volume, not by weight. Cheap ice-cream can contain up to 120 per cent added air. To judge the quality of any ice-cream, feel the weight of the

tub. The lighter it feels, the more removed from the real thing and the poorer the quality.

WATCHWORD: Organic ice-cream is made with a minimum of 95 per cent organic ingredients. Non-organic ingredients may include pasteurised free-range eggs; this is because there are no pasteurised organic eggs currently available.

The three *major brands* are:

Green & Black's organic dark-chocolate ice-cream Soil Association registered. Described as 'smooth, ultra-dark and deca-dent', this is one chocolate ice-cream you need never feel guilty about. Made from organic concentrated skimmed-milk powder, double cream, sugar, plain chocolate, cocoa powder and vanilla, plus permitted stabilisers and lecithin emulsifier and minimum added air. Excellent flavour.

Rocombe Farm Fresh Ice-Cream Ltd. The leading brand. See opposite.

Waitrose organic vanilla ice-cream Soil Association registered. A smooth, milky ice-cream made for Waitrose by Rocombe Farm Fresh Ice-cream. Available in most stores.

Also:

Stonyfield Farm Not ice-cream, but a new range of American low-fat frozen desserts, imported from Vermont. They are made by an established company, now entirely organic, using skimmed organic milk, sugar, organic cream and other ingredients and flavourings. Note that they also contain permitted stabilisers and emulsifiers, and some contain added rice syrup and whey protein concentrate. Part of the company's profit is donated to environmental causes. Flavours include: vanilla, vanilla and fudge brownie, strawberry, mango, mocha fudge biscotti, chocolate raspberry and double chocolate swirl, all in 473ml tubs. I find them too sweet and much prefer the real thing, but many disagree.

Star Performer:
Rocombe Farm Fresh Ice-cream

A small family company in Torquay, Devon, Soil Association registered, whose luxury ice-creams – praised by countless food writers – are an example of commercial ice-cream at its best, equal to home-made. Flavour and texture are superb. No emulsifiers or stabilisers are used in any of their ice-creams, which are made only with cream, full milk, eggs, fruit, real flavourings and sugar, and they contain a minimum of added air (35 per cent). They have recently become totally organic, and all their products – ice-cream, frozen yoghurts and high-fruit sorbets – are now either 70 per cent or 95 per cent plus organic. All their ice-creams are made from mainly organic Jersey milk. Flavours include vanilla, chocolate, cinnamon, strawberry, bananas, excellent cream and honey, irresistible crunchies and cream, and yummy 'Taste of Christmas'. More flavours are constantly being introduced. Their frozen yoghurts (p. 166) and sorbets are equally excellent. They also offer a mail order service, tel: 01626 872291/873800.

Buying and storing: It is important to have ice-cream well wrapped and to get it home as quickly as you can. Commercial organic ice-cream has a storage life of 9–18 months, depending on the brand; unless the box says differently, farm-made ice-cream is best eaten as soon as it is bought. Ice-cream should not be eaten straight from the freezer but allowed to soften and 'ripen' for a few minutes, to bring out the flavour.

- Ice-cream must be stored in the freezer at a minimum temperature of -18°C. It will keep unopened, but once opened should be eaten as soon as possible, as constant softening and re-hardening leads to deterioration of taste and texture
- To prevent ice crystals forming on top of the ice-cream, keep the tub covered at all times.
- Never refreeze ice-cream that has thawed; this can be a health hazard.

Price guide: Organic ice-cream sells at around the same price as premium ice-creams such as Häagen-Dazs, around £3.50–£3.80

per 500ml tub. Waitrose organic vanilla ice-cream sells at about £1 less than Häagen-Dazs vanilla ice-cream, and is a bargain. Stonyfield frozen desserts cost around £3.20 per tub.

Where to buy: Organic ice-cream is sold mainly through organic/wholefood/health food shops. Rocombe Farm ice-cream is also available in delicatessens and fine food shops. Sainsbury's sell Green & Black's organic chocolate ice-cream in selected stores; Waitrose sell their own in most stores. Stonyfield frozen desserts

What You Get

Where ice-cream is concerned, reading the labels is essential; only then can you see what you are getting for your money in terms of quality of ingredients used. Comparing the ingredients and prices of four vanilla ice-creams, two cheap ones, retailing at 95p and £1.13 per litre box, an expensive brand at £3.59 per 500ml tub, and Waitrose organic ice-cream at £2.49 per 500ml tub, reveals:

1 Neither of the two cheap ice-creams contains any cream, full milk or eggs. Both contain vegetable fats, whey solids, added sweeteners in the form of dextrose and/or glucose syrup, emulsifier E471, and natural flavourings. The three major ingredients are reconstituted skimmed milk, hydrogenated vegetable oil or vegetable fat, and sugar.

2 Both the expensive and the organic brand contained only real ingredients. The expensive one contained more cream, but does not state what kind of cream, egg yolks, sugar or 'natural flavouring' it uses; and it uses only skimmed milk, whereas the organic one contains full-cream milk, double cream, pasteurised free-range eggs and unrefined sugar, and lists vanilla essence as the only flavouring.

are sold through conventional outlets such as London food halls, delicatessens and independent shops.

Others A few farm shops, including Old Plaw Hatch, East Grinstead and The Barn, Penzance (p. 168), who both make their own organic ice-cream.

Also

Swaddles Green Farm tel: 01460 234387 and Home Farm Foods tel: 01380 722254 deliver Rocombe Farm ice-cream in London.

Mail order: Rocombe Farm's ice-cream mail order tel: 01626 872291/873800.

Organic Eggs

Organic egg–producing systems, like those of one or two independent egg-producers, aim primarily to maximise the health and well-being of the chicken, not to maximise egg production. As a result, fewer but better-quality eggs are produced which, at their best, offer a taste of how eggs used to be: free of artificial colourings, with a real flavour and an extra-thick yolk sitting proud of a soft, creamy white.

Though steadily increasing, the supply is very limited, and currently only a handful of pioneers are producing organic eggs on a commercial scale. They are more labour-intensive and far more expensive to produce. Organic feed alone, for example, adds over 40p extra to the cost of a dozen eggs. Though most major supermarkets now stock them, if you are unable to get hold of any I recommend either Martin Pitt eggs (p. 177) if you live in the south of England, or Richard Guy's Real Meat Company eggs (p. 184). I have visited both, and they produce high-quality eggs to the highest welfare and feed standards.

Organic egg facts

- In the UK, organic flock sizes are usually between 100 and 500, and rarely larger than 1,000, though draft EU regulations allow a maximum of 4,800 birds. This compares to flock sizes of 3,000–15,000 in conventional free-range systems supplying the retail sector generally.
- Unlike mass-produced conventional eggs, organic eggs vary, particularly those from small producers: the colour and richness of the yolks, for example, change with the seasons, becoming richest in summer, as do the number of eggs laid. This is an indication that the eggs are being produced in the best way possible.
- It is illegal to sell free-range eggs loose, whether organic or not, except from the farm direct; all must be boxed and labelled with the name of the grower or packer.
- Organic eggs are all free-range; the term 'organic free-range' is usually found on the box.
- The national average consumption of eggs is two per week; eating two organic eggs would cost an extra 6–15p only.

WATCHWORD: Unless you know the supplier, or the box says differently, the term 'free-range' generally has little meaning, either for eggs or for poultry. The majority of free-range systems are highly intensive. Flock sizes can be massive, and though 'free-range' birds have access to the outside through small pop-holes, conditions, including feed, are otherwise similar to those found in batteries.

Standards: organic eggs versus the rest

There is probably more agonising about standards of organic egg production than about those concerning most other foods. Debates over flock size, over permitted use of coccidiostats (opposite) for chicks when necessary, and so on, continue and have not yet been completely resolved. The fundamental problem is that conventional eggs have become so cheap that few consumers are prepared to pay the necessary extra for eggs produced in the best ways possible. There is further confusion currently because of differences between the egg production standards of the two main organisations concerned, the Soil Association and the Organic Farmers and Growers.

The debate mainly applies to commercial organic eggs, rather than to those from small producers or from organic farmers who keep a few chickens in the traditional way. In practice, it is what each organic producer actually does rather than which logo the eggs carry that is the most important factor.

Some compromises are inevitable. For the moment, the main differences between commercial organic and free-range eggs is that all organic eggs are produced in non-intensive systems; the hens have constant access to organic pastures, which are permanently covered with appropriate vegetation, and they are fed a natural diet comprising a minimum of 70–80 per cent organic feed.

Also:

- The birds have up to twice as much room. Stocking densities, both inside and out, are up to half that of free-range systems; some small producers have stocking densities up to one-third less.
- Prophylactic and routine medication of flocks is forbidden; if medication *is* used to treat individual hens, withdrawal time before the sale of eggs from hens thus treated is two or three times longer than with conventional systems.
- Birds are fed a natural diet. In-feed medication, growth-promoting agents, yolk-colourants and animal wastes, including feathers, are forbidden.
- Producers supplying organic eggs subscribe to organic farming principles.

NOTE: The use of coccidiostats is permitted, as a preventative measure, under UKROFS regulations in starter poultry rations for chicks and young birds up to four weeks old, as in conventional systems. This does not mean that coccidiostats are *necessarily* used. Under Soil Association regulations, producers cannot use them routinely, but only if they can demonstrate a real need. Artificial light to extend day length is also permitted under UKROFS regulations and is generally employed.

For pesticide and antibiotic residues in eggs, see Appendix 1, pp. 344 and 347.

Commercial producers

Produce eggs to either Organic Farmers & Growers or Soil Association standards, and have the largest flocks. The eggs are boxed and sold to wholesalers, who sell them on to retail outlets including supermarkets. All eggs carry the appropriate symbol on the box.

> **WATCHWORD:** Currently, the Soil Association permits flock sizes of between 100 (ideal) and 500 birds, forbids debeaking and permanent housing, and stipulates that pasture should be rested one year in three to prevent disease build-up, while Organic Farmers & Growers follow UKROFS standards, which permit larger flocks, permanent housing, and debeaking if necessary – though no organic producer does this. The amounts of non-organic feedstuff permitted are also different, being 20 per cent and 30 per cent respectively. Note, also, that both allow conventionally raised pullets up to sixteen weeks old to be bought in and managed organically for six weeks; thereafter, the eggs receive organic status.

Small producers

Independent organic farms, smallholdings and so on which keep very small flocks and sell directly to the public or to local shops in rural areas. If you get the chance, buy some of their eggs. They all carry the Organic Farmers & Growers, Soil Association or Demeter symbol, and are boxed. Some feed chickens with 100 per cent, or thereabouts, organic feed. To find your nearest supplier, or organic farm shop selling eggs, consult the Soil Association's booklet *Where to Buy Organic Food*.

Cherry Tree Eggs Carry the OF & G symbol and is a good example of eggs from a small producer. Featured on the BBC's 'Food and Drink' programme, the eggs are produced by Growing Concern, Loughborough, Leicestershire (p. 86), who have been producing top-quality organic eggs for many years. The hens are kept in movable houses, a hundred in each, graze on organic pastureland and are fed home-grown organic wheat. Their eggs are available at Planet Organic and Bumblebee health food shops in London, in local shops and from the farm direct.

Martin Pitt Eggs, *Marlborough, Wilts.* tel: 01672 512035 An independent, award-winning commercial egg-producer, with thirty-five years' experience, who produces eggs to his own exacting standards and who produces over a hundred thousand eggs a week. They are *not* registered organic eggs but are, I believe, every bit as good. The hens graze on organic pastures, fertility maintained with his own chicken and pig manure, and have easy access to the outside. Animal welfare is paramount. The hens have individual boxes, perches and ample room. They are not debeaked or given any form of prophylactic or routine medication, including coccidiostats, and are fed a natural diet comprising some home-grown organic feed and other natural ingredients mixed on the premises. Stocking densities are one-third that of other free-range systems; the hens are housed in large, airy barns, 1,800 hens per barn. He vaccinates his hens against salmonella and stamps each box with the date of lay. His eggs are widely available throughout the south of England and retail at between £1.50 and £2 per dozen, depending on the outlet. Send SAE for list of stockists.

Buying and storing: Stored properly, a fresh egg will keep perfectly well for a month. Keep cool at a constant temperature, or in the least cold part of the fridge. Allow to come to room temperature before using.

- The thicker the shell, the better the eggs will store and keep their eating quality. Conventional eggs tend to have thinner shells. Martin Pitt's and many other organic eggs have thicker shells on account of the quality of the calcium feed in the hens' diet.
- Avoid buying eggs in recycled egg boxes, which may be

contaminated with bacteria, including salmonella, or with broken egg remains from previous eggs.
- Keep egg shelves in fridge doors clean; so as to avoid contamination from, e.g., spilled yoghurt or dripping meat, which can cause bacterial build-up in eggs.
- Cracked eggs should be used only for cakes and for cooking where the eggs are cooked thoroughly, and should be used as soon as possible.

Price guide: The price of organic eggs represents the true cost of producing a first-class egg. They are twice as expensive as intensively produced eggs, but cost only 20p per half-dozen (or less) more than the 'farm-assured free-range eggs' to be found in supermarkets. £2–£3 per dozen, depending on where you buy them – organic eggs are likely to be cheaper in rural areas and when bought direct from the farm.

Where to buy: The availability of organic eggs is limited more by supply than by the number of outlets. Organic farm shops selling their own are one of the best sources. For examples, see p. 86. Major supermarkets stock OF&G registered organic eggs in selected outlets. Alternative supermarkets, organic/wholefood and some health food shops have regular supplies.

Others Local shops in rural areas. Plus some box schemes and home delivery services.

Mail order: The Fresh Food Company, Damhead Organically Grown Foods and Organics Direct. For telephone numbers, see pp. 98–101.

meat, poultry, game and fish

Meat

As one meat scare follows the next, and the writer Colin Tudge's vision of genetically engineered farmyard freaks and the Arnold Schwarzeneggers of the cattle world, Belgian Blue bulls, bred to have more muscles for consumers to eat than the Incredible Hulk, becomes a reality, animal welfare has never loomed larger.

Faced with such dilemmas organic meat offers consumers a saner, more humane choice. It is meat produced as meat traditionally used to be produced. In organic husbandry systems the overriding objective is not to force animals beyond their natural capacity for growth, but to ensure that they are as healthy as they can be and to respect their welfare needs. This starts with proper suckling and feeding and continues throughout the life of the animal, and includes the rotation and organic management of the land that it grazes. In this way, stress and disease of both animals and land are reduced to a minimum, thereby avoiding the need for routine drugs as well as most of the associated pollution problems. In organic systems this innate strength and health are passed on from one generation to the next – thus the vigour of the whole herd is progressively built up.

In addition, organic meat-producers tend to have smaller herds than many conventional farmers, often favour the more flavoursome, traditionally slower-growing domestic breeds, and use small local abattoirs where possible. At slaughter, everything is done to ensure that their animals experience minimum stress, which is critical to the eating quality of the meat. Most kill a few beasts, or just one, at a time; many have their own butchers and sell their own meat, which is usually hung for longer than conventional meat; and generally the whole carcass is hung in the traditional way, to help ensure optimum eating quality.

All organic meat conforms to UKROFS standards, which set out regulations and guidelines about how an animal should be reared and fed, what medication it should receive, how it should be handled in transit and how it should be slaughtered. UKROFS standards cover every aspect of husbandry, from animal welfare to the disposal of waste products, land management, environmental practices and pollution. Many producers voluntarily exceed these standards. The Soil Association's standards – which are the ones referred to in this section – are more detailed and, in some instances, stricter than UKROFS. No other farm-to-table system of producing meat is so rigorous, or can offer the consumer the same comprehensive, stringent set of guarantees and full legally binding traceability. In addition, only organic meat is guaranteed not to be genetically modified or to be fed GM feedstuffs.

Rest assured that Incredible Hulks, super-milky Friesians capable of producing four thousand gallons of milk a year, and chickens that can barely stand, have no role in organic farming systems.

Organic versus conventional meat: the basics

Though regulations differ slightly for each species, all organically raised meat shares the following fundamental characteristics. Save for occasional specific points peculiar to independent rearing systems that can be even more exacting, these characteristics also represent the major differences between the organic and the standard conventional systems of husbandry. When you buy organic meat, you can be assured that:

- Animals are raised in non-intensive systems and on land managed organically.
- Animal welfare is paramount; this includes extended suckling of the young, to develop optimum health.
- Depending on the species, animals are fed a minimum of 70–90 per cent organic feed.
- Manures, sawdust, fillers, solvent-extracted compounds and genetically modified foods are banned from feedstuffs.
- Routine drugs, antibiotics, growth-promoting agents, animal by–products and all other additives are banned. Antibiotics are used as and when necessary to prevent suffering; if used, withdrawal times, before the animal can enter the food chain, are a minimum of two weeks and two or three times longer than in conventional systems.
- Mutilations are banned.
- The keeping of animals on slatted concrete floors, common practice for conventional pork and beef, is banned.
- Permanent tethering is banned.
- Artificial fertilisers and synthetic pesticides on feed crops, grass and elsewhere, including OP insecticides for warble-fly in cattle and for sheep-dipping, are banned.
- The feeding of animal matter to ruminants is banned.

WATCHWORD: Wherever possible, all stock is born and raised on an organic farm. However, up to 10 per cent conventional stock may be brought in for replacement or expansion, provided the animals meet the strict welfare criteria and undergo the stipulated time for conversion before they can be classified as organic. Chickens must be raised entirely organically from one day old. Pullets for egg production may be brought in to organic systems up to sixteen weeks of age.

what they say . . .

'This farm has been converting to organic principles for the past ten years and is all now of [Soil Association] symbol status apart from the last couple of fields. One of these appears to be permanently blighted by one particular chemical used in the past, because it is still in the soil and refusing to break down, and nothing will grow there.

'The experience has been a rewarding one. Yields of grass for stock, and cereals for feed and other uses, especially from the more mature organic fields, are now almost on a par with those on intensive, chemical-based farms. They are weed-free, strong-growing crops, from a now very fertile soil, and the stock which feed off them mirror this – massively reduced vet bills, herds of cattle, sheep and pigs which look to have natural vitality, which grow at their own pace and which produce meat of the highest quality. We have a pig herd that is utterly stress-free and also, remarkably, smell-free; you'd be happy to have them in your garden.

'As with an athlete coming off drugs, the first few years are painful, but come through that and you start to realise your natural talents – which most farms possess if they choose to tune in to them.'
– *Tim Finney, Eastbrook Farm Organic Meats*

The eating quality of organic meat
Organic meat often looks and eats differently from much standard meat. Butchers who have experience of both wax lyrical about the difference in muscle tone and the sheen of the carcass. This is because the animals have been reared more slowly and have had more exercise. How much difference, however, depends on the age and breed of the animal and, most importantly, on the butchery skills employed, including maturation. Size and age, too, vary more than with conventional meat. This also makes buying organic meat more haphazard, and makes it important to choose it carefully.

fact Codes of practice for the welfare of conventional livestock published by the Ministry of Agriculture state that 'husbandry systems in current use do not equally meet the physiological and behavioural needs of the animals'.

To the thousands of people who now buy organic meat, its flavour is one of the main reasons why they buy it. Comments from satisfied customers all testify to this. Compared to cheap, mass-produced meat, all organic meat has incomparably better flavour and eating quality, particularly pork and poultry. Compared to the highest-quality conventional meat, though, this may or may not be the case. It is also fair to say that, in some cases, there is room for improvement.

Generally speaking:

- Organic meat is denser and less watery than most meat. When cooked, shrinkage is about 10 per cent compared to 30 per cent.
- Organic meat has a richer, more fulfilling meaty flavour and is often closer-grained, giving it a more toothsome texture. It is more satisfying to eat, and goes further.
- The fat is creamy and the meat has good marbling.
- It can be darker-coloured, and dulls more quickly from bright to dark red on the slab.

NOTE: Organic meat sold by supermarkets is hung using modern methods, in vacuum-packaging, for a shorter time. This gives it an eating quality more consistent with conventional meat stocked by super-markets.

All this is very good news for anyone who enjoys traditional meat. If, however, you prefer less robust, very lean, or conventionally tender meat you may find that some organic meat is chewier, or even has too much flavour. If so, organic meat sold in supermarkets, or organic meat raised from modern rather than traditional breeds, may suit you better.

Slaughter

How an animal is slaughtered is of prime concern to the organic producer. All abattoirs used must be approved by a registered organic certification body. The maximum travel time allowed before slaughter is eight hours. Organically reared animals are kept apart from conventional ones, are generally the first in the day to be slaughtered, and are slaughtered in small numbers rather than in hundreds. There is now a mobile organic slaughterhouse that slaughters animals individually. After slaughter, the organic ones are separated from non-organic animals and stamped with a seal certifying their organic status.

Other animal welfare systems

Animal welfare is becoming a critical concern for consumers and various meat-producing schemes have been developed which address this. The two best-known are:

Freedom Foods Developed by the RSPCA and supported by large retailers, this is a voluntary scheme with its own standards of husbandry; although these standards are not as strict as organic standards and have not won universal approval, the scheme offers the shopper traceability guarantees.

Richard Guy's Real Meat Company, *near Warminster, Wilts.* tel: 01985 219020 An independent company with exacting standards of animal welfare, producing high-quality meat. It is not organic; animals are neither fed organically nor managed on organic land, nor does the system purport to address any of the environmental issues that are an integral part of organic systems. But it has its own codes of practice and own inspection system, and offers the shopper full traceability guarantees. The meat is produced by its own farmers and sold through designated real-meat butchers, through independent butchers or through mail order. Regular use of antibiotics and growth-promoting agents is forbidden, and there has been no recorded case of BSE on any of their farms.

> **WATCHWORD:** Green-sounding labels such as 'Traditional', 'Farmhouse', 'Naturally Reared', and so on, are not organic. They are variations or improvements on intensive production systems.

The cost of organic meat

Organic meat costs more, undeniably. The price differentials mainly reflect the increased costs of production. But compare organic meat prices to those of other high-quality, non-intensively produced meat and you will find very little difference, if any in some cases.

Prices vary depending on the time of year, the demand, the cut and the supplier. A small local producer selling his own meat will invariably be able to sell it more cheaply than a specialist supplier, operating a professional mail order service. The same goes for retailers. A retailer sourcing organic meat direct from the producer is able to sell it more cheaply than a retailer who sources it through intermediaries. What this means is that organic meat prices are not standard, and you cannot expect to buy an organic steak for the same price everywhere you go.

How much extra *does* it cost?: Estimates of what it costs to make a direct switch to organic meat from meat sold elsewhere vary from an extra £5–£7 to £10–£12 per week for a family of four, depending on what you buy and where from. But by choosing carefully, perhaps deciding to eat less but to buy organic whenever possible, and to source the best deals, then organic meat becomes a realistic option for most people some or even most of the time, and an option for everyone occasionally. Because there are no fillers or added water in organic hams or bacon, and meat is usually hung for longer, weight for weight, you are also getting more for your money.

A few guidelines:

- The cheapest way to buy organic meat is direct from the producer at a farm shop.
- Braising joints are proportionally cheaper than the most popular cuts such as steak, chicken breasts, pork fillet and prime roasting joints.
- Mail order and home delivery services have regular special offers including family packs.
- Small producers are usually happy to sell half or a whole lamb, half a pig and sometimes a cow, which is far more economical for the customer than buying separate joints. You can usually arrange to have the animal cut as you want. This is a good option for people joining together to share the cost.

- Because organic animals live a more natural lifestyle, supply is not as consistent. Prices may come down when there are gluts and go up when supply is poor; when buying direct from a farm, check the best time to buy.
- If you are buying meat by mail order, shop around and get as many leaflets as you can before making your decision. Prices vary!

Finally, if you can buy large quantities, and have a freezer to match, Higher Hacknell Farm's mail order fresh meat boxes could be the answer. They offer outstanding value – high-quality meat at prices every serious meat-eater can afford. For details, see p. 107.

Buying: Buying organic meat can be a hit-and-miss affair and it is worth taking the trouble to check out your supplier first.

- The best source of organic meat is the expert, be he a butcher who specialises in organic meat, or a producer who understands the butchery side of meat production as well as the rearing.
- Buying organic meat by mail order is usually very reliable. Use the notes on p. 96.
- Try to avoid buying frozen organic meat: you cannot see the quality clearly.

Storing: My own view, borne out by experience, is that as long as you store it correctly, organic meat keeps better than most other meat.

- Unless it is in vacuum-packaging, always remove meat from its wrapper, put it on a clean plate and keep it in the fridge well away from any cooked meat or other food.
- Joints do not need to be covered, nor does chicken; cover small pieces, individual portions, with non-PVC film. A good idea for sliced meat, such as steaks, is also to rub both sides liberally with olive oil.
- Organic meat bought by mail order will come with full instructions on how to store and, usually, how to cook the meat.

● Organic chicken should be eaten within 2–3 days; remove any giblets immediately, wipe out the cavity with kitchen paper and keep the chicken on a clean plate in the fridge. Pork will keep for 3–4 days, lamb and beef for 5–7 days, depending on the cut.

Vacuum-packaged meat Joints or slices of meat will keep perfectly in the fridge for 7–14 days, depending on the meat; you will find that meat 'ages' in the pack and in time develops a stronger smell and a slightly richer flavour. This applies only to meat where the seal is airtight; if the seal has been broken, take the meat out, wipe it dry, put it on a clean plate and store it in the fridge in the usual way. It does not apply, either, to vacuum-packed sausages or to minced meat products, which should be used as soon as possible or frozen.

Where to buy: The major source of organic meat is direct from the producer, either through farm shops or by mail order. Producers often have local retail outlets, too. Supermarkets sell very limited quantities of organic meat, and in selected stores only. Sainsbury's sell the most; see p. 69. Organic shops usually sell organic meat, as do alternative supermarkets, including that of well known producers such as Graig Farm and Eastbrook Farm Organic Meats, or that of local producers. Organic markets in London, Farmers' Market in Bath and a few other markets elsewhere have meat stalls.

Organic butchers There are very few dedicated organic butchers, though an increasing number of independent ones, especially Q Guild butchers, an association of high-quality butchers, sell some organic meat, including that from Prince Charles' organic farm, Highgrove Estate. A list of these, together with the eight butchers registered with the Soil Association, can be found on p. 202; Pure Organic Foods and Black Mountain Foods (p. 203) supply to independent butchers and are happy to tell you the name of your nearest supplier. Planet Organic in London has an exceptional meat counter.

Others Home delivery schemes.

Meat by mail order: You will find organic meat in over a hundred shops up and down the country, and in many farm shops. For detailed descriptions of the major suppliers who operate a mail order service, see pp. 96 and 104.

Organic Meat and Health

Common sense says that meat produced from animals that receive a natural diet and graze organic pastures, that are not stressed or constantly dosed with antibiotics, has to be better for you; that inherently healthy meat makes for healthier people. For example, one paper I was given explained how intensive agriculture reduces the mycorrhizal fungi that grow in the soil on the roots of most plants and increase plant mineral content, and how minerals such as zinc, copper and selenium are further reduced by the use of artificial fertilisers.

Deficiencies in minerals affect animal as much as human health. Furthermore, application of certain minerals such as zinc and copper to fields in which sheep are raised has been shown to result in increased lambing, to halve early mortality and to double the lambs' growth rate. Other correspondents pointed out that OPs bind selenium in the soil, leading to selenium-deficient meat (a lack of selenium has also been implicated in falling sperm counts in Western males); that kiln dust containing carcinogenic waste has been used as a fertiliser and as a cattle-feed binder; that excess free nitrogen may trigger some forms of cancer; and that it has now been shown by a group of EU scientists that hormonal growth-promoters in beef can also be carcinogenic. Unfortunately, too little work has been done in this field, and meat production methods and their effects are currently not a factor in scientific investigations on health. We are now being told that eating too much red meat causes stomach and colon cancer. Is it beyond the bounds of scientific probability that intensive practices may be a contributory factor, or that animals raised organically or by similar systems are safer?

BSE and all that: the organic facts

Organic meat offers one of the best chances of BSE-free meat. Indeed, if all beef were raised organically, BSE would almost certainly never have happened. Unfortunately, the conversion of conventional herds and replacements coming into organic herds from outside sources to meet rising demand have meant that cases of BSE have occurred in a small minority of herds – though such cattle could never have been sold as organic meat, because only animals born and reared organically can be sold as organic meat.

These are the facts:

- The feeding of animal proteins to cattle and sheep raised organically has been banned since 1983 by the Soil Association, five years before the Ministry of Agriculture took action.
- Since before 1985, there has been no recorded case of BSE in any herd on farms managed organically; neither has there been any case subsequently, in closed herds – that is, in herds where no animals have been brought in from outside sources and where all replacement stock has been raised on the farm.
- The only cases of BSE recorded in organic herds are those from recently converted farms where the animals were exposed to contaminated feed before entering an organic regime.
- The use of OP insecticides is banned. These compounds have been cited as a possible causal factor in BSE.

As in conventional herds, any animal suspected of BSE must be immediately removed and destroyed. Any offspring are also destroyed. In addition, current regulations offer safeguards that ensure a complete purge of any herd which undergoes conversion, or any herd where conventional replacements are brought in, namely:

- In herds where animals have contracted BSE, or where animals have been brought in from other herds in which BSE has occurred within the last six years, all contemporary animals born into those herds – that is, born three months either side of a BSE case – and sharing the same food, as well as offspring of such cases, must be removed from the herd and cannot be sold as organic.

● Only animals of known origin can be brought into an organic herd. Any animals of unknown BSE history must be treated as a contemporary and removed from the herd.

what they say . . .

'Having seen various documentaries on intensive farming methods, I have converted to only organic meat and dairy products.'
– *Mr A. Frullo, Hampshire*

'I always try to buy organic meat as I believe that all animals should live their life in dignity and be shown respect, even if – and especially if – they end up as the food on our children's plates.'
– *Mrs J. Golding, Brighton*

'I buy organic produce whenever I can find it, as I know that it has not been drenched in pesticides . . . I like pure food and meat brought up naturally, which always tastes better and, of course, is much more healthy.' – *Mr R.H. Grassam, Leicestershire*

Individual Meats

Beef

Since the BSE crisis, sales of organic beef have soared. Organic beef, conceived, born and reared within an organic system, comes with a BSE-free guarantee. The eating quality varies, but can be glorious. This is particularly true of traditional breeds, which do not mature until two to two and a half years old or older – they have a pronounced rich flavour and a firmer texture.

NOTE: Since BSE, all beef animals must be killed at a maximum age of thirty months. This means that organic producers raising traditional breeds are having to kill their animals before they are ready, and before their flavour and fat conformation have fully developed.

Until very recently, most organic beef came from specialist beef suckler herds, where the mother rears her own calf for up to eleven months before it is weaned. It is then fed on a natural 90 per cent organic forage-based diet (grass, hay, silage), supplemented with home-grown cereals and protein such as soya. Specialist beef breeds have large backs and rumps, where the prime joints are. Though such breeds are still the main source, because of the demand for organic beef, increasingly beef also come from dairy calves; interestingly, in blind tastings these have performed very well. All are allowed to develop at their natural pace, so they grow more slowly, and they are not killed until 20–24 months old, or 30 months in the case of a traditional breed. Most conventional beef is killed at 12–15 months old.

Star Performer: Kite's Nest Farm

Situated near Broadway, in Worcestershire, this is one of the UK's foremost organic beef farms, run by Mary Young and her son and daughter Richard and Rosamund. The farm is totally organic, has been featured often on TV and is renowned for the rare wild flowers and wildlife that thrive there. Cattle are raised in family groups, usually three or four generations together, and each animal is known by name. They are free to wander, and spend a good deal of their time in the farm woods as well as on the grazing pastures. The herd has been 'closed' since 1987, and is given only home-grown organic feed. No feed concentrates or bought-in feed have ever been given. The herd is, and has always been, completely BSE-free. Their farming system is unique, even by organic standards. Their richly flavoured beef is sold through the farm shop only, and is excellent value. It is butchered and hung on the premises, can be cut to particular requirements and is available fresh when butchered and frozen at other times. The shop also sells suet, their own stoneground flour, and wool from their own sheep. Visitors are made welcome tel: 01386 853320.

Also, see Domini Quality Foods, Diss, Norfolk, p. 152.

Veal

Organic veal is produced the way veal *should* be produced. Unlike with 'welfare-friendly' veal, organic calves are suckled entirely with their mother or replacement mother, and are given freedom throughout their lives; they are kept inside in small groups in roomy pens when the weather is too bad for them to go out, but otherwise range freely. Their diet comprises whole organic milk and organic pasture. They are killed at between three and six months old and hung for around 10–14 days. The result is a deep-pink meat, best thought of as beef-veal, which offers a very different eating experience from intensively raised veal. Because the animal has spent its life running around it has a much firmer texture, and can have a far more 'beefy' flavour.

Not surprisingly, veal is also the most expensive organic meat you can buy, and you can expect to pay up to 50 per cent more than for crate veal. It is currently available from three main sources: Eastbrook Farm Organic Meats, who are the major producer, Swaddles Green Farm, and Meat Matters who sell Eastbrook Farm veal. For telephone numbers, see pp. 96, 105–6. Individual producers, such as Domini Quality Foods (p. 152), may have the occasional veal calf from time to time. Loin and escalopes are extremely expensive. Pot roasts are more manageable; minced veal is usually good value, and makes excellent hamburgers, and ragù for pasta and risotto.

Lamb

Because sheep are still largely raised extensively, there is far less difference between the way conventional and organic lambs are produced than with other meats. Nor can it be said that the flavour differences are marked; here it depends more on whether the sheep are upland (more flavour) or lowland (milder flavour), and which breed they are.

However, keeping sheep more intensively inside, on pelleted feed, is becoming more common, particularly for raising lambs.

Also commonplace is sheep-dipping with OP pesticides, as well as the use of antibiotics, both routinely and as growth-promoting agents. By contrast, organic lamb is more expensive to raise, in terms of both feed and labour, and the lambs grow more slowly.

- Lowland organic sheep graze on organic pastures that receive no artificial fertilisers. They do not stay on the same pasture, but are rotated to ensure no build-up of parasites or disease. Stocking densities for organic sheep are lower, permanent indoor rearing is banned, and travel time to slaughter, as for all organic livestock, is limited to eight hours.
- Worming with Ivermectin and similar compounds is forbidden. Sheep-dipping with OP pesticides is forbidden.

Mutton

Produced in small quantities, mainly by Graig Farm. It comes from lambs raised organically that are over two years old, and is good value. Mutton at this age is not tough. It has a richer flavour, is less fatty and therefore a drier meat. You can cook it in exactly the same way as lamb, and you will find that it roasts just as well – roast at a moderate temperature until slightly pink. It responds to gentle cooking and is excellent for braised and spiced dishes.

Pork

If you have never bought organic meat, and have forgotten what pork should taste like, then try organic pork.

- Unlike conventional pork, most organic pork is raised by small producers; many use traditional breeds such as Gloucester Old Spot, Berkshire, Tamworth and British Saddleback, favoured for their flavour and ability to thrive when reared in natural ways.
- Organic pigs grow more slowly and are killed at an older age, typically four and a half to six months instead of 14 weeks.

- Organic pigs are fed a diet containing a minimum of 80 per cent organic feedstuffs, which includes 60 per cent fresh green food or unmilled forage.
- Growth-promoting additions such as zinc, copper and antibiotics, common in conventional feed, are banned.
- Outdoor organic pigs are not kept permanently on the same land but are moved around, as part of the general organic land management to prevent build-up of disease and to ensure soil fertility.
- The use of concrete slatted floors is forbidden. Pigs raised inside must be bedded on straw in warm, well ventilated sheds, given ample room and access to the outside, and toys to play with.
- Tail-docking, routine teeth-clipping and nose-ringing are banned.
- Organic pigs are kept in small groups, a maximum of thirty animals for fattening and ten breeding animals per group.
- Farrowing crates are forbidden. Piglets are weaned for six–nine weeks instead of two–three weeks, until their digestive systems are sufficiently well developed. Sows have only 2 litters a year instead of an average of 2.5.

The result of all this is pork with real flavour, that has a good texture, that is neither pappy nor wet, that has a creamy rather than a pasty white fat, and which smells wonderful while it is cooking.

Wild Boar pork Also known as wild blue pork, this is a cross between wild boar and Gloucester Old Spot or Tamworth pig. It has a richer, slightly more gamey flavour than usual, and is very lean with a closer-grained texture. An excellent meat, well worth a try; the animals are much smaller and slower growing, which means smaller joints, and are killed at around six months or older. It is available from Cusgarne Organics, Cusgarne, near Truro tel: 01872 865922. Prices are similar to pork and good value. Mail order on request.

Pork sausages Most producers make their own pork sausages, using only organic minced pork, organic rusk or organic ground rice, and organic flavouring ingredients and natural casings. Unlike most other sausages, they contain no artificial flavourings or additives, no preservatives, polyphosphates, nitrates, nitrites, soya proteins, carcass scraps or mechanically recovered meat (MRM), fillers, or added water. Though I have had one or two that I have not enjoyed because they were too fatty, most are delicious, moist, succulent and meaty.

Organic pork sausages have a short shelf life and should be eaten as soon as possible, within three or four days, or frozen. Because they are meaty they go further, and two per person is usually enough. They are superb on the barbecue, especially with aïoli (garlic mayonnaise). Finally, don't forget that sausage meat – remove the skins from sausages if you have none – is excellent for pâtés and rissoles, and for stuffing vegetables.

Bacon, Gammon and Ham Produced from organic pork and cured in traditional ways, using salt or brine; or, in the case of a special cure, using salt, organic sugar and herbs or spices. Artificial preservatives such as nitrates and nitrites that keep bacon and ham pink are banned, as are polyphosphates to increase water content. The result is a full-flavoured bacon that does not ooze water or tell-tale whitish scum when cooked, and ham that is moist and meaty. They are available from most major organic meat producers who operate a mail order service. Note that organic bacon and ham do not stay pink, once cooked.

fact

Chickens and pigs are cannibalistic when reared under stress in crowded conditions. Pigs are also highly intelligent animals and readily suffer stress, to the extent that mutilations – tail-docking, teeth-clipping and nose-ringing – are necessary in intensive conditions.

Poultry

Chicken

Ironically, the nation's most popular meat is the most expensive to produce organically, in terms of labour, welfare and feed costs. Apart from those of a few independent producers, organic chickens are the only ones that are properly free-range and reared naturally. Organic standards are not always superior to or different from the exacting standards by which other high-quality free-range chickens are raised: the major difference lies not necessarily in 'quality', but in the fact that organic producers subscribe to organic farming systems which are environmentally sustainable in a wider context. Also, as you would expect, their chickens enjoy a mainly organic diet. Inevitably, it comes down to size. A small producer raising a few chickens is obviously in a different situation from that of the producer trying to satisfy public demand by producing large quantities.

That said, the major differences between organic chickens and the vast majority of others are:

- Because they are reared more naturally and growth-promoters are banned, organic chickens grow more slowly, and are not killed until they are usually twice as old as conventional chickens, from 9–12 weeks or older, instead of only 6–7.
- Flock sizes are small, the birds are given at least three times as much space as their conventional counterparts, as well as regular fresh bedding; older birds have constant access to free-range organic pastures, and are fed a diet containing a minimum of 80 per cent organic grain. Organic birds eat more, approximately doubling the food costs. Non-organic feedstuffs are strictly controlled. Under Soil Association regulations, this includes no animal by-products such as feather meal, poultry offal meal, blood and bonemeal and animal fat, which are permitted in conventional animal feedstuffs.
- Mutilation – decombing and debeaking – is forbidden under Soil Association standards.
- Prophylactic in-feed medication is forbidden; coccidiostats are permitted, to control coccidiosis in

chicks, if necessary (p. 175), though I have not found any producer who uses them.

● Most organic chickens are killed on the farm, and in small numbers. Evisceration is done by hand when the chicken is cold, not by machine when the chickens are still warm.
● They do not have up to 5 per cent water injected into them.

NOTE: As with free-range eggs, remember that the term 'free-range chicken' means very little. Unless the label specifically says otherwise, apart from access to the outside and slightly more space, a standard free-range chicken does not enjoy any other extra welfare, feed or rearing benefits.

All this makes for chicken that has real flavour, and a moist, succulent texture; it is satisfying to eat, is just as good hot as cold, and is sensational on the barbecue. You will also find that you want to cook organic chicken on its own or in very simple ways, saving you time and extra ingredients.

Remember:

● Organic chickens are not standard, and vary in size, depending on their age. Large birds generally have a slightly firmer texture and meatier flavour.
● The most economical way to buy organic chicken is to buy a whole one and joint it yourself; don't forget to make chicken stock with the bones.
● All mail order producers sell whole chickens and chicken joints; some supply carcasses very cheaply for stock.

fact

The industrial production of fishmeal, used extensively in conventional poultry and pork feeds, from small fish and sand eels hoovered out of the oceans, causes significant ecological damage and depletion of fish stocks.

● Prices vary from supplier to supplier and from shop to shop.

NOTE: Some producers hang their chickens for a few days, to develop the flavour further; I find these easily the tastiest of all, though if you are unused to them you may not like the smell and you may find they have a slightly more gamey taste.

WATCHWORD: Some mail order organic producers, such as Graig Farm, also produce a non-organic additive-free chicken. These have been reared in exactly the same way as organic chickens, and graze the same pastures, but have not received organically grown grain. They represent very good value. They are labelled 'additive-free'.

Some suppliers of organic chickens are:

Brillbury Hall Farm Food Company, Brill, Bucks. tel: 01844 238407 OF&G registered. An organic farm supplying their own beef, pork, lamb and traditional Light Sussex poultry, including cockerels; available at the farm shop or through their home delivery service. Their cockerels have recently won the 1997 Organic Food Award for poultry and are to be commended. They have a real farmyard flavour and texture and have been highly praised. Do not expect a plump-breasted bird, though. Cockerels are smaller and leaner than chickens and have a darker skin.

P.J. Onions, near Newark, Notts. Organic Farmers & Growers registered. The largest specialist organic producer of award-winning chickens and turkeys, with many years of experience, and a long-standing member of OF&G. His chickens are all killed on the farm, hand-eviscerated and hung for three days. They are sold at Planet Organic and Lidgate butchers in London, Out of This World, alternative supermarkets and selected Sainsbury's stores; they are also widely available through other mail order and meat companies such as Eastbrook Farm Organic Meats (p. 105) and Meat Matters (p. 96). Their large chickens made an excellent festive bird.

Rushground, Campsea Ash, Suffolk tel: 01728 746928 A small specialist chicken producer, registered with the Soil Association, producing a few birds per week. The chickens lead an idyllic life free-ranging on organic pastures and fed organic grain including lucerne, which gives the skin a yellow tinge. No coccidiostats or other drugs are used. Colony sizes are very small – no more than a hundred. They live in movable houses, with fresh bedding every day, and are moved every two weeks on to fresh ground. The birds are not killed until 10–12 weeks or older, are hung for three days, are large (2.5–5kg), and have an excellent flavour. Sold through Planet Organic in London, or from the farm direct as whole birds or portions. Highly recommended.

Springfield Organic Poultry, near Leominster, Herefordshire Another specialist poultry producer, registered with the Soil Association, whose label you may see on organic chickens. Flock sizes are no more than five hundred, the chickens receive organic feed and no antibiotics or other drugs, and are hung for from one to seven days, depending on customer requirements. Sold via wholesalers and independent butchers, and available widely in the south but also elsewhere.

Welsh Haven Poultry, Whitegates Farm, Little Haven, Pembrokeshire tel: 01437 7815521 OF&G registered. Situated in an enviable position, in the Pembrokeshire National Park. An experienced specialist poultry producer who has recently converted to the organic system, supplying chickens, ducks and geese. They are also one of the leading producers of ostrich, which also range on organic pastures. The chickens live in movable houses, are raised in small flocks of two hundred, range on grass and receive no coccidiostats or other antibiotics. They are killed and prepared on the farm at 10 weeks old and hung for 3–7 days. Large Christmas ducks and geese are a speciality – these are fed organic corn, are dry-plucked and wax-finished and hung for seven days. Available as whole birds or as portions through Black Mountain Foods (p. 203), at their own farm shop, or direct by mail order. They also operate gastronomic weekends featuring local foods, and short breaks.

Also Graig Farm, Longwood Farm and Swaddles Green Farm produce their own organic chickens, available widely or through mail order; mail order meat suppliers all stock chickens. For telephone numbers, see pp. 104–107.

what they say . . .

'Under modern intensive conditions, up to forty thousand birds may be crammed, two birds to a square foot, into a single, windowless building, with almost continuous low levels of artificial light. It is no wonder that they need to be debeaked, that stress levels are high and that continuous use of antibiotics is needed to keep them alive. Growth-promoting agents force the rate of growth such that very often their legs cannot support their bodies.

'The organic system is an extensive one. The primary aim is to produce healthy, content birds by minimising stress and by ensuring that they have a more natural life and a quality diet. In this way, the bird's own immune system can fight off disease, doing away with the constant need for drugs. Our poultry, for example, is reared from one day old on a specially formulated feed containing cereals, vegetable protein, and a vitamin/mineral supplement. They are given no routine drugs, growth-promoting agents, antioxidants or any other additives, including coccidiostats, which are given continuously to most other chickens.

'Our birds are kept in small groups to allow them to establish a social or 'pecking' order. By doing this we avoid feather-pecking – each bird knows its place in the hierarchy. In the barns, they have plenty of space to move around and older birds have constant daytime access to pasture. They are finally slaughtered on the farm at nine to twelve weeks, ensuring a quick end without any undue suffering.' – *Bob Kennard, Graig Farm*

Turkey

Turkeys are semi-wild birds and are naturally more aggressive than other poultry, especially when kept in confined conditions. Most are raised as intensively as chickens. Modern varieties are bred to have super-huge breasts, because this is what consumers prefer; unless they get regular exercise, they are so large that they have difficulty in walking. Traditional farm-fresh turkeys have much higher welfare standards. Organic turkeys, bronze- and white-feathered types, are raised to the same standards as organic chickens and cost more than other high-quality turkeys primarily because of the extra feed and labour costs involved. They enjoy natural daylight and ventilation and are kept in much smaller flocks – one tenth the size of intensively raised flocks. They may be killed at around four months, or, as in the case of P.J. Onions turkeys, when fully mature at twenty-two to twenty-three weeks. They are generally hung for seven to ten days, to acquire maximum flavour. Available from all meat mail order specialists.

> **NOTE:** Scientific studies at Bristol University have shown that hanging turkeys in this way is the safest way to produce a Christmas turkey: the gut becomes acidic and inhibits the growth of bacteria.

Geese
Organic geese are generally available at Christmas from mail order meat suppliers and a few independent organic farmers who raise a few to sell locally. They are raised outside on organic pastures, fed organic grain and receive no routine antibiotics. Also available from Cusgarne Organics (p. 194), Longwood Farm (p. 106) and Meat Matters (p. 96).

Ducks
Organic ducks are delicious. Available from Swaddles Green Farm (p. 106) and Welsh Haven Poultry (p. 199), whole or jointed. Eastbrook Farm Organic Meats and Graig Farm (pp. 104–105) supply excellent free-range additive-free ducks, fed a natural though not organic diet.

Quail
No one is producing organic quail. The next-best thing is additive-free quail, from Graig Farm (p. 104), produced on a local farm.

Offal

Eating organic offal when you can makes very good sense. Liver and kidneys are the excretory organs, which have to deal with toxins (most of the testing for antibiotic residues is done on offal). A cocktail of OC residues has been detected in the kidney fats of sheep, lambs and cattle, where residues are generally present at up to three times the levels in other tissues. OC residues have also been detected in pâté samples, for example, and antibiotic residues are found in a tiny proportion of liver and kidney samples every year. Eating organic offal minimises these.

Organic chicken, lamb and pork livers, and lamb, pork and ox kidneys, are readily available from mail order meat specialists (p. 104) and are usually excellent value. Organic calves' liver has a darker colour and a stronger flavour than conventionally reared Dutch, and commands the same premium.

Organic butchers

More and more butchers are beginning to sell organic meat. The following are registered with the Soil Association. Telephone first to check opening times and the choice of organic meat available.

Bell's Butchers, Leicester, Leics. tel: 01162 2896119
S.R. Cowell Butchers, Morpeth, Northumberland
　　tel: 01670 513447
Eastwood's of Berkhamsted, Berkhamsted, Herts.
　　tel: 01442 865012
Heard's, Wigston, Leics. tel: 01162 8804444
S. & A. Rossiter Traditional Family Butcher, Bournville,
　　Birmingham tel: 0121 458 1598
Michael F. Wood, Leicester, Leics. tel: 01662 705194
Wood's Butchers, Heanor, Derbyshire tel: 01773 531613

Q Guild butchers: The following butchers sell Highgrove Aberdeen Angus beef and Highgrove lamb and may sell other organic meat.

R.A. Byford & Sons, Rayleigh, Essex tel: 01268 742021
Eastwood's of Berkhamsted, Berkhamsted, Herts. tel: 01442 865012

D. & G. Hepburn Ltd, Mountnessing, Brentwood, Essex
  tel: 01277 353289
C. Lidgate Ltd, Holland Park Avenue, London W11
  tel: 0171 221 5878
M. Newitt & Sons, Thame, Oxon. tel: 01844 212103
Randell's, Wandsworth Bridge Road, Fulham, London SW6
  tel: 0171 736 3426
Wincheap Butchers, Canterbury, Kent tel: 01227 462938

Also Tetbury Traditional Meats, 31 Church Street, Tetbury, Glos.
tel: 01666 502892

Finally, two companies who specialise in buying and preparing
organic meat to sell to independent butchers and other outlets.

Pure Organic Foods Ltd, near Leiston, Suffolk tel: 01728 830575
A label you may see in many butchers, including Q Guild
butchers, selling prepacked fresh organic meat, and in some
London stores such as Selfridges, Fortnum & Mason, Partridges
and some Cullens stores. Based in Suffolk and Demeter-registered,
the company are wholesalers of organic meat, poultry, charcuterie,
dairy products, Dutch cheeses and Crone's apple juice. They have
their own organic processing and packing plant, where they
mature and prepare a wide range of meat cuts, including kebabs,
chicken tandoori and plain and speciality sausages. They source
meat from certified farms in the UK and Europe. Their charcuterie
range includes salamis, pâtés and smoked turkey, as well as hams
and bacon. Their pies, made by a Demeter-registered butcher in
the Midlands, include beef in beer and venison in wine. They also
supply Domini Quality Foods with untreated Jersey milk and
cream (p. 152). Telephone direct for details of how to buy this,
and where to find their other products.

Black Mountain Foods, Talyllychau, Dyfed tel: 01558 685018 An
Organic Farmers & Growers registered organic meat wholesalers,
who purchase meat from selected small producers which is then
aged and prepared by themselves and sold to around twenty independent high-quality butchers, primarily in London and along the
M4, and to home delivery companies. They also make sausages
and burgers. They produce a leaflet, available at the butchers they

supply, and supply by mail order on demand. To find your nearest stockist, telephone direct.

For pesticide and antibiotic residues in meat, see Appendix 1, pp. 344, 346.

Game

Apart from game reared on organic estates, there is no organic game to speak of – only wild or farmed game. Farmed venison is reared extensively, but this is not necessarily the case with farmed pheasants, which account for about half the pheasants we eat. Though the majority are reared and released birds, managed by gamekeepers, the Farm Animal Welfare Network (FAWN) reports on instances of game being kept in large numbers, where debeaking, routine medication, growth-promoters in feed and other practices associated with intensively reared chickens are found. Because wild game is 'natural', we also presume it to be 'pure'. Alas, this is not so. As the Game Conservancy Trust are aware, game are in the front line when it comes to environmental pollutants. The increased use of pesticides, for example, has been partly responsible for the severe decline in wild partridge numbers. Pesticide residues have been detected: for instance, DDT has been found in pigeons, which are migratory birds and can pick up pollutants between here and Scandinavia. Antibiotic residues in pheasant and partridge are also monitored.

Organic sources of game

There is currently no one raising farmed game to organic standards; indeed, there are no standards for organic game, so strictly speaking the term does not yet apply. The best alternative is to buy game from organic estates and farms when you can. The Old Dairy near Reading (p. 87) sell pheasants and rabbits from their own organic estate. Brillbury Hall Farm in Brill, Bucks. (p. 198) is another, and supplies wild rabbit. Graig Farm near Llandrindod Wells (p. 104) sells additive-free quail raised non-intensively in humane conditions by a local farmer, available by mail order.

Fish

Up to now, fish has had an admirable health profile – but for how much longer is anyone's guess. Pollution of rivers, of seas such as the North Sea and of oceans with toxic chemicals including pesticides is a major international concern. Britain is considered to be 'the dirty man of Europe' in this respect. Chemical pollutants are believed to be affecting the fertility of whales, porpoises and dolphins. Reports of deformed fish, as well as of pesticide residues in fish, are also increasing. Another dilemma is that modern techniques trawl fish in such vast numbers that stocks are being severely depleted; and once-common species, including cod, are becoming endangered, which threatens the sustainability of fish-farming worldwide. Currently no code of sustainability exists, though an international body, the Marine Stewardship Council, is addressing the issue and expected to form such a code.

Meanwhile, in the UK farmed fish are neither reared naturally nor fed a natural diet. The use of pesticides such as dichlorvos on salmon farms poses a significant problem for the aquatic environment, while the genetic engineering of salmon and carp is already a reality. In response to this, the Soil Association is grappling with the task of establishing organic standards for the fishing of wild and farmed fish – standards which will address the question of the purity of fishing grounds and of sustainable methods of catching fish that do not severely deplete stocks, as well as the issue of sustainable rearing and feeding practices for farmed fish that will not damage the environment and will address welfare needs. No one should underestimate the enormity of the task. What do you do about migratory fish, for example, and can any fish really be said to be organic? But something has to be done, and a growing body of consumers now want to be able to buy fish that has an organic seal of approval.

The German certifying body, Naturland, has drawn up standards for farmed salmon and other fresh-water fish, and they represent an excellent start. Meanwhile, though available in limited quantities and from very few outlets, organic farmed salmon and Glenarm Salmon from Ireland, St Helena fish and pure Blue Mountain fish from the USA, are the first positive examples of the provision of 'purer' fish and, as such, they point the way for the future.

Blue Mountain Fish A taste of the future. Imported from Oklahoma, these environmentally pure fish are raised in self-contained high-tech 'aquasystems' using pure oxygenated water, and fed natural feedstuff comprising corn, GM-free soya and minced fish. No chemicals or pollutants are used. Arctic char and Atlantic salmon (raised at sea in unpolluted waters), yellow perch, steelhead trout, tilapia and striped bass are also available. Each fish comes with its own Blue Mountain tag. Smoked Arctic char tastes like a mild and delicate smoked salmon. Available only from Planet Organic, London.

Clare Island Irish organic salmon Certified by Naturland in Germany, these salmon are reared off the west coast of Ireland, in Connemara, in conditions similar to Glenarm salmon; they are fed a natural diet, receive no routine medication and grow slowly. Sold primarily to Germany, France and Belgium, but expected to be on sale in the UK shortly. For more information tel: 00353 9533 501.

Glenarm High Seas-reared Salmon from Northern Ireland A unique source of farmed salmon, produced to the highest possible welfare and environmental standards. Everything is done with a view to mirroring the conditions of wild salmon. Fish are kept out in the open sea at very low stocking densities, and in single large nets rather than cages, where they can swim freely in strong currents and where salinities and temperatures do not fluctuate abruptly – a cause of stress in fish. They are fed by hand with high-quality feed, produced locally from whole fish rather than offal. No chemicals, antibiotics, artificial pigments or extra oil (which makes salmon grow faster) are used. The strong currents keep the sites clean, and ensure that parasites and pollutants do not accumulate. The result is a superbly flavoured, healthy fish with firm flesh and natural colour which eats like wild salmon. It is gener-

fact
An estimated 150,000 man-made chemicals are dumped in the oceans each year. This number is increasing by 2,000 per year.

ally available in London, at retailers including Planet Organic, Selfridges and Harvey Nichols as well as a few good fishmongers; smoked and fresh Glenarm salmon is available by mail order from Severn and Wye Smokery, Glos. tel: 01452 750777. A detailed leaflet on the production process is available on request from Glenarm tel: 01574 841691.

Also:
Alaska Salmon Canned Alaska salmon is produced from wild salmon. Brands include John West, Prince's and own-labels such as ASDA, Co-op, Safeway, Sainsbury's and Tesco.

Fish by mail order

If you have no local fishmonger or have to rely on supermarkets, and presuming you have a freezer and don't mind freezing fish, mail order solves the dilemma of sourcing local fish in quantity.

Two examples:

Cornish Fish Direct, Newlyn, Cornwall tel: 01736 332112 Set up by fish expert William Black to supply spanking-fresh seasonal fish direct from Cornish fish markets nationwide. The fish is sent in chilled polystyrene boxes and arrives the next day. There's a choice of either the standard 'inshore' or the 'gourmet' box, both containing 4kg of fish, costing around £29 and £45 respectively, plus £9 carriage; or a customised order service, including preparation, minimum order £30. Full storage details, preparation hints and recipe suggestions are included. Though not organic, the company are committed to sourcing fish from boats using sustainable fishing methods, and they actively encourage local handliners. All fish comes from inshore boats. They also supply Ryton Gardens Restaurant near Coventry.

The Market Fish Shop, Dartmouth, Devon tel: 01803 832782 Run by Jenny Rothery, who supplies local restaurants. Specialises in local caught fish including wild salmon, dived scallops, crabs, lobster and John Dory in season, and offers customised mail order service at shop prices. Fish is prepared as you want – gutted, filleted etc. – then vacuum-packed in chilled polystyrene boxes, to

Fish from St Helena

From the clear, unpolluted fishing grounds surrounding the tiny British island of St Helena in the South Atlantic, a unique source of pure fish, available by mail order, and now certified by the Soil Association. The fish are individually caught using hook and line by the local fishermen, landed within four hours and processed and frozen immediately on the island, then shipped to the UK via the island's main link with the outside world, the Royal Mail ship. The fish is caught using sustainable methods, in small quantities that do not upset the natural balance of fish stocks, and because it is processed on the island it supports the local economy.

The range comprises several varieties of tuna, plain or smoked, wahoo, plain or smoked, grouper, bull's-eye and smoked mackerel. All offer instant meals as they need no preparation and either require no cooking or take little time to cook. The tuna is excellent and comes as prime steaks that, being quite thin, need a minute each side on a hot griddle. Bull's-eye fillets, a delicate white fish with a texture like that of Dover Sole, are excellent steamed. The wahoo is similar to swordfish and the grouper can be used like cod. The smoked tuna won the 1997 Organic Food Awards for fish; thicker than smoked salmon and quite dry, try it cut into strips and used in salads, or with lime juice or organic crème fraîche. Prices are very reasonable. Imported exclusively by Graig Farm, and also available in Planet Organic, London. Detailed leaflet available tel: 01597 851655.

arrive next day. This is the shop I use; both fish and service are splendid. There is no minimum order, but remember carriage costs are around £10.

> **TIP:** Fish freezes much better if vacuum-packed. Ask if this is possible when buying fish that you intend to freeze.

Also Nationwide organic fresh produce delivery service, the Fresh Food Company tel: 0181 969 0351 supplies a fresh fish box from Cornwall. See p. 100.

For pesticide and antibiotic residues in fish, see Appendix 1, pp. 345, 347.

chapter seven

bread
and flour

Organic Bread

For most people, bread is the most important staple. Apart from health considerations, organic bread offers many other advantages. Most is made by small bakers dedicated to producing the best loaf they can using traditional bread-making methods, which include long fermentation to ripen the dough and develop the flavour. Organic bread does not contain the plethora of chemical improvers, dough-conditioners, additives and artificial flavourings that are standard in much bought bread. Sink your teeth into an organic loaf made by any of the bakers listed here and you will again discover bread with real flavour and texture, and twice as satisfying to eat.

These days most supermarkets and bakers stock an organic loaf of some kind. The range available includes everything from everyday white and wholewheat loaves to country bread made with natural leavens, Irish soda bread, hefty sourdough ryes, mixed seed breads, Italian breads, enriched breads and fruit breads, long-life breads, breads made from sprouted seeds and imported continental breads and crispbreads. You can even buy organic pizza bases and crostini. The image of the classic wholesome but dense organic loaf is also changing, as lighter breads, speciality breads and special-occasion breads come on stream. The other fast-growing sector is organic breads for special diets.

It is impossible to talk of bread without these days wondering what pesticide residues they might contain, especially as cereals are sprayed so regularly. Over twenty pesticides are monitored every year, and are generally found, in individual and multiple residues, in twice as many samples of wholewheat and grain breads as in white breads, about a quarter of which can be expected to contain residues, including OPs. Residues have also been found in organic bread samples (p. 4). Over the last decade residues have declined, and OC traces are now rarely found, which is encouraging. Not so encouraging is the fact that it has recently been discovered that post-harvest insecticides, including OPs, and fumigants such as methyl bromide, bind to cereals in store, including wheat, and can remain active when ingested. Such 'bound' residues are now causing international concern. The Food and Agriculture Organisation (FAO) of the UN has declared: 'It is common knowledge that such residues do exist, often in large quantities, and no one can attest to their safety or lack thereof.'

Organic bread facts:

- All organic breads contain 95 per cent or more certified organic ingredients. Savoury and fancy breads, and baked goods made with 70 per cent certified organic ingredients, must be labelled 'Made with organic . . .'. If ingredients are not certified, 'organic' cannot figure on the label.
- A small number of approved baking agents such as ascorbic acid, citric acid, calcium carbonate and raising agents are permitted. These must be clearly listed with their chemical name on the packaging. The vast majority of organic breads contain none of these, and none of the bakers listed below uses them in their own breads, except in soda bread.
- Organic breads carry a double guarantee. Both the bakery, and each individual organic bread, are certified by an approved certification body, usually the Soil Association.
- Many organic/wholefood/health food shops sell fresh organic bread; though a few make their own, it is usually made for them by an outside registered baker.
- Only unbleached white flour can be used in organic white bread.

WATCHWORD: Many shops and small bakers, and some supermarkets, sell bread made with organic flour. This may be excellent bread, but it is illegal to sell it as 'organic bread'; it has not been certified, and it may contain other, non-organic, ingredients and non-permitted chemical agents.

TIP: White (and brown) organic bread is a much better bread to cook with than standard, pappy breads. This is because it has real flavour, less air and a firmer structure which holds up more, absorbs oil and other liquids better, and does not go squishy or tacky. Use for bread-and-butter puddings and summer puddings, in stuffings and meat balls, and to make croûtes, croûtons, breadcrumbs and bruschettas.

Organic bakers

Bakeries producing organic bread must be registered. To qualify for organic status they must use only certified organic ingredients in their organic breads, except for a few permitted added agents, and must not use hydrogenated fats or refined white sugar; they must also keep detailed records providing a full audit trail from ingredients bought to the finished bread. Most such bakeries produce non-organic breads and other non-organic baked goods as well. All of their organic ingredients must be kept separate at all times – by using separate storage facilities, and by shutting down the bread-making process and cleaning down the units before baking organic breads. In addition to the premises having to be registered, so must every different organic bread and baked good. This is to avoid any confusion with other loaves, and to provide the consumer with an extra guarantee. There are over twenty-five independent bakeries registered with the Soil Association who bake organic breads. Some of the best-known brands and specialist organic bakers to look out for are listed below.

Primary organic bakers: Bake *only* organic breads and other organic goods, or are primarily organic bakers who use only

More Good Reasons to Eat Organic Bread

1 Non-organic wheat is one of the most intensively farmed crops, and receives repeated sprays throughout its growth; once in store, the wheat grains are subjected to insecticide sprays; once milled, chemicals may be added to the flour to improve its keeping quality; at the bakery, more chemicals are added to make the bread. A standard loaf has thus received constant exposure to chemicals throughout its life. For details of pesticide usage on conventional wheat, see p. 340.

2 Eighty per cent of British bread is industrial bread, made in bread plants producing over 6,000 loaves an hour using the high-tech, computer-controlled 'no-time' Chorleywood Bread Process. Invented in 1961, this process enables more water to be absorbed into the dough, and replaces traditional fermentation with high-speed mixers such that it takes three and a half hours from start to finish to produce a cooled, sliced loaf ready to eat. Almost all organic bread is made in small bakeries by craftsmen bakers using traditional methods.

3 Genetically modified yeasts and all other GM ingredients are prohibited in organic breads.

organic flour and other organic ingredients in their goods wherever possible:

The Authentic Bread Company, Newent, Glos. tel: 01531 890348 Winner of 1996 Soil Association food awards for their olive bread, this is a small baker using traditional methods and Shipton Mill flours (p. 230). They offer a range of twenty-three different organic breads, including French sticks, onion bread, malted-grain loaf, black olive and pumpkin seed and rye and wholemeal.

Available locally and nationwide through organic/wholefood shops and delicatessens; also through several box schemes via the Organic Marketing Company, Hereford.

The Brilliant Bread Company, Wigan, Lancs. tel: 01942 768803 A small organic baker producing breads with Shipton Mill flours (p. 230), using traditional methods. The range comprises white and wholemeal bread with or without sesame or sunflower seed toppings, baps, granary and rye loaves, and fresh white and wholemeal pizza bases. He supplies wholefood shops and delicatessens in Liverpool, Manchester and Warrington. His breads can now be enjoyed in sandwiches from the Organic Sandwich Company (p. 290).

The Celtic Baker, West Hendon, London NW9 tel: 0181 202 2586 Another small organic baker, fast gaining wide acclaim for his delicious and richly flavoured traditionally hand-made breads using flour, minimum yeast, salt, water and long fermentation. The range comprises twenty-seven different breads and rolls, including barley bread, natural sourdough ryes, olive and pumpkin and cheese and onion bread, wholemeal croissants and a dairy-free Irish soda bread without salt; they also produce organic cakes (p. 276). All breads are certified by the Soil Association or Demeter. Available widely in London and the south-east from wholefood/health food shops, delicatessens and Cullens, and from their own stall at Greenwich and Spitalfields markets; from the Organic Shop, Stow on the Wold; and from a few outlets around Cardiff, including Jenkins Grocers in Cowbridge.

The Engine Shed, 19 St Leonard's Place, Edinburgh tel: 0131 662 0040 A community workshop based on Rudolf Steiner principles that includes a small organic bakery and tofu processing unit, registered with the Organic Food Federation. Produce around a dozen different organic breads, using strictly traditional methods, including Demeter loaves, oat and herb breads, a five-grain bread spiced with star anise, fennel and coriander, and sourdoughs. No improvers or additives of any kind are used. They also make organic flapjacks, oatcakes and other baked goods using organic ingredients served in the Engine Café, a vegetarian café that uses only Demeter and organic vegetables and other organic ingredients. Breads also available for sale in their wholefood shop at 123

Bruntsfield Place and throughout Scotland through Sundrum Organics (p. 121) and Greencity Wholefoods (p. 99).

Paul's, *Melton Mowbray, Leics.* tel: 01664 60572 Small baker and tofu-producer. Makes an impressive range of traditionally baked fresh breads and other baked products using organic flour from local miller Nigel Moon, ionised water and sea salt. All their products are either 100 per cent organic or 100 per cent organic except for cooking oils. All breads are available salt-free, and sliced to order if required. The range includes excellent white and other yeasted breads, rolls, baguettes and tea-cakes; fancy breads, foccacia, olive and basil breads, and sourdough or yeast-free breads including barley bread and pain de campagne. They also bake three yeast- and gluten-free breads, including a chick-pea, rice and corn bread. Their breads are widely available in independent organic/wholefood/health food shops throughout greater London, Essex, Cambridgeshire, Lincolnshire, Leicestershire, Nottinghamshire and the West Midlands; Ryton Organic Gardens (p. 83), and through local home-delivery and box schemes.

Sunshine Organic Bakery, *Stroud, Glos.* tel: 01453 763923 A small family-run bakery registered by the Soil Association, using only traditional methods to produce bread and other baked goods for their shop, Sunshine Health Shop in Church Street. The range includes thirty different certified organic lines baked daily, including wheat, rye, oat, spelt, multi-grain, sprouted-wheat and soda breads, rolls and baguettes. The mainly organic lines – 75–90 per cent organic ingredients – include focaccia, Bara Brith and cheese bread; vegetarian savouries, cakes and biscuits. Selected breads available also in the Cheltenham Nutrition Centre in Bath Road and in Malmsbury Wholefoods in Winchcombe Street.

The Village Bakery, *Melmerby, Cumbria* tel: 01768 881515 The leading bakery for speciality organic breads, cakes and other baked goods, it has won countless awards as well as national recognition. See Star Performer, p. 218.

Other bakers producing organic breads, or other fresh organic breads generally available include:

Camphill Village Trust Communities, Larchfield, Middlesbrough and Botton Village, Botton, N. Yorks. Produce a range of excellent breads made with Demeter-registered organic flour. Available direct from the bakery and through local outlets.

Cranks, London A popular vegetarian restaurant chain selling four organic breads – wholemeal, honey and sunflower, wheat and rye, and malt and brown granary-style – certified by the Soil Association and made for them by a traditional bakery in London and another small baker in Devon. The bread is used in their restaurants and widely distributed in major supermarkets and organic/wholefood/health food shops and delicatessens in London and the south-east, and locally around Brixham, Devon.

Doves Farm, Hungerford, Berks. A well known organic millers (p. 229) who sell organic white and wholemeal loaves made for them by a traditional baker in London. Widely available in major supermarkets and shops throughout London and the south-east.

Duchy Originals, London Have introduced two organic brown breads certified by the Soil Association, and made for them by La Fornaia bakery, London. Widely available from independent stores and in selected branches of Waitrose and Sainsbury's.

St Fagans, Museum of Welsh Life, St Fagans, Cardiff Though not organic, has a reconstructed bakery producing fresh bread in the old-fashioned way using organic flour in a wood-fired oven. You can see the bread being made and buy it in the tiny bakery shop next door.

Hobb's House Bakery, Chipping Sodbury, Glos. A Soil Association registered baker, producing bread by traditional methods including organic white and wholewheat loaves and rolls, widely available in shops in Bath, Bristol and south Gloucestershire.

Neal's Yard Bakery, London WC2 Produce an organic wholewheat bread certified by the Soil Association plus a range of breads made with organic flour. All their breads are made with filtered water. Available from the bakery and from Portobello Wholefoods, 266 Portobello Road, London W10.

Finally, **Penrhos Court Organic Country House** *at Kington, Herefordshire* tel: 01544 230720 Their delicious home-made bread was made joint winner, along with Botton Village rye bread, at the 1997 Organic Food Awards. The hotel is registered with the Soil Association and runs vegetarian cookery courses.

Star Performer: The Village Bakery

The most successful organic baker in Britain, based in Melmerby, Cumbria, for twenty years, has a varied and mouthwatering selection of organic breads and other baked goods in which taste and integrity go hand in hand. All their goods are baked in a wood-fired oven, and the bakery and attached restaurant have won many awards. They have started their own box scheme, supplied by the Organic Marketing Company, Hereford, from their restaurant in Melmerby, and an outside organic catering service. Their contact number is 01768 881515. E-Mail Admin@village-bakery.com. Website www.village-bakery.com.

Their products are widely available throughout Britain in supermarkets, shops, coffee houses, tea rooms and even butchers, and via box schemes. They run bread-making courses and have a separate mail order brochure and booklet containing a full list of stockists, all available free of charge. All their goods are made with organic flour, and other organic ingredients wherever possible; are suitable for vegetarians; are coded 'suitable for vegans', 'no added salt', 'wheat-free' or 'yeast-free'; and are graded according to their organic status, be it certified, over 70 per cent, or not certified. They do not use hydrogenated fats or refined white sugar, and use less sugar than usual. The total number of lines exceeds seventy.

The bakery is registered with the Soil Association, and their organic range is certified by them. It comprises:

Breads Nineteen, including their now famous Campagne country bread and Rossisky and Borodinsky sourdough rye breads, sesame plait, caraway bread, hazelnut and fennel and Pane Toscano, and a new one, Cobbett bread.

Wrapped rolls and buns Ten, including spicy buns, scones, croissants and pain au chocolat, made with Green & Black's organic chocolate.

Trenchers Tomato and olive, wild mushroom and garlic.

Cutting cakes Hazelnut and apple, carrot cake with cream cheese.

Wrapped cakes Nine, including Borrowdale tea-bread, carrot cake, gingerbread, Cumberland Rum Nicky, three fruit-cakes and a new simnel cake.

Cake slices Date, Westmorland parkin, flapjack, Grasmere gingerbread, apricot and new brownies made with Green & Black's chocolate.

Biscuits Oatcakes, butter shortbread fingers, florentines, date and coconut slices, Grasmere gingerbread, flapjacks and crunchy cookies.

Christmas goods Christmas cakes, mince pies, Christmas pudding, plum pudding, mincemeat.

Chocolate cake Their latest organic cake, made with Green & Black's chocolate, organic almonds, eggs and sugar, topped with chocolate icing and toasted almonds; superb.

Also A range of organic jams and conserves: blackcurrant, damson, plum, raspberry, Seville orange and three-fruits marmalade, green tomato chutney.

Other Organic breads

A wide range of other types of organic breads, many of which have a longer shelf-life, are available. They include:

Kjaers Food for Life, London W1 tel: 0171 723 0091 A small company producing organic foods specifically to meet the needs of food-sensitive and food-intolerant diets, which involve an estimated five million of the UK population. The range includes breads, cakes and biscuits: namely, a yeast- and salt-free organic buttermilk soda bread; a wheat- and yeast-free light, moist, sprouted-rye loaf; a yummy wheat- and dairy-free, no-added-sugar pineapple fruit-cake; gluten- and dairy-free chocolate cake slices; wheat, dairy and egg-free flapjacks; gluten and egg-free chocolate-orange shortbread slice. All have detailed nutritional breakdowns, are made by the Village Bakery, and are available nationwide or direct via the Village Bakery mail order service (p. 218). In addition, Kjaers operate their own mail order service, including a catalogue for gluten-free hampers and food-sensitive recipe booklets.

Sunnyvale Breads The leading brand of long-life breads and breads made with sprouted seeds. With denser textures and earthy wholefood flavours, long-life breads are a different eating experience from fresh breads. Sprouted breads have a similar taste to malt loaves, but are chewier. The range includes six different yeast-free rye sourbreads and a mixed-grain gluten- and yeast-free loaf; plus seven varieties of sprouted-wheat breads including fruit and almond, stem ginger and date; and two traditional tea-breads, malt loaf and their Fruit-T-Loaf. Their breads are pasteurised, giving them a shelf life of eight months at room temperature. The company is registered with the Organic Farming Federation; all products carry their logo and have full information on the packaging. Available nationwide through wholefood/health food shops.

Whole Earth organic breads A fresh mixed-grain wholewheat bread made for them by Goswell's bakery and certified by the Soil Association; and Natural Balance bread, a long-life naturally leavened 800g loaf, sealed in an airtight bag flushed with nitrogen. Both have been formulated for optimum nutrition by the addition of sesame seeds, carrot, sea kelp, flax seeds and sunflower seeds to provide extra calcium, beta-carotenes, selenium, iodine and soluble fibre. Available nationwide through wholefood/health food shops.

Supermarkets' own-label organic bread tends to be lighter and more uniform. It contains permitted bread-improving agents such as ascorbic acid and may contain extra ingredients such as added wheat protein.

Bake-off breads A range of long-life breads, baguettes, rolls, croissants and Danish whirls produced by Biona. The breads, made with Demeter flour, require five minutes in a hot oven.

Pizza bases Wholemeal pizza bases produced by Whole Earth Foods, La Bio-Idea, Biona and Pronto Pizza. The Brilliant Bread Company produces fresh pizza bases for sale locally.

Pitta Long-life Golden Temple wholewheat pittas in packs. Evernat wholewheat pittas, sealed under nitrogen, come in boxes of eight, and taste as good as home-made. They are also made by Eghoyans Pitta Bakery Ltd, sold in packs of eight.

Continental seed breads Dark, dense, distinctive German-style vollkornbrot breads, including pumpernickel (Molen Aartje), long-life sourdough rye and linseed (Rapunzel), wholemeal rye and sunflower seed bread (Mestemacher).

Crisp breads The main brand is De Rit. Others include Finn Crisp, and amaranth crispbreads from Allos.

Crostini Sweetish-flavoured wheatgerm crisp rolls produced by Eu Vita.

Organic breadcrumbs Dried wholemeal breadcrumbs produced by Just Wholefoods.

Organic croûtons Wholemeal soup croûtons made by Biona.

Buying and storing: Except where it is baked on the premises, organic bread is usually wrapped and clearly labelled. Most keeps fresh for 3–4 days; rye loaves keep well for up to a week, as do naturally leavened breads.

- Organic breads are good to eat both fresh and a few days old, and do not go stale so much as grow old gracefully.
- The best way to store bread is to freeze it; divide large loaves into smaller portions and you can be sure of very fresh bread, every time.

- Don't keep bread in the fridge; this will make it dry out sooner.
- To refresh bread, place it in a hot oven for 7–10 minutes.

TIP: Never throw away organic bread. Use old bread to make breadcrumbs or baked croûtes. Breadcrumbs have many uses, such as strewn over gratins and baked vegetables, and in stuffings. Fried breadcrumbs are excellent with pasta or scattered over salads. Caramelised breadcrumbs – breadcrumbs and a little organic sugar, toasted under the grill – make a delicious topping for poached fruit and fruit fools.

Price guide: Organic breads are very good value. They are no more expensive than the equivalent conventional premium breads, and can be considerably cheaper than top-of-the-range 'gourmet' hand-baked breads. Glance along the supermarket shelves and compare prices, and you will find virtually no difference between the organic wholewheat loaf and the conventional equivalent. Organic white bread is more expensive than organic wholemeal bread, because only 70 per cent of the grain is converted into flour, as against 100 per cent for wholemeal – so as well as being more expensive to buy, supplies are more limited. Expect to pay 55–75p for most small loaves, 85p–£1.30 for most large loaves, and £1.10–£1.75 for most fancy breads. Supermarket own-label breads are cheaper – in fact, they are usually the cheapest organic breads you can buy. Doves Farm large wholewheat loaf at £1.05 is excellent value.

WATCHWORD: Do not compare the price of organic bread with the standard sliced and wrapped mass-produced loaf. This is often sold as a 'loss-leader' at below production cost in order to attract customers to the store.

Where to buy: Organic bread is widely available everywhere. When you can, buy it fresh from a local organic baker, or a shop that sells it freshly baked. Most major supermarkets stock at least one organic loaf. Sainsbury's stock Doves Farm, Cranks, Duchy Originals and three Village Bakery breads in selected stores; they also sell own-label Nature's Choice white and wholemeal organic bread, certified by the Soil Association. Safeway sells Doves Farm and Whole Earth bread in selected stores; Waitrose sell Doves Farm, Duchy Originals and Cranks honey and sunflower bread in selected stores, and four Village Bakery breads in all their stores. Tesco sell their own-label pre-sliced white and wholemeal organic bread, certified by the Soil Association, in selected stores. Alternative supermarkets have a good selection, and Planet Organic (London) has an excellent one. Organic/wholefood and most health food shops stock organic bread, as do many conventional shops and delicatessens; plus Selfridges, Harvey Nichols and Bluebird food halls in London.

Others Organic markets (London). Organic farm shops, box schemes and home deliveries often supply organic bread.

Mail order: The Village Bakery (p. 218) has an extensive mail order list for all its products. Organics Direct and Sundrum Organics supply fresh breads; Damhead Organically Grown Foods, Organic Health, and Longwood Farm supply sprouted-grain and long-life prepacked breads. For telephone numbers, see p. 98–106 and 121.

what they say . . .

'The organic bread and baked goods market is good news for consumers, because it means they now have the choice of a wide range of proper breads again, made by craftsmen bakers who are breathing life and character back on to the bread shelves.'
– *Claire Marriage, Doves Farm*

fact | Most commercial bread contains substances to lengthen shelf life, including enzymes, which may be genetically modified.

'By choosing organic bread, the consumer is joining the growing number of people who think that bread – the staff of life – should be made in a way which respects the integrity of the people who eat it and the earth from which it comes. And the best way to encourage people to eat organic bread – which we strive very hard to do – is to make the best bread possible.'
– Andrew Whitley, the Village Bakery

Organic Flour

Nothing illustrates the results of modern methods of farming as clearly as the production of conventional wheat and other cereal crops. Though yields may have increased and prices are low, intensively grown cereal crops are responsible for much of the soil erosion now threatening most of Britain, the decline in bird species and in native wild flowers, 17 per cent of which used to flourish in cornfields, and in all the associated insects and butterflies which contributed to what was once our traditional landscape. Cereal farming has significantly contributed to the nitrate pollution of waterways. Pesticide use is intensive, post-harvest chemical treatment of cereals in store is commonplace; and residues are detected every year in cereals, flour and baked goods such as biscuits.

The alternative is to choose organically grown wheat, flour and other cereals. Generally they have a depth of flavour and character absent from mass-produced cereals and flours. This is partly due to the fact that they are grown more slowly, and yields are not artificially increased with nitrogen fertilisers. Organic millers also mainly use traditional techniques, which grind wheat slowly to preserve maximum flavour and nutrition, and bleaching agents in organic white flour are prohibited. If you eat bran or bran-based products you should be aware that this is where any chemical residues in wheat and grains are highest.

There is an excellent range of organic flours to choose from. They are produced by registered organic commercial mills, who frequently employ traditional milling techniques and whose flours are available nationwide; and by small independent traditional millers, often open to the public, who mill flour on a small scale sold at the mill or locally. A few operate a mail order service, which works well, is economical and gives you the opportunity of buying freshly milled flour – a real treat if you bake bread – without having to lug it home. Most supermarkets these days stock organic flour; note that own-brand organic flours are usually milled using modern techniques.

How conventional wheat is grown

Conventional wheat is grown with maximum reliance on chemical inputs, which inevitably allow little regard for the environment or wildlife. The use of chemicals enables the wheat to be grown on the same land continuously, with minimum manpower (one man per 500–600 acres) and on a prairie scale. It could not be grown this way without heavy reliance on a wide range of pesticides, and large subsidies. Land used for the same crop continuously becomes impoverished, so it needs nitrogen fertilisers – these days targeted scientifically, so that the wheat plant produces the largest ears and the highest protein content possible. Research shows, though, that when nitrogen fertilisers are applied to poor soils the uptake of valuable minerals, including magnesium, can be poor or erratic. Nitrogen also makes plants grow lush and heavy, which means that they fall over in the wind and are not easy for combine harvesters to get to grips with. To combat this, growth-regulators are sprayed on to the crop to make the stems (the straw) grow shorter and stiffer. Modern breeding of wheat varieties also aims to produce semi-dwarf wheats and maximum protein content; such varieties match the needs of intensive systems, but do not necessarily have any other desirable qualities, such as a good flavour. Once in store, the wheat is treated with insecticides, including OPs. For more on pesticide usage on wheat, see p. 340.

Wheat flour

For general use, organic wheat flours perform exactly the same as non-organic flours. From a bread-making point of view, they fall into two broad groups, native organic flours and blended ones:

Native organic flours Milled exclusively from English wheat which, because of our climate, has a lower protein content than 'hard' organic wheats; they vary with the season, the variety of wheat used, and the part of the country in which the wheat has been grown. The flours are full of character, have a beautiful sweet flavour but make a less buoyant, less well risen loaf than blended flours. Protein content is typically 9–11 per cent. This is the flour commonly found in small independent mills.

Blended organic flours Milled usually from a blend of English wheats and imported Canadian, North American, East European or Australian organic wheats. They are physically harder than the native kind and have a higher protein content, so are termed 'hard' wheats. These flours make the well risen, lighter bread that everyone has become accustomed to, and are blended so as to be consistent and thus satisfy consumer demand and commercial baker alike. Protein content is typically 11–13 per cent. All commercial organic millers produce these flours, and they are the ones you will mainly see for sale in the shops and supermarkets.

> **WATCHWORD:** Do not confuse 'conservation-grade' flour with organic flour. Conservation-grade wheat is grown using fewer chemicals, but is not organic.

Will it bake the same?

The quality of organic flour, especially that from well-known commercial organic millers, is excellent, and generally you can expect the same results as with your normal brand. The major difference you may find is in bread baked from flours milled from native English wheats, which do not rise as well and produce a different kind of loaf. Such flours, however, make wonderful biscuits. If in doubt, seek advice from your supplier as to which flour is best for your purpose.

How organic wheat is grown

Organic wheat is grown using natural, sustainable methods which avoid the need for chemical sprays and other external inputs or heavy subsidies. The wheat is not grown continuously on the same land but as part of a crop rotation – usually as part of a mixed farm – which helps to sustain natural fertility. More labour is involved, and the wheat is grown on a smaller scale. Instead of timed artificial fixes of nitrogen fertiliser, the wheat takes up, at a steady, natural rate, the nitrogen that has been naturally fixed into the soil by the previous crop of legumes. Growth-regulators are not applied; indeed, long straw is an advantage as it shades the weeds and provides protection for wildlife. In addition, the burning of straw and stubble is forbidden, more space is left at field margins to encourage wildlife, and cultivation techniques are timed to create as little disturbance as possible to ground-nesting birds. Traditional wheat varieties like Maris Widgeon, renowned for its flavour, give lower yields but are naturally tall-growing, so keep out weeds. Genetically engineered seeds are forbidden. Insecticides in grain stores are banned. Instead, stores are thoroughly cleaned and natural pest control methods used.

> NOTE: Organic cereal crops cannot always be protected from spray drift and occasional residues have been detected by the WPPR in organic flour. If residues are found, the organic authorities are notified and further investigations are carried out to check that no fraud has taken place.

Other flours

Organic barley, rye, buckwheat, millet, maize, potato, spelt, brown rice, corn, soya flours and oatmeal are all available, and are grown to the same organic standards as wheat. Many are gluten-free. Many, too, have a delicious nutty depth to their flavour; organic oatmeal, for example, is a revelation compared to the

> **fact**
>
> Farmers spend around £50 per acre each on chemical sprays and fertilisers. In 1996 they received £108 per acre in subsidies under the Arable Aid Scheme. Meanwhile, the annual bill for cleaning up pesticides from drinking-water is estimated at £121 million. Source *Killing of the Countryside*.

ordinary packet stuff. You cannot buy these flours in conventional supermarkets. The best place to find them is in wholefood shops and shops specialising in organic food. Infinity Foods, the major brand, has the best selection. Others include Kitchen Garden (soya flour) and Essential (brown rice, maize flour). The Stamp Collection have recently introduced an organic wheat-free flour made from a blend of organic barley, rice, millet and maize.

Also Joannusmolen and Shipton Mill make a gluten-free baking mix.

Buying and storing: Organic flour has the same shelf life as non-organic. Organic wheat and rye flours are often available in small bags, loose, or in bulk bags; if you bake bread, bulk buying is much more economical. If buying loose, buy from a shop with a good turnover and check the date stamp on the bag. This is most important; ideally, aim for a date stamp which has six months to go for white and three months for wholemeal. If you use a lot of flour, buy from the miller direct. Always store flour in a cool, preferably dark, place and in paper bags or sacks. The same applies to all cereals.

- Remember that any flour which contains the germ of the grain – and so this applies to grains too – is perishable, and that though starch is stable, the oils in the grains deteriorate fairly quickly.
- White organic flour stores better than wholemeal, and can be kept for 6–8 months, from the time it was milled.
- All wholemeal and wheatmeal flours should be used within three months, because their flavour and nutritional quality deteriorate.
- Speciality flours keep for 3–6 months, depending on the kind of flour and whether it was milled from whole grain.

Price guide: Given that most people use comparatively little flour, buying organic flour instead of conventional is an easy switch. If you make bread, it is especially good value. Remember, flour is sold in 500g, 1kg and 1.5kg bags, and bear this in mind when comparing the prices of brands. Standard organic whole-wheat flour bought in supermarkets will cost you the same as, or a few pence more than, equivalent non-organic flours. Otherwise, expect to pay 10–20 per cent extra, usually 10–20p or so per 1.5kg bag, which costs around 90p–£1.20; speciality blends and flours cost more. Loose flour is cheaper than ready-bagged flour. Flour bought by mail order direct from the miller is the best value; bulk orders can be 30 per cent cheaper. Note that prices also vary slightly depending on the retail outlet, and on whether the flour has been bagged by the wholesaler or bought direct from the miller.

> **PRICEWISE:** Do not compare the price of organic flour, especially white flour, with cheap mass-produced flour. This is another product that is often sold as a loss-leader and that bears no relation to its actual cost.

Where to buy: Just about most places, including supermarkets, many conventional food shops, and farm shops. Doves Farm organic flour is available from selected branches of Booths in the north, Safeway, Sainsbury's, and Tesco. Allinson's organic whole-wheat flour is available from Tesco. Tesco and Waitrose do own-brand organic flours.

Mail order: See the entries above. Most shops offering mail order supply flour, including Damhead Organically Grown Foods, Longwood Farm and Organic Health. For telephone numbers, see pp. 98–107.

Others Some box schemes and home delivery services.

Organic Millers: Star Performers

Doves Farm, Hungerford, Berks. tel: 01488 684880 Soil Association registered. They produce a large range of stoneground flours and baked products, widely available nationwide, including supermarkets. Their organic flours include home-grown organic grain, and are specially blended to give optimum baking qualities. The range comprises seven different stoneground wholemeal fours, five different white flours, organic wheat grain and bran, and organic stoneground spelt flour, which has an intense wheaty flavour, contains more protein, fat and fibre and can be tolerated by some with gluten allergies. Spelt is an ancient variety of wheat and spelt flour can be used for bread and cakes. Food writer Annie Bell is a fan, and recommends it for cheese scones and pizza bases. Doves Farm also produce a range of non-organic gluten-free and other speciality flours. All are available through mail order; recipe leaflets provided, and there are recipes on the packaging also. Other products include Doves Farm organic bread, biscuits and cornflakes.

Shipton Mill, Tetbury, Glos. tel: 01666 505050 Soil Association registered. Established in 1981, Shipton Mill produce a wide range of traditionally stoneground flours in a restored eleventh-century mill, and are the leading speciality bread flour millers. Their flours, specially blended from home-grown and imported wheats to give optimum baking quality, are used by many master bakers. They have recently introduced a gluten-free baking mix and a range of children's baking mixes to encourage children to bake. They operate a mail order service, Flour Direct, featuring over twenty speciality flours, including their organic range comprising white and wholewheat flours, oatmeal, and light and dark rye flours, available in 1kg, 1.5kg and 2kg bags. Carriage included, minimum order 5kg. Full descriptive leaflets are included, and personal advice on bread-baking given. Contact Sue Perrett or, for bread-baking queries, Clive Mellum. Their organic wheat flours are widely available nationwide in organic/wholefood/health food shops and in independent delicatessens and fine food shops.

Five millers producing flour from native-grown organic wheats available nationwide are:

Maud Foster Mill, Boston, Lincs. tel: 01205 352 188 Soil Association registered. Run by James Waterfield, chairman of the Traditional Cornmillers' Guild, and his parents, it is one of only four commercial windmills in the country. All their flours are organic, milled from local grain. They produce a range of flours including wholemeal, white and rye; plus maize meal, pancake and chapati flours; and organic muesli, available at Bluebird, London, and in their own delightful vegetarian tea room.

Little Salkeld Watermill, Penrith, Cumbria tel: 01768 881523 Soil Association registered. One of a few traditional working water-powered mills which specialise also in mail order; in addition, they produce a newsletter and run baking courses. They mill only British organically grown grain, of either Soil Association or Demeter standard, and produce a wide range of specialist stone-ground organic flours including white and wholemeals, Four-grain Blend, Granarius malted flour, semolina, oatmeal, porridge oats, barley flour, wheat and rye grain for sprouting, and muesli. Flour is freshly milled to order. The mail order catalogue also includes organic dried fruits, pasta, pulses, nuts and seeds, chocolate, sugar, herbs, spices, tea, coffee – all available from their mill shop and tea room.

Perry Court Farm, Chartham, Canterbury tel: 01227 738449 A Rudolf Steiner bio-dynamic farm which produces its own Demeter-standard stoneground wheat flour and bread, which can be bought at the farm shop on Fridays. The farm also produces its own beef, for sale in the shop at Wincheap Butchers in Canterbury, and runs a subscription vegetable box scheme.

Pimhill Mill, Lea Hall, Harmer Hill, Shrewsbury, Shropshire tel: 01939 290342 Soil Association registered. A pioneering organic family who have been milling their own home-grown grain exclusively for nearly fifty years. The stoneground 'soft' flour, which produces a bread renowned for its flavour, is freshly milled to order. Their full range (including Pimhill organic bread) is for sale at the mill shop and is distributed nationwide. It comprises organic wholewheat and fine brown (85 per cent extraction) flour; organic bran; organic wheat grain; organic groats, oatmeal, porridge oats and jumbo oats. They also produce Pimhill muesli,

> **fact**
>
> In nitrogen-sensitive areas (NSAs), where nitrogen pollution is worst, farmers are paid to use fewer fertilisers – up to £240 per acre for those who switch from arable cropping to ungrazed grassland. Outside special areas, farmers are free to use as much artificial fertiliser as they want. Source *Killing of the Countryside*.

which is not certified organic but is made with organic grains and no added sugar, and a range of organic cakes. All Pimhill products can be added to basic bread recipes to create different loaves, and can also be used in biscuits, tea-breads and cakes.

Rushall Mill, Rushall, Pewsey, Wilts. tel: 01980 630335 Soil Association registered. Produce stoneground wholewheat flour from their own home-grown organic wheat, available from the farm shop and by mail order. They also bake a wide range of breads, tea-breads, scones, pizza bases and garlic croûtons using their organic flour, for sale at the farm shop, which stocks their own meat and local produce.

fact
In 1996, five arable farmers each received £1 million in subsidies, the same as the total amount of subsidies received by organic farmers as a whole.

chapter eight

organic
baby food

Babies and toddlers are especially vulnerable to chemical toxins, including pesticides, and it is probably more important that they, rather than any other single group, should be given an organic diet. Compared to their body weight, they consume far more food than older children or adults, which means that they could easily be ingesting up to five times more residues than an adult. Most importantly, they eat far more of fewer foods. A baby's diet mainly comprises fruit juices, fruit and vegetables, and milk – precisely those foods where residues are detected most, at a time when he or she is least able to deal with them.

Given all of this, it is not surprising that the market for organic baby food in Britain and throughout Europe is booming, such that now in the UK one in every twenty jars of baby food sold is organic – and in some supermarkets the figure is higher. First introduced into Britain in 1992, it now has a market share of around 5 per cent, and that share is growing at ten times the rate of the overall baby food sector, with sales increasing at a rate of well over 50 per cent a year. There are several brands to choose from, and more in the pipeline. All sell at approximately the same price, with a few pence difference at most on individual items. They include meat and vegetarian meals, both dry and wet; drinks; desserts; cereals and pasta meals; plus yoghurt and formula milks. Baby pasta shapes – alphabets, stars, animals and ducks – are tops with babies!

Organic baby food offers mothers everything they could hope for: in particular, convenience, and the peace of mind that they are giving their babies the best nutritional start in life. It also offers the purest food available – free, for example, of the nineteen or so processing aids and emulsifiers, ingredients such as hydrogenated vegetable fat, demineralised whey, thickeners, added starches and sugars and approved flavourings that are included in most conventional brands of baby food, especially the cheaper ones, and which have no health benefits, dilute the nutritional value and affect the flavour. It's perhaps worth stressing, however, that the best and most economical way to feed your baby organic food is to make your own, using branded foods as a supplement. Baby books and the Baby Organix brand provide many simple recipes.

Finally, babies and toddlers drink far more water for their weight than any other age group. Because drinking-water these days contains so many chemicals, including pesticide residues, it's wise to give them still mineral water (one that is not highly mineralised) wherever possible or to use filtered water.

- Organic baby food contains 95–100 per cent certified organic ingredients and is produced with minimum processing.
- Most stockists sell a selected range of given brands; ask for a list of their full range, or contact manufacturers for the nearest stockist.
- Packet and jar sizes vary from brand to brand; bear this in mind when making price comparisons.

Major brands of organic baby food are:

Baby Organix The leading brand, produced by a small award-winning UK organic baby food company, the first to launch organic baby food in the UK; certified by the Soil Association, and with more than a 60 per cent share of the organic baby food market. Widely available at supermarkets including Waitrose, Sainsbury's, Safeway and some Boots stores. See Star Performer, p. 237.

Range Over forty products, including vegetarian baby meals enriched with iron and vitamin B12. The first company producing dried pasta (the dinky shapes mentioned above), pasta sauces and whole-milk organic yoghurts – natural, apple and blueberry, banana, and strawberry, all sold in four-pot packs. They produce Christmas dinner and Christmas pudding each December. Their latest addition is a range of ten high-quality sweet and savoury infant cereal mixes, free from maltodextrin and sugar, and are currently the only range to declare ingredient percentages.

Popular lines Garden vegetables, apple and blueberry, pasta vegetarian, pear (reckoned to be the best), apple and oats babymeal jars, banana (a particular favourite) and strawberry porridge, pasta stars and pasta alphabets.

> **NOTE:** Since babies need maximum nutrition, they should always be fed whole-milk, not low-fat, yoghurts; and their yoghurts, like those of Baby Organix, should be as pure as possible, containing no unnecessary flavourings, additives or other ingredients.

Boots Introduced organic baby food in 1994 under their Mother's Recipe range, which is made in Germany for them and certified by the Soil Association. The majority of stores sell selected lines; larger stores (two hundred of them) have a more extensive selection.

Range Over twenty-five products, including baby pasta and fruit and muesli breakfast.

Popular lines Baby rice, wholemeal breakfast; spring carrot and potato, creamy vegetables and noodles; spaghetti bolognaise and apple and peach dessert.

Cow & Gate Introduced their 'Organic Choice' wet baby foods in 1996. They currently offer four choices, namely apple and banana (the most popular), banana and apricot, carrot and apple, and spring vegetable medley, though more are planned; all have added vitamin C. Produced by Cow & Gate in Germany, each jar carries the German organic registration number. Available nationwide at Safeway, Sainsbury's, Tesco, Morrison's, Superdrug, Mothercare and most major pharmacists and retailers.

Hipp A well known award-winning German company that has been making organic baby food since the 1960s. Introduced into the UK in 1994, Hipp is the fastest-growing brand, with 25 per cent of the market. Strict controls and the highest standards ensure purity of ingredients, sourced primarily from their own growers. Certified by the Soil Association.

Range Over thirty products, including organic toddler

meals. The only company producing juices – apple, grape and raspberry, and apple and carrot – and a chocolate dessert (containing organic sugar). Their latest addition is follow-on formula milk.

Popular lines Mixed vegetables, vegetables with rice and chicken, creamed vegetables with wholemeal pasta, banana and peach, and apple and blueberry dessert. Available nationwide from larger branches of Boots, Co-op, Leo and Pioneer stores, Safeway, Sainsbury's, Tesco and good health food shops. Follow-on formula is available in Waitrose.

> NOTE: Though organic formula milks are made to very high standards, infant formulas, whether organic or not, are not generally recommended by nutritionists – except for mothers who are unable to breast-feed – as they lack vital elements that breast milk has, such as antibodies, digestive enzymes and the long-chain fatty acids necessary for brain development. For more information, consult *The ABC of Healthy Eating for Babies and Toddlers*, by Janette Marshall, published by Hodder & Stoughton.

Also

Babynat French infant milk formula, 0–4 months; follow-on milk formula, 4–12 months.

Bio-Korn Bis kids, rusk-type biscuits for infants (6 months).

Eco-Baby Muesli with apple and nuts, apple rice. Their products are wheat-free.

Holle Baby cereals, rusks.

Johanus Demeter-registered vegetable purées, fruit and cereal jars.

L'Origine Demeter-registered baby pasta; 4 cereals, wheat- and gluten-free light pasta; complete pasta.

Price guide: Organic baby food costs approximately 20–30 per cent more than standard commercial brands, but generally no more than 5–7.5 per cent more than premium brands. In practice this works out to around 4–10p extra per jar. When used to supplement home-made baby food made with fresh organic ingredients, it is not an expensive addition. Expect to pay 55–99p per jar, depending on the size, and £1.75–£2 per 150g packet. Look out for offers in mother and baby magazines and women's publications, special promotions, offers of the 'two for the price of one' kind, and coupon offers.

Where to buy: Organic baby food is widely available nationwide through major supermarkets and multiples, independent retailers, Boots, wholefood/health food shops and shops selling organic food. Supermarkets are usually a good place to buy, and often have a choice of brands. Large pharmacists and shops specialising in organic food usually have the most complete range.

Others Farm shops sometimes stock organic baby foods.

Mail order: Baby Organix offers mail order on selected products (below). Mail order specialists usually offer at least one brand of baby food; Damhead Organically Grown Foods (p. 98) have the best selection and offer Hipp, Eco-Baby, Baby Organix, Holle and Johanus. Shops offering mail order also usually offer baby food.

Star Performer: Baby Organix

Founded by Lizzie Vann and Jane Dick who, concerned about the quality of commercial brands, started producing organic baby food in their own kitchens and thus single-handedly created the market for organic baby food in the UK today. Committed to organic farming, they work alongside organic farmers and have all their produce grown for them. The food is produced to the highest quality and nutritional standards, and regularly tested for absence of residues. Their dry products contain no fillers, milk powder or added sugar. Their wet meals contain no unnecessary water, are not thickened with starchy fillers or gelling agents, and contain no emulsifiers or flavourings. Their excellent free information service 0800 393511 provides advice by health experts, offers detailed literature on feeding and weaning, and recipe cards. They operate a mail order service for dry products and publish a regular newsletter containing money-off vouchers.

what they say . . .

'Our recipes are based on getting babies into good feeding habits. We produce food with fresh vivid tastes and only use simple recipes. To ensure the best taste, highest nutrition and minimum processing times, we make smaller volumes than large baby-food companies, cooked as soon as possible after harvesting. Parents are closely involved in every aspect, and recipes approved by a panel of fifty babies before going into production. We encourage parents to make as much of their own food as possible, and share our recipes.' – *Lizzie Vann, Baby Organix*

Why Feed Your Baby Organic Food?

The growing infant is extremely vulnerable to any foreign substances – known collectively as xenobiotics – that is, substances not natural to the human body. Babies and toddlers are many times more sensitive to pesticides than are adults, and are more exposed to pesticides from food and water than are adults. This is why it is important to protect them, and to give them an organic diet wherever possible.

Research shows that:

- Infants develop quickly, needing relatively large quantities of food at a time when their eliminative organs – blood, kidneys and liver – are not fully able to excrete complex chemicals such as pesticides. Their body cells divide much more rapidly than adults', and have a different ratio of water to fat and of protein to minerals, which research suggests increases the length of time residues are stored in the body. The most rapid rate of growth is from conception to one year old, while the brain does not complete its development until four to six years old. Evidence also suggests that infants' nervous systems may show an increased vulnerability to neurotoxic pesticides during these periods of rapid growth.

- An infant's immune, reproductive and endocrine systems are not fully developed and may be particularly sensitive to toxins. Their developing tissue barriers are more permeable to toxins, and they are less efficient at excreting them.
- Many pesticides can mimic and interfere with sex hormones, which could have effects on the immune and reproductive systems in later life.
- As a result of increased exposure to pesticides and other toxic substances, children are more likely to suffer from neurotoxic effects, endocrinal problems and impaired immune-system function. Pesticide exposure could potentially cause cancers to develop later in life.

Also:

- Infants and toddlers need optimum nutrition. Food that has been over-processed or watered down or had 'improvers' added does not provide optimum nutrition.
- Contrary to accepted opinion, babies are very sensitive to taste. Their senses of smell and taste are developing throughout the first twelve months of life. Research shows that weaning-foods affect food preferences later in life; so bland, starchy, sugary, adulterated food, for instance, may affect food choices later. Maltodextrins,

> **fact**
>
> Over 70 per cent of four hundred baby-food products tested by the Food Commission were found to have been bulked out with low-nutrient starches such as modified starch and maltodextrin.

for example, present in many commercial brands of baby food and permitted in formula milks, are partially broken-down carbohydrates used extensively in food processing. They provide bulk and enhance the flavour of other, often cheap, ingredients, have no nutritional function, and their presence helps familiarise infant taste buds with poor-quality synthetic foods.

Chemical mixtures

When it comes to chemical mixtures, it seems that the cocktail effect may be greater than the sum of the parts. This could have profound implications, especially for babies.

The science is complicated and only just beginning to be understood, but it has recently been discovered that some combinations of hormone-disrupting chemicals are much more powerful than any of the chemicals individually, and that combinations of two or three common pesticides, that may be found at low levels in the environment, are anywhere from 160 to 1600 times as powerful as any of the individual pesticides alone.

Hormones are particularly important during the growth and development of the egg, the embryo, the foetus and the baby. Since 1992, at least fifty synthetic industrial chemicals have been shown to interfere with hormones. Hormone-mimicking chemicals, which include many pesticides, have been shown to have serious effects on normal growth and development and on the reproductive health of many species, including man. Results of this interference include small penises, diminished sperm count, various cancers, nervous-system disorders, birth defects and damage to the immune system.

One last word: it's thought that the toxic effect of some groups of bioaccumulative substances can be subtle, and may have their maximum effect on the next generation while they are in the womb. Research is also showing that mixtures of organic pollutants, which cause effects such as immunosuppression and hormone disruption, can have an additive or a synergistic effect, and that the foetus may be most at risk to these.

Source Material supplied by Dr C.V. Howard, Foetal and Infant Toxico-Pathology, Liverpool University; Green Network papers on hormone-mimicking chemicals; *Our Children's Toxic Legacy*.

what they say . . .

'Children aged one to five eat about three times more food per unit of body than the national average, and they consume large volumes of water and reconstituted juices so that the amount of pesticides they encounter is also larger. Many foods that children eat contain multiple pesticide residues. Most research, however, is done on single pesticides, and combinations are not usually studied because interactive effects are not easy to discern. But we have often found six or seven pesticide residues in our patients, some of them in very large quantities.

'The EPA [US Environmental Protection Agency] sets safe tolerance levels for individual pesticides, on the assumption that they occur only one at a time in a serving. But in fact there are often more, and often they are neurotoxic substances. We have found that some people, including children, are more vulnerable to pesticides than others, because they have an impaired metabolic detoxification system. Almost 25 per cent of children now have asthma. How many are being exposed to pollutants in their food which they cannot degrade and which are therefore going to poison them because the backlog will inevitably be a neurotoxic effect.' – *Dr Jean Munro, Medical Director, Allergy and Environmental Medicine Ltd (Breakspear Hospital), Hemel Hempstead*

'You've no idea what's in the products you buy. You get a picture on the jar of a smiling little brat, glugging away. It's the equivalent of battery eggs being sold with a picture of a farmhouse on the box. Buy organic meat and vegetables and purée them yourself.' – *Shaun Hill, chef, the* Independent on Sunday

'I was pleasantly surprised when I discovered organic baby food – the different makes, but also the range of recipes (Toby's favourite is squash and apple). There is no doubt that organic food is more expensive, but not by a great deal, and the peace of mind it gives me outweighs any price difference.' – *Mrs Emma Read, Coventry*

chapter nine

sugar and spice, tea and coffee

Organic Sugar, Honey and Other Sweeteners

All organic sugars, honeys and other sweeteners can be bought from organic/wholefood/health food shops and are available by mail order. Although produced only in very small quantities, organic sugar and honey are becoming more widely available and can increasingly be found in supermarkets that stock organic food. You can also buy organic molasses and maple syrup. Whole Earth produce organic barley, maize malt and brown rice syrups, popular in macrobiotic diets. These thick, glossy syrups have a deeper flavour than sugar, with earthy, malty tastes and, like honey, they can be used as a spread, to sweeten desserts and for baking certain cakes. One friend, for example, prefers them for her Christmas pudding and cake and for making flapjacks. Only organic sugar, honey or other sweeteners are used in organic manufactured foods including cereals, cakes and confectionery. Note where organic sugar is used, it does not affect the flavour in any way.

Sugar

There are two kinds of sugar in this world: refined white sugar, much of which is produced from sugar beet, but also from sugar cane; and unrefined cane sugar of various hues, from pale-golden granulated to dark, sticky molasses, much of which comes from Mauritius. Both are grown with intensive use of fertilisers and pesticides. Unrefined sugar contains B vitamins, potassium and other minerals which refined white sugar does not. All organic sugar is produced from unrefined sugar cane but instead is grown on separate plantations that have undergone a five-year conversion period, without any applications of synthetic fertilisers or pesticides. Organic sugar cultivation is more labour-intensive – weeds are controlled manually or by using blow lamps, for example, and yields are 40–50 per cent lower than on conventional plantations. Organic sugar is extracted from the cane in exactly the same way as is ordinary sugar. The machinery is always cleaned first, if it is also used for conventional sugar, to avoid contamination. The only processing aid allowed is lime, in the form of calcium hydroxide. Organic sugar tastes the same and can be used in the same way as the ordinary sugars, including preserving, though of course it does not give a colourless syrup and so produces darker, duller results.

Billington's The only UK brand of organic sugar, which carries the Soil Association symbol. A mild, pleasing, crunchy granulated sugar, and a natural alternative to white. The colour varies slightly from golden to pale brown. Widely available, including at selected Sainsbury's and Waitrose stores.

> TIP: If you need organic caster sugar, whizz Billington's organic sugar briefly in a food processor.

Rapunzel Produce Rapadura cane sugar, which is a muddy brown colour, has a slight fudge flavour and is not granulated, but powdery with tiny pebble-like lumps, giving it a gritty rather than a crunchy texture. It is made by pressing sugar cane to release its juice, then heating the juice gently in large pans until it dries into cakes. These are then finely grated to produce Rapadura.

Other sweeteners include bio-molasses (Biona), maple syrup (Shady Farm, Morgenland) and organic barley, maize malt and brown rice syrups (Whole Earth, Fertillia).

Price guide: Because organic sugar is far more costly to produce and grown in tiny quantities, it is about a third more expensive than equivalent unrefined sugars and twice as expensive as refined white sugar. Expect to pay around £1.20–£1.40 per 500g bag; Rapadura costs around £2.30–£2.50 per 500g. Organic molasses sells for around £2 per 450g tin, and non-sugar syrups for around £2.30–£3.50.

Honey

The major organic honey-producing country is New Zealand, which has pioneered it to exacting standards. Mexican and Tanzanian are the other two most common organic honeys, and you may occasionally find Italian and French. Waitrose have introduced an excellent pine forest honey from Turkey.

Though all honey is natural, not all of it is pure. Most commercial honey is a devitalised product that has been flash-heated to 70°C for cosmetic reasons so as to keep it runny, a process that destroys the individual flavour of a honey as well as its nutrients. It is then passed through very fine filters to make it clear, which removes its valuable pollen grains. Standard honey is often a blend of honeys from various countries. Most organic honeys, by contrast, tend to be individual rather than blended, and are produced with minimum heat treatment and filtering. The flavour will depend on the country it comes from and the flowers from which the bees collected the nectar.

Other major differences between organic and other honeys are:

- Organic honey must be taken from bees that forage in organically cultivated areas, or in areas of natural vegetation free from pesticides and that have been so for a minimum of two years; and from hives situated well away from major agricultural or commercial sites and any possible pesticide contamination – a minimum distance of five kilometres (three miles), the average roving distance of bees.
- Feeding the hives with sugar is forbidden, except in emergencies. This means that sufficient honey must be

left in the hives for the bees to overwinter. If sugar *is* used, the resulting honey cannot be used within four weeks of starting to flow.

- Chemical wood preservatives for treating hives are forbidden, as is the use of commercially prepared wax.
- Treating colonies with antibiotics is forbidden, as is the use of OP or other chemical traps to control the varroa mite, *Varroa jacobsoni*, a major pest which feeds on bee larvae.
- Pasteurisation of honey is forbidden. Heat treatment must not exceed natural hive temperature, 35°C. At all stages, care must be taken to minimise heat damage.
- Strainer sizes must not be less than 200 microns; this allows debris to remain behind but pollen grains to pass through.
- Honey must be tested for residues for the first two years of organic production, to ensure purity.
- Beekeepers, processors and packers must be registered with an approved organic body.

NOTE: These standards represent those of New Zealand. They vary slightly in other countries but the important guidelines remain the same: namely, hive management and honey extraction methods are aimed at the production of pure honey and the preservation of the colony, which must not be destroyed when the honey is harvested. The Soil Association's standards for honey production forbid any feeding of sugar, or anything at all other than organic honey and natural pollen supplements. The comb used in the production of comb honey must be made with organically produced beeswax.

The HMF factor

HMF is a refined glucose molecule present in honey that increases as honey is heated. It is used as a measure of how much degradation honey has undergone due to heat treatment and, broadly speaking, the lower the HMF factor the better quality the honey. New Zealand organic honey has one of the lowest HMF ratings, at 8 mg/kg; most EU countries allow 40mg/kg, while UK regulations allow 80mg/kg to be present. A revision of these is currently being considered. Major organic producers test for this in their honeys, and include the HMF rating on the label.

Wild honey Wild honey – that is, honey collected from out-of-the-way places – is deemed to be organic by virtue of its isolation, and may be certified as such as long as it meets other organic requirements.

British organic honey There are as yet no registered British organic honeys. Some organic farmers have their own hives and sell their honey, but it does not necessarily qualify as organic. The Old Dairy, near Reading (p. 87), is one example.

Flavour

The majority of organic honeys are strongly flavoured; African honeys, for instance, may seem strangely strong. Forest honeys are also very strong, as they contain a high proportion of honeydew. If you prefer a milder-tasting honey, try Tawari, described as delicate and buttery, or most other New Zealand honeys; or named monofloral honeys such as acacia and lime blossom.

The *major organic honey producers* are:

Allos A specialist honey company. High-quality honeys, cold-extracted, unblended and with a maximum HMF factor of 15. All their honeys undergo testing for residues and radioactivity, the results of which can be obtained from Allos by quoting the number on the jar. They offer an extensive range comprising ten different honeys, including Eucalyptus, Canadian, Maya and Argentinian Wildflower, and Bio Blossom.

De Rit Another specialist honey company. It claims to be the best honey money can buy, because of the unique process its honey undergoes, which guarantees that it is pure, unblended and cold-extracted, and that its natural enzymes and nutrients are all retained. Though fully organic, it is not certified because De Rit prefer to maintain their own independent standards. The HMF content is a maximum of 10mg/kg. The range comprises twenty-one different honeys, from acacia and wildflower from Hungary, to lavender, sunflower and fruit blossom from France, and forest honey from Greece, all supplied to them by known producers in various countries.

New Zealand Food Company The major specialist supplier of organic New Zealand honeys, which have a distinct floral aroma. All of their honeys are untreated and of the highest quality. Available only through independent health food stores, their range comprises Biogro Tea Tree, Honeydew, Native Flower, and Tawari honeys and honeycomb. They also offer a mail order service tel: 0181 961 4410.

Also
BHC (British Honey Company) New Zealand.
Campo Italian wildflower, Millefiori.
Epicure a mild and clear and a pleasant set honey, available in Safeway.
Equal Exchange Forest honey, Mexican.
Forest Harvest Tropical forest.

Buying and storing: If you have never tried organic honey and are used only to commercial brands, New Zealand organic honey is a good one to start with. Waitrose pine forest honey, distinctive but not strongly flavoured, is another. As the flavour of honey is very much a question of personal taste, seek advice and try different ones. Natural honey lasts for ever. Store at ambient temperature, not in the fridge.

fact

The poisoning of honey and wild bees by pesticides is a worldwide problem. Honey losses due to reduced crop pollination in the US alone are estimated at $150 million per annum.

Three things to know about honey

1 As a general rule, the darker the honey, the stronger the flavour.

2 Different honeys crystallise at different rates. Some honeys, such as acacia, are naturally runny and will not crystallise for a couple of years; others, like rape, crystallise almost immediately. This is a sign that the honey has not been over-processed.

3 If your honey has gone cloudy, or starts to set when you want it to be runny, immerse the jar in hot water for a few minutes.

Price guide: Most organic honeys cost about a third more than the cheap commercial brands, but are no more expensive than other unprocessed up-market honeys. Expect to pay £2–£2.50 per 500g jar of regular honey, and up to £4.50 or so for honeycomb and rarer honeys. New Zealand Natural Food Company honeys range from £3.50 to £7. Waitrose organic pine forest honey, at £1.79, is a bargain and cheaper than many of their other honeys.

Honey products

Honey is used as a sweetener instead of refined white sugar in many organic cakes and biscuits – look out for honey cakes and waffles especially – in confectionery and in some jams and spreads. De Rit, Allos and Biona are the major brands. Honey marzipan, made with organic ground almonds and honey, is produced by De Rit and Davert Muhle. Organic mead, brewed from Tropical Forest honey, raisins and cane sugar, by Broughton Pastures, is available exclusively through Vinceremos wine merchants (p. 103).

Organic Herbs and Spices

Organic herbs and spices provide the final touch to enliven your cooking. They are available mainly in dried form, though producers of organic vegetable box schemes often have fresh organic herbs in season, and some supermarkets are beginning to stock organic parsley. Fresh organic culinary herbs are not available all year round; they are limited to what grows well and is easy to grow for each supplier – traditional favourites such as sage, thyme, mint, rosemary and parsley, plus perhaps tarragon, chervil, oregano, dill and occasionally the ultimate treat, basil, and even coriander.

Herbs and spices have a healthy image, and it would be nice to think that all of them were grown naturally. Unfortunately, this is not so. Fresh glass-house herbs are grown hydroponically, in water flushed with chemical nutrients; field herbs and spices are grown using a range of herbicides and insecticides. Dried spices may receive post-harvest chemicals, and both dried herbs and spices may have been irradiated. As one organic grower has said, 'How many consumers know that their ginseng has been treated with powerful chemical solvents, or that their garam masala has been fumigated with methyl bromide?'

One of the reasons pesticides are used is because of the demand for cosmetically perfect herbs, by retailer and consumer alike. This makes it extremely difficult for growers. The UK commercial herb growers I have spoken to are sympathetic to organic methods, and assure me that they use pesticides only very infrequently, and as a last resort. Nevertheless, the 1995 WPPR report showed that, of the ninety-five-plus different pesticides sought, residues were detected in two-thirds of samples tested.

Herbs and spices are nature's healers, and their efficacy, as well as the concentration of their natural oils and hence their flavour, depend on the way they are grown. Organic herbs and spices, for example, are able to draw up naturally a pot-pourri of trace elements from the soil. For this reason, many believe that organic herbs and spices are more potent; certainly, this is borne out by the organic spices I have tried. The organic herb industry is in its infancy – and this is even more the case with fresh herbs. This is why, though dried herbs and spices are common enough, you will not yet find fresh organic herbs generally available.

The *main brands* of organic dried herbs and spices are:

De Rit Bio-dynamic herbs, spices and spice pastes, including pizza, pasta and Provençal herb mixtures, garlic and chilli powder.

Hambleden Herbs A specialist company who operate a mail order service. Their herbs are widely available. See Star Performer, p. 252.

Kitchen Garden Fair-traded organic herbs and spices, produced in Zimbabwe, on company-owned farms, by small-scale farmers who use composts, manures, legume rotations and natural mineral supplements. The herbs and spices are processed on site, and are sold in packets and jars. There is an extensive dried range, including Italian seasoning, crushed chillies, piripiri and pickling spices, plus herbal condiments such as minced garlic, fresh minced basil, coriander, oregano and tarragon and chamomile, lemon grass, apple and cinnamon and variety pack herbal teas. Widely available.

Lebensbaum A full range of organic herbs and spices including Herbes de Provence and curry powder, a mixture of organic and Demeter.

Buying and storing: Stored properly, somewhere cool and dark – keep them in a cupboard, not on show – dried organic herbs and spices have a long shelf life, around 18 months for dried herbs and two years or longer for spices. Ready-ground spices and powders have a shorter shelf life, 12–18 months maximum. Fresh herbs should be picked over, and any damaged or rotting leaves removed. Store green fleshy herbs in a thick plastic bag or box lined with kitchen paper in the fridge; they will keep for 7–10 days. Tougher-leaved herbs such as thyme, rosemary and sage can be stored in the fridge, or they will keep well in a jar of water.

fact Less than 0.1 per cent of herbs consumed in the UK are home-grown; less than 0.1 per cent of these are certified organic; and less than 0.1 per cent of these are produced in the UK.

Price guide: Dried organic herbs and spices are not expensive – no more so than those you can buy in fancy jars and packaging. Expect to pay around 75p–£1.50, depending on the herb or spice and the quantity. With the exception of the parsley sold in supermarkets, fresh organic herbs are not sold prepacked and are excellent value, being weight for weight cheaper than the prepacked supermarket herbs.

Where to buy: The best places to buy organic dried herbs and spices are organic/wholefood/health food shops and alternative supermarkets. Being light, they are ideal to send off for via mail order – they are a popular mail order catalogue item, either direct from Hambleden Herbs or from mail order suppliers such as Damhead Organically Grown Foods, Organic Health and Longwood Farm. For telephone numbers, see pp. 98–106. Fresh organic herbs are available through box schemes when in season, and through local outlets including some organic farm shops. Sainsbury's and Waitrose sell organic parsley in selected stores.

Star Performer: Hambleden Herbs

Winners of four awards in 1997, the country's only specialist organic herb supplier, experts in their field, registered with the Soil Association and based in Milverton, Somerset tel: 01823 401 205. They source worldwide, have their own drying barn, and offer the most comprehensive range of dried organically grown herbs and spices in the UK; over 450 species in total, including a range of organic herbal (unbleached) tea-bags, loose herb infusions, culinary herbs and spices, vanilla pods, cinnamon sticks, organic chilli braids and mulling spices. They also sell a comprehensive range of medicinal herbs, including caisse herbal formula, rose petals, organic flower remedies, comfrey products and pot-pourri and incense mixtures, and have begun to grow their own herbs. New products include green tea and China spice. They produce an excellent informative catalogue and a newsletter, and have a gift service.

Their organic herbal tea range comprises: chamomile, elderflower, fennel seed, hibiscus, Lemon Heaven, lemon verbena, lime flower, peppermint, rose-hip, Spice Delight and Crimson Glory. For anyone who likes citrus, lemon verbena is a winner. Their Lemon Heaven and Crimson Glory have both recently won awards.

Herb plants

The other way of having a constant supply of fresh organic herbs is to grow your own. Most herbs are accommodating plants and grow well in pots.

Two producers of organic herbs who operate by mail order are:

Jekka's Herb Farm, Alveston, Bristol tel: 01454 418878 Owner of a well known herb nursery, best-selling author and Chelsea Flower Show gold-medallist, Jekka McVicar is the leading herb mail order specialist registered with the Organic Food Federation. Extensive catalogue available. Plants are mailed during June–October; they can also be bought at Ryton Organic Gardens tel: 01203 303517.

Grange Cottage Herbs, Nuneaton, Coventry tel: 01530 262072 Soil Association registered. A small herb nursery, garden and shop selling a small range of local herbal products and Hambleden Herbs teas. Plants are sold direct and by mail order.

Also Look out for organic herb plants and fresh-cut herbs in organic/wholefood shops and some greengrocers, and on market stalls. Wye Valley Herbs, Chepstow, Monmouthshire tel: 01291 689253 sell pot-grown organic herbs; Hillside Herb Farm, near Leominster, Hereford & Worcester tel: 01568 613023 sell herb plants and cut herbs; Abbotts Vegetable and Herb Garden, Birkenhead, Wirral tel: 0151 608 4566 sell cut herbs; Tamar Organics, Tavistock, Devon tel: 01822 618765 sell cut herbs and plants from their market stall in Tavistock (Fri.); Yorkshire Garden World, Haddlesey, near Selby tel: 01757 228279 are not

> **fact** Herb plants in flower are major attractants for bees, butterflies, hover-flies and other beneficial insects.

registered but are committed organic growers and sell plants. If you're in the area, don't forget Marshford Organic Nursery, near Bideford in north Devon (p. 87), have a herb garden and fresh herbs for sale.

what they say . . .

'Organic herbs and spices are grown without the use of pesticides and herbicides; instead, producers rely on good husbandry to build soil fertility and protect crops. These do not receive any post-harvest treatments such as fumigation, irradiation or nitrogen-flushing, and are not treated with the chemicals routinely used in herb-processing such as etherol (a ripening agent sprayed on at harvest time), ethloxyquin (an antioxidant) and chlorine (a cleaning agent).

'Organic herbs contain no colouring, flavouring or preservatives and are, in our experience, usually of superior quality. With the absence of agrochemicals to fall back on, producers have to apply far greater attention to each stage of the production and processing of the herbs, and the results of this are obvious.

'We also distinguish between wild-crafted herbs and wild-harvested herbs. A dandelion root harvested from some waste ground near Chernobyl at the wrong time of the year can be called wild-harvested, but it is certainly not wild-crafted. "Wild-crafted" means the conscientious collection of correctly identified herb species from areas unpolluted by roads, industry or conventional farming. Gathering takes place at the peak of each herb's growing cycle, is effected without depletion of the natural plant populations or damage to their habitats, and is monitored by ourselves, by overseas colleagues or by recognised organic organisations.'
– Gaye Donaldson, Hambleden Herbs

Organic Herbal Teas

Herbal teas are becoming as popular as mineral water, and are a natural alternative to tea and coffee as they contain no caffeine or tannin. Organic herbal teas are made with only certified organic herbs and natural flavourings and are guaranteed free of irradiated herbs. They are sold in non-chlorinated tea-bags, and are of excellent quality. The difference, incidentally, between herbal tea-bags and loose herb teas is that the herbs for tea-bags are very finely cut, whereas in loose tea you can expect the whole leaf or flower, or large sections. Which you choose is a matter of preference and convenience. Like ordinary loose tea, the flavour can be better from loose herbal teas; also, it enables you to see the quality of the flowers or leaves better.

The *main brands* are:

Evernat Four herbal teas: chamomile, nettle leaf, peppermint, rose-hip.

Golden Temple, Yogi Bhajan's ancient herbal-formula teas A Dutch brand of unique Ayurvedic herbal teas blended from different herbs and spices. Eleven formulations including Detox, Women's, Men's, Stomach Ease, and Revitalise tea. Their ginger tea is especially recommended by one devotee. See p. 258.

Hambleden Herbs and *Kitchen Garden Herbs*. See pp. 252 and 251.

Piramide A specialist Dutch herb company who work with small-scale organic growers worldwide and import organic herbs direct. Their herbs carry the SKAL, ECO or Demeter symbol. In addition, they operate their own independent quality controls and every batch is checked for purity. Their extensive range includes chamomile, fennel, liquorice, peppermint, maté, lemon grass and Child, fruit, Spicy, Star (with star anise) and Sunny Mix teas. Loose herbal teas include Baby Tea, nettle and lemon grass, maté and five different healing teas.

TIP: Use herbal tea-bags to flavour fruit compotes. Use chamomile as a rinse for fair hair.

Price guide: Expect to pay the same or slightly more than for up-market and other high-quality herbal tea brands, around £1.50 to £1.95 per box of 20/24 tea-bags. Loose teas are boxed in different sizes, so it's difficult to give price guides. As an example, chamomile tea costs around £2.20 for a 40/55g box. The number of bags per box, and the size of boxes of loose herb teas, vary. Be mindful of this when comparing prices.

Where to buy: As for herbs and spices. They can also be bought from selected delicatessens and fine food shops.

Organic Tea and Coffee

Though not generally thought of as 'front-line' organic purchases, tea and coffee are part of the basic global organic shopping basket that is coming under increasing scrutiny. Working conditions often leave a lot to be desired. Most crops are grown with intensive use of pesticides, including OPs and paraquat – classed as one of the Pesticides Action Network 'dirty dozen' most harmful pesticides – which are a major health hazard for the plantation workers. So, as with all tropical food commodities, though residues may not be a problem for those drinking the tea and coffee, they are a major problem for those growing them.

Organically produced tea and coffee address all of these issues and offer a much better and fairer choice all round. Quality these days is generally excellent. Organic teas have clean, pure flavours and coffee a fine, rich flavour. Most organic coffee, including instant brands, is made from arabica beans, which are the best quality you can buy and better for your health. Remember that organic tea-bags are made from non-chlorinated paper and are therefore duller in colour.

The market is small, but growing rapidly; in the USA, for example, organic coffee sales are booming and are shortly expected to reach 5 per cent of the retail market. Supermarkets have started to stock both, and the range – from everyday tea-bags and instant coffee to rare and exotic fine teas and speciality coffees – grows daily.

IFOAM standards for organic tea and coffee

Growing tea and coffee organically means far more than not using artificial fertilisers and synthetic pesticides. It embraces everything from the prevention of soil erosion, the use of legumes to improve soil fertility and shade plants to protect the crops, and the selection of the tea and coffee varieties suited to local conditions, to the living standards of the workers.

Guidelines produced by the IFOAM, which apply to cocoa as well, state that:

- The tea, coffee and cocoa should be produced as part of a sustainable farming system that observes conservation practices. The whole farm should be organic.
- Clearance of land must be selective, so that it does not adversely affect the environment or the local population. The demand for firewood, used to provide fuel for processing, must not lead to deforestation, and the use of fossil fuels and other non-renewable resources must be minimised. Any by-product – coffee and cocoa pulp, tea stalks – is recycled back into the fields.
- Only natural fermentation and mechanical and physical processes are allowed in the processing. As far as possible, processing and packing should be done in the country of origin. Crops should aim to be residue-free, and samples may be taken for residue analysis.

Finally, pesticide residues, including fumigants, are frequently found in conventionally grown green coffee beans, but they decrease in storage and all but disappear, it seems, when the beans are roasted, so they are rarely detected and are not a problem.

Daily cuppas: organic tea

Organic tea comes primarily from India, the Seychelles and Sri Lanka, and a small amount comes from Japan. Assam, Darjeeling,

Earl Grey and Breakfast Tea are available, loose and in tea-bags. As with conventional tea, there are different grades and leaf sizes, and this is reflected in the price. There are several organic brands, including Clipper, Evernat, Hampstead Tea & Coffee, Luaka, Nature's Garden, Ridgeway, and Simon Levelt. Clipper, TopQualiTea and Seyte brands are both organic *and* fair-traded (see p. 260).

Japanese teas There is a small range of these very special teas. In Japan, Sencha green tea is a prized commodity served in high-class restaurants and to honoured guests. Clearspring is the major brand; their Nagata Sencha green tea, grown by the Nagata family on a remote mountain-top plantation, is available loose in foil packs and as tea-bags, and has an exquisitely delicate flavour and a lovely calming influence. Also available are Kukicha, loose and in tea-bags; Hojicha tea-bags (Clearspring), Kukicha tea-bags (Lima) and Kukicha loose (Western Isle).

Flavoured teas These are black teas – that is, the fermented kind with which we are most familiar – with natural flavourings. The main brand is Seyte, who offer vanilla, orange, mint, cinnamon and lemon-flavoured.

Green teas Green tea – tea leaves in their natural unfermented state that have simply been dried, then rolled or cut – is being promoted as the latest health drink, as having powerful antioxidant and anti-bacterial properties as well as the ability to lower blood cholesterol. It is also said to have anti-cancer properties and to help reduce tooth decay; it contains very little caffeine and is a rich source of vitamins and trace elements. It is a costly tea, most of it Japanese; some organic green Darjeeling (Hampstead Tea & Coffee) and fair-traded tea (Rapunzel, TopQualiTea) is also available. Green tea is drunk on its own. As with black tea, the larger the leaf, the better the quality.

Golden Temple Natural Products These specially blended Ayurvedic organic green teas and herb tea-bags are extremely pleasant to drink. Three formulations are available: Green Balance, Green Power and Green Guardian. Ayurvedic Yogi teas, blends of organic green tea and Ayurvedic spices – a personal favourite –

offer something different from the normal flavoured teas; they include Classic (cinnamon), Licorice (Egyptian spice blend), Jamaica (mocha spice blend) and Choco (Aztec spice blend).

Star Performer:
The Hampstead Tea & Coffee Co.

A small company, supplying finest-quality, top-grade (first two leaves and buds) Darjeeling tea from a single estate – Makaibari – currently the only Demeter-certified tea in the world. The estate, personally managed by the owner, who also looks after the welfare of his workers, is remarkable in several ways. Natural sprays prepared from plants grown on the estate, and ladybirds, encouraged and collected by the workers, are used to control pests, while permanent legume crops between the tea bushes provide shade, mulch and fertility. Herbal preparations such as chamomile, valerian and dandelion, applied to the bushes, promote health and vitality. The tea has a fine, delicate flavour and is among the best I have drunk. It is available as black and green whole leaves in selected stores; 250g packs can be had by mail order tel: 0181 731 9833.

what they say . . .

'When tea was first planted in Darjeeling in 1852 by the British, the hills were covered with dense forest. The pioneers, while clearing the forest for tea plantations, saw to it that some balance was maintained in the ecosystem. After Independence most of these jungle areas were encroached upon and destroyed. Next, it was the turn of the beautiful shade canopies to be destroyed, and by the late 1960s the tea gardens were virtually denuded, resulting in the destruction of flora and fauna, besides continuous soil erosion causing heavy landslides. During the Green Revolution in the mid-1960s, heavy usage of artificial pesticides and fertilisers was promoted as the future of agricultural production. However, despite these apparently beneficial changes, the crop and yield remained

static. Thus the logical conclusion is that the use of chemicals and artificial pesticides in Darjeeling has had no effect towards increasing the crop, thus hastening the switch over to an organic system of cultivation with an improved soil structure, the re-establishment of shade, the replanting of the forest and the full restoration of the balanced ecosystem.'
– *Brij Mohan, veteran tea planter, Darjeeling [Quoted with permission from TopQualiTea literature]*

Daily cuppas: organic coffee

Most organic coffee comes from Mexico, where coffee represents three-quarters of the organic produce grown, and from Peru and Nicaragua. A small amount, grown at high altitudes and reckoned to be the best, comes from Papua New Guinea. It is usually fair-traded. The full range – beans, ground, espresso and decaffeinated – is available, and Simon Levelt has them all. Other brands include Ashby's, Café Latino (from Oxfam), Café Organico, Equal Exchange, Fertillia, Molen Aartje and Percol. Mount Hagen produce premium-quality bio-dynamic arabica filter coffee from Papua New Guinea. Finally, not registered yet, but fully organic – the world's rarest and most expensive, St Helena coffee, sold by the East India Company and available from Harrods and Whittards in London.

Instant coffee Two major brands are available, Mount Hagen (Demeter-registered) and Natura (freeze-dried).

Organic and fair-traded

Fair-traded organic teas and coffees offer the best of both worlds: as well as being organic, they are guaranteed to have been produced under conditions that offer maximum benefits to the employees and their communities – above-average wages, training, protective clothing, housing, a clean water supply, good living conditions, health and safety, profit-sharing and a pension scheme. Companies who buy fair-traded products pay above the market price, part of which goes into a social fund for the workers and their community.

Two to look out for are:

Seyte Part of the Kitchen Garden range of fair-traded products (look out for their handshake logo). The tea is produced in the Seychelles, at Port Glaud, a small tea garden and factory that has been producing tea for thirty years. The isolated situation and climate enable the tea to be grown organically.

Equal Exchange A fair-traded company, founded in 1979 and based in Edinburgh, selling organic fair-traded tea and coffee. Their organic tea, sold under the TopQualiTea label, is certified by Naturland of Germany, comes from tea gardens in Darjeeling (Seeyok and Selimbong) and Assam (Banaspaty), and is packed in India. The Darjeeling is single-estate first-flush Golden Broken Orange Pekoe and carries the seal of the Tea Board of India, signifying that it is 100 per cent unblended Darjeeling. Assam, English Breakfast (80 per cent Assam and 20 per cent Darjeeling), Earl Grey (100 per cent Assam blended with bergamot oil) and Green Darjeeling tea from the Samabeong estate are also produced. All available loose or as tea-bags.

Their organic ground coffee, certified by the Soil Association, is sold under the Equal Exchange label and is easily recognised from its stylish silver packaging. The coffee comes from small-scale co-operative plantations in Nicaragua and from the Cecooac Nor co-operative in Chiclayo, north-west Peru, high up in the Andes. It is available as medium, dark-roast and decaffeinated multigrind, or as medium-roast coffee beans.

Price guide: Pack sizes and prices vary quite a bit, making it difficult to make value comparisons. The best advice is to shop around. As more organic tea and coffee become available, so prices are getting more competitive. Compare prices with well known brands of conventional tea, and you may be pleasantly surprised. For example, Seyte and Ridgeway's organic teas are cheaper than Twining's. The same is true of coffee. Supermarkets often have the keenest prices and promotional offers are regularly to be had in them and independent shops.

Tea Tea-bags range from 89p to around £1.20 for breakfast blends, up to around £1.60 for best-quality Darjeeling and some

Japanese and green teas. Loose organic teas range from around 90p to £1.99 per 125g packet.

Coffee Organic coffee is good value. Generally costing around 15 per cent more than other premium or arabica coffees, it can be had for less. Expect to pay around £4.50–£5 per 500g of beans and around £2.25–£2.50 up to £3.50 per 225g pack of ground coffee.

Where to buy: The best source is organic/wholefood/health food shops or mail order. Major supermarkets stock organic tea and coffee in selected branches: Safeway sell Lyons organic tea-bags and coffee; Sainsbury's sell Ashby's organic coffee and Ridgeway's organic tea; and Waitrose sell own-label organic tea-bags and Percol organic coffee.

Others Though they have been the slowest to respond, conventional tea and coffee merchants are beginning to stock organic tea and coffee. Also available from good delicatessens, farm shops, the London food halls, Oxfam and Traidcraft shops.

Mail order: The Tea & Coffee Plant tel: 0171 221 8137 offer Assam, loose and as tea-bags; fine- and medium-ground arabica filter and espresso coffees from Colombia, Mexico, Malawi and Papua New Guinea. Mail order specialists include Longwood Farm and Damhead Organically Grown Foods. For telephone numbers, see pp. 96–106; for Hampstead Tea & Coffee, see p. 259.

What makes organic coffee special?

Growing coffee organically is not easy. The coffee tree takes eight years to mature and is subject to a multitude of pests and diseases. For any chance of success, the plantations need to be isolated and generally at high altitude, which makes transport more difficult and costly. Organic growers do not use pesticides, defoliants, fungicides or synthetic fertilisers, a combination which produces a 50–100 per cent increase in yields and that is offered to growers under various low-cost buy-now-pay-later schemes. With organic coffee-growing there are no economies of scale, the conversion period is a minimum of three years, and land, compost and beans have to pass the purity test before official organic status by either the Organic Crop Improvement Association (OCIA) or Demeter is granted. A full audit trail from plantation to processor to importer has to be set in place, and at no stage in its production may the coffee, as beans or in any other form, be in contact with any non-organic coffee or any other non-organic products.

Unlike conventional coffee plantations, which are very large, organic ones are small. Farmers use natural composting, natural animal manures and mechanical weed-control, and make maximum use of forest shade. Other crops are grown alongside the coffee, such as bananas, maize and pineapple and, in Peru, potatoes. Biological pest-control methods are used. On the estates, good drainage, sanitation and hygiene are essential.

what they say . . .

'In St Helena I use guano – seabird waste, extremely rich in nutrients, especially nitrogen – which is diluted with water and applied manually to each tree. Otherwise I use only manure from my own animals, fed organic feed grown on my own farms. For irrigation and for processing the coffee, only pure spring water is used, from the island peaks, and/or low cloud cover. St Helena is very fortunate in not suffering from the various coffee diseases that other coffee-producing countries experience. Damage such as ring-barking of the trees by slugs etc. is prevented by keeping mulch material a few inches away from the stem of the coffee tree and through good tree husbandry practices.

'Heavy organic mulch material is used, legume crops are grown as a windbreak, and intercropping waste material from banana and maize production provides mulch and food, but also windbreaks and shade for the coffee. Other simple methods that are implemented daily on my farms are the burning of waste such as weeds, old tree stumps etc., with the ashes being utilised as a ground cover. Water is boiled in drums on the waste fires and then poured on to cut weeds in paved areas. The immediate areas around coffee trees are kept weed-free in order to reduce food competition for the tree, though not the ground between the rows, as this would cause soil erosion during heavy rains. We use irrigation trenches to prevent soil erosion and to encourage the tree root system to develop uphill, creating a stronger-anchored tree with access to a greater food source.'
– *David Henry, coffee grower, St Helena*

Organic coffee substitutes

Various 'no-caff' organic coffee-look-alike drinks made from blends of grains, chicory roots and sometimes figs and chick peas are available; most have roasted flavours. They include Bambu (Bioforce), Malt Fit (Mount Hagen) and Yannoh (Lima). Nocaf and Wakecup (Whole Earth) taste similar to the real thing, but you need to make them strong.

chapter ten

the complete organic store cupboard: from baked beans to salsas

Branded Organic Goods: the Major Players

This chapter describes all the other kinds of foods – everything from breakfast cereals to vegetarian burgers – of which you can buy organic brands and which are readily available on the shelves. For anyone new to organic food, you will be more than pleasantly surprised for the range is truly staggering. The main categories have been dealt with in detail, including price guides. At the end of the chapter is a list of other store cupboard items, including vegetarian products.

The quality of manufactured organic goods is usually extremely high, and I find the flavour generally better than that of their conventional counterparts. The difference can clearly be seen by reading the labels: organic foods have no artificial anythings, no fillers, no added water or unhealthy ingredients. Hydrogenated fats, refined white sugar and GM ingredients are banned. This, and the fact that many contain less salt and sugar, or use natural fruit sugars, honey or other natural sweeteners, make them a healthier alternative.

All the foods here can be bought in shops specialising in organic foods and in good wholefood/health food shops. London's food halls (p. 75) have a reasonable range. Box schemes and home delivery services (p. 107) increasingly offer a range of store cupboard goods. They are also available by mail order (p. 91). Except for the occasional item, you will not, as yet, find these foods in major supermarkets selling organic food. Many are imported from Europe, and American brands are beginning to arrive. Prices are tumbling fast. Keep your eye on the shelves and watch out for bargains and promotional offers.

These are some of the names you will find most often on the shelves when looking for dried or manufactured organic foods.

UK brands:

Clearspring The major importer of Japanese wholefoods, buying from small traditional producers. Their Onozaki miso, for example, is made by the Onozaki family, and is one of the few remaining authentic misos. They also import excellent organic Japanese teas (p. 258). Other lines include sea vegetables, said to contain more minerals than any other food, and macrobiotic specialities, Celtic organic sea salt, Danival products and Rice Dream. Two of their sea vegetables, arame and hijiki seaweed, now have organic certification, and are collected only from special certified unpolluted and isolated beaches. Full information and recipe leaflets available   tel: 0181 749 1781.

Evernat 'Organic foods that don't cost the earth' The Evernat range of organic foods is part of Brewhurst Health Foods, a major manufacturer of health foods and fast becoming one of the leading UK brands. All products are fully organic and carry either the Soil Association symbol or an EU equivalent, and are manufactured in France. The range comprises breakfast foods, cereals, flours, pasta, pasta sauces, oils, juices, organic ravioli, grains and pulses, rice cakes, dried fruit, nuts, seeds, milk powder, breads, corn and rice cakes, tomato ketchup, mayonnaise and mustard, peanut butter, cider vinegar, vegetable stock cubes, teas, biscuits, muesli bars, chocolate, tortilla chips and salsas; and organic crisps made with unpeeled potatoes, fried in organic sunflower oil. Their chilled and frozen foods include milk, soups, tofu, cheeses and frozen rice meals. New lines are constantly being introduced. A general product leaflet and an organic food recipe leaflet containing twelve recipes are available from health foods shops or tel: 01932 334501. A reliable, consistent brand.

Infinity Foods Infinity Foods Co-operative Ltd began as a small wholefood shop in Brighton in 1970 and is now a major supplier of wholefoods for London and the south-east, though their products can also be found nationwide. They have the most extensive selection of organically grown foods available, especially dried foods, which all carry the Soil Association symbol. The retail shop, now expanded, includes a wholegrain bakery and cash-and-carry. Their policy is to endeavour to sell only foods processed by natural methods.

Meridian Foods Founded in 1974 and based in Wales, Meridian Foods specialises in a range of high-quality natural foods produced with minimum processing and no artificial additives. Their organic range currently comprises olive, safflower, sesame and sunflower oil, pasta sauce with herbs and garlic, apple juice concentrate and six different excellent fruit spreads.

Suma An ethical registered workers' co-operative, Suma is the UK's largest supplier of wholefoods, and has been selling organic food since it was first set up in 1974. All their products are vegetarian and contain no unnecessary additives. They actively support and promote fair-trade and environmentally sound products, and do not sell products they believe to be harmful to the environment or which have unnecessary packaging. Their range is similar to Infinity Foods.

Whole Earth Foods Whole Earth Foods are an independent, award-winning, family-run business, which started in 1967, committed to expanding awareness of healthy eating. They are now a major brand of convenience wholefood vegetarian and vegan foods, sauces and drinks. They support and buy from over two thousand organic farmers worldwide, support environmental and fair-trade charities and seek to apply the highest ethical standards. Ingredients are strictly controlled: GM and irradiated materials, hydrogenated fats and refined sugar are excluded from all their products. Green & Black's chocolate is a separate company but part of the same family business.

Their Whole Earth organic range carries the Soil Association symbol, is constantly expanding, and currently comprises organic baked beans, hummus, peanut butters; All Your Fibre award-winning breakfast cereal and Swiss-style muesli; Italiano organic spaghetti sauces; pizza bases; Ready Rice (pre-cooked tinned organic brown rice); Russian Cookies, Fruit Waffle Cookies and honey gingerbread; pure-fruit spreads and salad dressings. They also produce organic brown rice, maize malt and barley malt syrups; Wakecup and Nocaf, substitute coffee drinks. They have a chilled range of soya-based Organic Harvest suppers; chilled pâtés, tempeh burgers and rashers; and have recently introduced the first range of frozen organic vegetables. About to be launched is a range of frozen organic dinners.

Some lines can be found in most major supermarkets. They also publish free recipe guides and newsletters for customers and retailers tel: 0171 229 7545.

Imported brands:

Allos A specialist Dutch honey company, producing high-quality honeys and an extensive range of honey confectionery, biscuits, honey-based spreads, fruit spreads and fruit sauces. They also specialise in honey-sweetened amaranth grain products including breakfast cereals; and also produce crispbread, pasta and vegetable bouillon with amaranth.

Bio-Korn A Belgian organic biscuit company offering a wide range of biscuits and wafers with various fillings. Their products are sugar- and dairy-free and are manufactured under the Biogarantie label.

Biona A German company that concentrates on speciality organic rices – red Camargue, jasmine, black Thai and risotto rice; organic grains and seeds, long-life breads and rolls, pizza bases, organic croissants, a large selection of hand-made cookies, waffles and honey cakes, and fruit and vegetable juices. They also produce organic sunflower margarine, cider vinegar and bio-molasses.

Bonvita A Netherlands firm producing organic chocolate and carob, chocolate- and yoghurt-coated organic rice cakes, excellent organic liquorice sweets and other confectionery.

Campo A small farmers' co-operative from the Marche region of Italy, exclusively organic for twenty-five years, producing high-quality pasta, pasta sauces, excellent canned tomatoes and passata, olive oil, red-wine vinegar and wines. Their canned tomatoes and passata are to be commended, are single-processed and really do retain their fresh taste. Their pastas are made from freshly stoneground home-grown durum wheat, manufactured in the traditional way and dried slowly.

Cereal Terra An Italian firm producing a gourmet range of organic antipasti and condiments including sun-dried tomatoes, pesto, black olive pâté, capers in oil and cream of artichoke.

De Rit A specialist Dutch honey company established for twenty years, and the major producer of Demeter-registered (bio-dynamic) products, with a broadening range of organic foods. For their honey range, see p. 247. They produce five different honey cakes and a range of biscuits, waffles, rice cakes and organic honey marzipan, plus other honey products including royal jelly, toiletries and beeswax candles. Organic honey is the sole or prime sweetener used in their products. Their other lines are Demeter-registered pasta, Bio Knackerbrod rye crispbread, Demeter bottled baked beans, vegetables and apple purée; Demeter herbs and spices and De Rit tomato purée, ketchup, barbecue sauce and mustard, and De Rit organic fruit conserves and marmalade sweetened with honey. Their organic products carry the ECO, SKAL and Grund organic labels.

Eunature An independent Italian company, based in Turin, one of the major producers of organic pasta and tomato products in Europe. They produce six different varieties of wholewheat and white pasta, whole and chopped tinned tomatoes, tomato passata and tomato sauce with basil. They also sell short- and long-grain brown organic rices.

La Terra E Il Cielo 'Naturally to your table' La Terra E Il Cielo – Heaven and Earth – is an Italian farmers' co-operative venture in the Italian Marche region, set up in 1980. They are committed to organic agriculture and grow, process and market high-quality organic products, notably an extensive range of award-winning dried and speciality pastas – the best certified organic pasta in Italy – including pasta made from spelt and an ancient rarity, Etruscan grain. All products are fully certified by Garanzia Biologico Marche. Other products sold by them are Millefiori honey, organic wines, beer, couscous, olive oil from Tuscany, tomato passata and barley coffee. They publish a charming traditional recipe and information booklet, available from the sole UK importers, Country Organics tel: 01707 660066 who will also supply details of stockists.

Their pastas Great care is taken, in making the pastas, to preserve the maximum nutritional content. They are made from stoneground wheat and spring water, and dried slowly for 24–40 hours at very low temperatures, never exceeding 50°C. The full range comprises 20 different white pasta shapes, 15 wholewheat and 12 speciality wholewheat pastas including spelt; plus nettle, red chilli, seaweed and buckwheat spaghetti.

Rapunzel One of the foremost Dutch companies manufacturing organic foods, with a commitment to organic fair-traded products. One of the labels you will most frequently come across, their range is one of the most extensive, covering everything from long-life breads, biscuits and confectionery to dried foods, seasonings, condiments, nut butters, oils, margarine, cheeses, chocolate, tea and beers and their own fair-traded Rapadura cane sugar.

Other imported labels you will find include:

Eu Vita Pasta and pasta sauces.

La Bio Idea Pastas, passata, pesto, pizza bases and olive oil.

Lima Grains, breakfast cereals, kamut pastas, rice cakes, soya desserts, salt.

Molen Aartje Savoury snacks, snack bars, biscuits, sweets and crispbreads.

Morgenland Dried and bottled fruits, nuts, seeds, pulses, grains and fruit juices.

TerraSana Varied selection, including biscuits, peanut butter and tinned refried beans.

Organic Breakfast Cereals

An organic start to the day has to be the best one. And if you thought that meant limiting yourself to seriously worthy mueslis, think again. The range of organic breakfast cereals includes cornflakes, puffed rice, malted wheatflakes and the healthy organic alternative to bran cereals, Whole Earth's All Your Fibre. More unusual lines include non-wheat cereals such as puffed amaranth, buckwheat and spelt, and amaranth, hemp seed and rice mueslis. As with organic cakes and biscuits, health is a top priority. Generally speaking, they are less sweet and sickly; all I have tried thus far have been good.

With organic breakfast cereals you can be sure you are getting optimum natural nutrition as well as maximum flavour. Pesticides also survive processing and can and do find their way into 10–30 per cent of conventional breakfast cereals. Taste-wise, there is something for everyone – from cereals that cry out for milk and sugar such as plain puffed rice, to Evernat Tropical Krunchy which you will find difficult to resist snacking on at any hour of the day or night. A fan of honeyed puffed rice likens them to healthier Sugar Puffs. There are several brands of cornflakes, each tasting slightly different from the next. They come in two broad types: those made from whole corn, such as Whole Earth's and Doves Farm, with a much higher fibre content – they contain natural B and E vitamins and minerals – and with a delicious nutty flavour that everyone appreciates, including children; and those made from refined organic maize, which look and taste more like regular cornflakes. Two other tasty, moreish flakes that are distinctly different are Nature's Path Heritage cereal, made from spelt, quinoa and kamut, and their equally nutty millet and rice flakes. Breakfast flakes – rye, malted wheat, barley flakes – can be bought loose; uninteresting on their own, they are for making your own muesli. Mornflake oats, available in supermarkets, are easy to cook and a popular favourite. More lines are constantly being introduced, especially from Europe, while the range I like the most and am impressed with is Nature's Path from Canada.

Major brands include:

Cornflakes *Biona, Billington's, Doves Farm, Essential, Evernat, Familia, Kallo Foods, Lima, Nature's Path, Whole Earth.*
Puffed rice, honey puffed rice *Evernat, Kallo Foods.*
Malted wheatflakes *Community Foods, Evernat.*
Puffed wheatflakes *Evernat.*
Wheat Poppies with maple syrup, and wheatflakes with Rapadura sugar *Rapunzel.*
Multigrain, multigrain and raisins, millet and rice, and Heritage flakes *Nature's Path.*
Puffed amaranth, buckwheat with honey *Allos.*
Puffed spelt *La Terra E Il Cielo.*
Amaranth Crunch, Honey Raisin Crunch; Honey/Hazel Crunchy, Choco/Coco Crunchy *Biona.*
Fruit Crunch *Essential.*
Original, Choco and Tropical Krunchy *Evernat.*
Cocoa Crisps, Rice Crisps, Honey Hoops *Sillbury.*

Organic mueslis

Organic mueslis come in many different varieties, standard or deluxe, with or without added sugar, as a base for you to add your own extras, and so on. They are available prepacked or may be mixed by a particular wholefood shop and sold loose. Organic millers – Little Salkeld, Maud Foster – sometimes offer their own mueslis, and they are a popular item in mail order catalogues. The ingredients vary slightly from one mix to the next – so read the label carefully to see if it is to your taste. For instance, some include salt or milk powder. Boxed mueslis are more expensive than pre-bagged ones.

Major brands are:

Alara, Billington's, Community, Essential, Evernat, Familia Swiss Muesli, Infinity Foods, Kallo Foods and *Whole Earth Swiss Muesli. Neal's Yard* and *Little Salkeld Mill* also produce mueslis. Sundrum Organics has an award-winning tropical muesli. Whole Earth Swiss muesli is a great-tasting crunchy one.

Nature's Path A specialist Canadian organic breakfast cereal manufacturer offer Heritage muesli with raspberries and hazelnuts, blueberry and almond, and 'tropical' mueslis, packed in attractive boxes. A bit short on the fruit and nuts, but otherwise an excellent flavour and good value.

Alternative grain mueslis include rice muesli with apple (Lima), quinoa chocolate muesli (Quinoa Real), hemp muesli (New Earth), hemp crunchy muesli (Davert Muhle), amaranth fruit muesli (Allos).

Price guide: Organic breakfast cereals compare very favourably to 'health food' or up-market brands of breakfast cereals – and are occasionally cheaper. Prebagged organic mueslis, for example, at around £2.20–£2.60 per kg, cost only 25–75p more. Most brands of organic cornflakes cost around £1.59–£1.99, depending on the size of the box. The Nature's Path range cost around £2.40–£2.65. In most cases, the extra cost per serving is minimal. It also pays to shop around, as prices do vary. Organic/wholefood/health food shops which buy in bulk and repack their own should be cheapest. Mornflake porridge oats sell for around 99p, slightly less than Scotch porage oats.

Organic Cakes and Biscuits

Organic cakes and biscuits are made with full integrity: integrity of ingredients and baking methods, and with respect for the environment. Because they contain no artificial flavours or additives and virtually all chemical processing aids are prohibited, they are as near to home-made as you can get. Though limited to a few specialist suppliers, the range is expanding rapidly, imported biscuits especially. The Village Bakery, Doves Farm, Sunnyvale and Whole Earth Foods are the major UK brands. Imported brands include Allos, De Rit, Biona, Bonvita and TerraSana. Otherwise, you will find organic cakes and biscuits made locally in organic bakeries and restaurants and organic and wholefood shops that have goods baked for them. You will also find a wide selection which, though not fully organic, are made with a fair proportion of organic ingredients.

The eating appeal of any cake or biscuit is largely a personal matter that tends to be based on what you're used to and how sweet a tooth you have. There was a time when most organic cakes and biscuits catered primarily for the wholefood market or for vegetarians, rather than for either the general or the gourmet market. This is changing fast. Many taste delicious in their own right, but don't expect them all to have mass appeal or necessarily to taste just like their conventional equivalent. They can be denser, for example, and some are drier. But unlike conventional cakes, which vary enormously in quality of ingredients, organic cakes and biscuits are all of a good quality; it's a question, rather, of which takes your fancy.

Which organic cakes and biscuits shall I try?

When I began to write this book I listed the following items, as similar to the conventional equivalents but usually less sweet and sickly, more satisfying, nuttier and fuller-flavoured: moist, dark, fruity fruit-cakes; tea-breads, carrot cakes, honey cakes and gingerbread; and traditional biscuits – oatcakes, digestives and flapjacks. Twelve months later I would add continental biscuits, including the ever-growing range of chocolate-covered and -flavoured wafer biscuits, and especially waffles and lebkuchen, which are different, good to drink with coffee, and more elegant than the standard British biscuit.

Particular examples scoring high on the yummy scale among friends are:

The Village Bakery cakes and biscuits See Star Performer, p. 218. In particular, their florentines; butter shortbread; and chocolate and almond cake, a super deluxe seriously-to-be-swooned-over cake made with Green & Black's chocolate, available in two sizes, small and large. Though expensive, at around £11 for the large size, it costs far less than many luxury conventional cakes.

Barbara's Double chocolate cookies.

Biona Danish pastries with maple syrup, organic apple and raisin rolls; a hand-made cookie range with no added sugar, including lemon and coconut, and butter and almond shortbread; plus blueberry, raspberry and Choco-cream cookies.

The Celtic Baker Lemon and orange cake.

Ceres Bakery Chocolate digestive biscuits, plain and milk; reckoned to be the best organic chocolate digestive biscuit.

De Rit Bio Kringler biscuits.

Doves Farm Lemon and chocolate chip cookies. Their new 100 per cent organic plain digestive biscuit, on sale in Sainsbury's, the first to be labelled GM-free, is made to a traditional recipe, is quite delicious and will have you reaching for the packet.

Duchy of Cornwall Elegant, high-class traditional biscuits: oaten, ginger, orange, lemon; pure butter Highland shortbread. Carry the Soil Association symbol. Note that these biscuits are not labelled as organic, but qualify for the 75 per cent organic status. They are made from organic flour or oatmeal, but the remaining ingredients are non-organic.

Evernat Chocolate and nut cookies, petit beurre biscuits. If you have a sweet tooth, try their new blueberry and award-winning raspberry rounds.

Molen Aartje Honey waffles.

Pimhill Delicious orange Jamaica, old–fashioned date and walnut cake; and Welsh Bara Brith.

Rapunzel Chocolate wafers.

Sunnyvale Malt loaf, Fruit-T-loaf, carrot cake, fruit-cake.

Others This is what else you can expect to find to tempt you as you scour the shelves for branded organic cakes and biscuits:

Sunnyvale date and pecan, stem ginger, choc and cherry, choc and orange, fig and orange, carrot with raisins, and almond cakes. Choc and orange, fruit and cinnamon, date and pecan cookies. *Whole Earth* Russian waffles. *The Celtic Baker* tea-bread, tea-buns, Bara Brith. *Ceres Bakery* honey gingerbread. *Doves Farm* oat and honey, Roman, muesli and seven-seed cookies. *Evernat* fruit triangles. *Allos* organic amaranth and muesli biscuits, Jumbo spelt, chocolate spelt, plum and cinnamon cookies; honey and apricot and almond lebkuchen; plain and chocolate wafer rolls; pausenkeks. *Braycot* apricot and sesame, pear and rum biscuits. *Biona* rye, raisin, mixed peel, and ginger honey cakes; organic hazelnut, raisin and coconut, muesli, sunflower, and cannabiscuit cookies; apple and pear, apricot, hazelnut, maple and malt syrup waffles. *Bio-Korn* Jams Jams (described as 'a kind of organic Mr Kipling's') and chocolate muesli biscuits. *Bonvita* Frou Frou, coffee and mélange wafers, Chocosticks, Chocopenny biscuits. *Ceres Bakery* organic honey gingerbread. *Tods of Orkney* and *Stocken and Gardens of Stromness* Orkney organic oatcakes. *De Rit* honey and hazelnut waffles; sliced honey, raisin honey, and rye flour honey cake; sponge fingers, Vanilla Slims. *Molen Aartje* Bio-honey, hazelnut, malt, and rice syrup waffles; bio-honey, malt, carob, and chocolate biscuits and waffles. *Rapunzel* lemon, orange, and vanilla wafer biscuits. *TerraSana* carob chip cookies; carob coconut, and fruit and nut biscuits; malt syrup, hazelnut, and honey waffles. *Tra'fo* honey and malt waffles, honey cake.

Also Look out for Christmas specialities – cakes, mince pies, and so on, from the Celtic Baker, Doves Farm, Pimhill, Sunnyvale, the Village Bakery and others. Organic plum puddings and Christmas puddings are another personal favourite.

TIP: The best and easiest way to store cakes is in an airtight plastic box; keep them cool. Otherwise, keep them well wrapped. Carrot and apple cakes, which have a high moisture content, do not store well; store in the fridge and eat within two or three days.

Price guide: Organic cakes are not cheap, but nor would you expect them to be. The price depends critically on the ingredients: any cake made with organic almonds, for example, is bound to be a luxury cake. That said, organic cakes cost no more, and often less, than other premium high-quality cakes, and less than many pâtisserie ranges. Prices range from £2 to £5, with luxury cakes fetching up to £12 and more. Organic biscuits are all high-quality

What you get for your money

As with ice-cream, it's important to read the labels when buying cakes. Generally, the cheaper they are, the less 'real' the ingredients. By law, cake ingredients are listed by weight in decreasing order, so you can easily compare the relative quantity of each ingredient in each cake.

Take, as an example, the Village Bakery organic carrot cake, which is made from carrots, stoneground wholemeal flour, raw cane sugar, cold-pressed sunflower oil, raisins, free-range eggs, coconut, cinnamon, bicarbonate of soda and sea salt, and retails at around £2 for 300g. Mass-produced carrot cakes typically found on the shelves have very little carrot, comprise mainly flour, sugar, and hydrogenated vegetable oil, and a cocktail of minor ingredients such as glucose syrup, humectant (vegetable glycerine), pasteurised egg white, soya flour, lactose, yoghurt powder, salt, whey, modified starch, emulsifiers and preservatives, citric acid and flavourings. They retail at approximately £1.50.

and range from just a few pence more than conventional premium biscuits to no more than 50p or so more for the luxury ones. Prices range from 50p to £2 per packet. For what you get, they're very good value. Prices for freshly baked cakes and biscuits vary according to type and baker; generally they cost a little less than, or the same as, branded baked goods. Pimhill cakes and Biona hand-made cookies qualify as bargains.

> **PRICEWISE:** When you compare the price of organic cakes and biscuits with mass-produced ones, remember that the latter are made with cheap ingredients. A comparison of ingredients listed on organic and on conventional cakes and biscuits will quickly illustrate which is better value for money (see box on p. 277).

Others Farm shops. Box schemes and home delivery often include baked goods.

Mail Order: The Village Bakery (p. 218). Mail order specialists such as Longwood Farm, Organic Health, Damhead Organically Grown Foods. For telephone numbers, see pp. 96–106.

Organic chocolate

The UK is one of the highest consumers of chocolate in the world and some £3 billion worth is eaten every year, three-quarters of it by women and children. Yet cocoa production is heavily dependent on agrochemicals, and the health and working conditions of workers in cocoa plantations, many of whom in some countries are also female, give considerable pause for thought. One food-writer friend who has visited cocoa plantations described 'a fog of pesticides, and plants and cocoa pods sticky with residues'; it is these cocoa beans that go to make all conventional chocolate, including the high-quality kind. Traces of pesticides, especially the OC lindane, crop up frequently; they were present in over three-quarters of UK and two-thirds of imported chocolate samples analysed in 1995. And cocoa production inflicts environmental damage in other ways, such as deforestation and erosion of land. Monoculture leads to the destruction of the natural ecosystem, which means that plantations cannot function without pesticides. In comparison, organic cocoa production is tiny, confined to small-scale plantations employing traditional methods of cultivation and disease control, and is often fair-traded – and, incidentally, is said often to produce better-quality cocoa. The organic standards applied are for those of tea and coffee outlined on p. 257.

Comparing organic chocolate to your average bar of choco-late is to compare two quite different substances. Mass-produced chocolate contains up to 50 per cent refined sugar, hydrogenated vegetable fats and artificial flavourings, and far less of cocoa butter solids (the ingredient that makes chocolate chocolatey). Organic chocolate is up to twice as high in cocoa butter solids, has less (unrefined) sugar and no hydrogenated fats, and contains only natural flavourings; it tastes delicious and is better for your health. Being high in cocoa solids, a little goes a pleasurable long way.

For anyone who enjoys chocolate, then, making the switch to organic, and fair-traded, chocolate makes sense; as the same friend who went to see for himself put it, it's better to feel good about eating less organic chocolate than bad about eating too much ordinary chocolate. The same applies to cocoa powder.

- Organic chocolate is made from cocoa beans, milk, sugar and natural flavourings, and must contain a minimum of 95 per cent organic ingredients. The only permitted emulsifier is soya lecithin made from non-genetically engineered soya.
- Organic chocolate typically contains double the amount of cocoa solids found in many conventional brands:

fact

At least thirty different pesticides are known to be used on cocoa; many, such as paraquat and lindane, are highly hazardous, and are applied without proper equipment or protection for the workforce, who sometimes mix them with their bare hands.

dark, 55–70 per cent instead of 30 per cent; milk, 30 per cent instead of 20 per cent or less.

Organic chocolate and chocolate products

Chocolate cakes, biscuits, spreads, ice-cream and drinks are becoming more and more popular; indeed, as far as chocolate is concerned the world is going green, organic and fair-traded fast, with an ever-growing selection of brands and products to choose from. To give you some idea, organic chocolate comes plain or milk, with nuts and with all kinds of flavourings, in large bars and in small. You can buy organic chocolate mints, chocolate truffles, buttons, chocolate-covered raisins, organic chocolate Father Christmases and Easter eggs – and a lot more besides, including hand-made chocolates from Holland. New brands are constantly being introduced to tempt you, and non-dairy organic chocolate, too. As with conventional chocolate, the flavour and 'mouth feel' of the different brands vary. To take two extremes, Evernat dark chocolate is grainy and earthy, while Green & Black's is smooth and satiny.

Major brands and products to look out for are:

Allos Produce a wide range of chocolate confectionery, mainly sweetened with honey, including chocolate wafer rolls, plain and milk chocolate Crunch, chocolate spelt lebkuchen and honey chocolate spread.

Bonvita A specialist chocolate and carob company from the Netherlands. Dark and milk chocolate, dark chocolate with hazelnuts, chocolate figures; chocolate wafers; Chocosticks.

Chocoreale Milk; bitter-sweet; hazelnut chocolate; and milk praline chocolate bars.

Evernat Milk and dark chocolate, with the Soil Association symbol.

Green & Black's Chocolate, hot chocolate and chocolate ice-cream (see p. 170).

Plamil The first UK company to manufacture organic chocolate, they specialise in non-dairy foods all suitable for vegans. Produce dairy-free organic plain, mint and orange chocolate, and chocolate drops. Certified by the Soil Association.

Rapunzel Produce the widest range of fair-traded organic chocolate bars, sweetened with organic Rapadura unrefined dried sugar cane juice (p. 244). Dark chocolate: bitter-sweet, bitter-sweet with almonds, dark with hazelnuts; milk chocolate and truffle creams, and hazelnuts; Rio! milk chocolate and truffle bar; Swiss chocolate and truffle, nut truffle, and hazelnuts; Tango! chocolate nut bar; Coco! chocolate coconut bar. Also, chocolate buttons, raisins, chocolate-covered almonds and hazelnuts.

The Stamp Collection Designer, hand-made, dairy-free dark chocs carrying the Soil Association symbol and with a celebrity tag, launched by Terence Stamp. The range comprises irresistibly good chocolate-coated sultanas, sun-dried apricots and sunflower seeds. Not fully organic (and therefore not labelled organic) but almost so: all the ingredients are certified organic except for fructose, plus the processing ingredients – namely, lecithin, acacia gum and shellac (natural wax). They are also more expensive than other brands.

The Village Bakery Florentines and luxury chocolate cake. See p. 218.

Organic chocolate powder, spreads, drinks and cocoa

Several brands exist: cacao and chocolate powder (*Rapunzel*); chocolate spreads (*Allos, Chocoreale, Rapunzel and Voegel*); choco-cream and chocolate hazelnut spread (*Molen Aartje*); chocolate drinks and hot chocolate (*Rapunzel, Tra'fo, Molen, Aartje, Whole Earth*); and cocoa (*Infinity Foods*).

And finally,

Jeannette's Organic Chocolates A popular continental brand of mouthwatering hand-made organic dark and milk chocolates, containing minimum sugar and maximum cocoa solids, made by a family firm of chocolatiers in Holland, certified by SKAL, recently introduced into the UK and sold by Hampers Hampers (p. 99). The last word in luxury, and available loose or boxed, there are over twenty tantalising filled chocolates to choose from, at around £2.95 per 100g or £3.25–£4.95 per box of eight or twelve different chocolates. Full ingredients breakdown, including carbohydrate content (for diabetics), is available. The range also includes Christmas chocolate decorations, chocolate bars and chocolate covered marzipan bars, chocolate hazelnut spread, and chocolate covered nuts and raisins. Available in selected organic/wholefood/health food shops and delicatessens and from Hampers Hampers direct tel: 0181 800 8008 who will also advise you of your nearest stockist.

Price guide: The price of organic chocolate is not exorbitant – it reflects the price of real chocolate. It retails at around the same price or at slightly more than other luxury chocolate brands, about £1.50–£2 per 100g bar. Small bars (a treat for yourself) are around 30–40p each.

fact

In a recent analysis, over three-quarters of UK-produced chocolate (milk, white and plain) and two-thirds of imported chocolate samples contained traces of pesticide residues. *Source* 1995 WPPR report

Star Performer: Green & Black's

Green & Black's award-winning chocolate has become synony-
mous with high-quality chocolate that is also organic. They trade
directly with over two hundred organic cocoa-producers in Belize
and six hundred in Togo, who receive a premium for their cocoa
beans. Green & Black's milk chocolate uses organic milk from
farms in the Bavarian Alps. Their dark chocolate contains 70 per
cent cocoa solids; their milk chocolate, 34 per cent cocoa solids
and 27 per cent whole-milk powder. All their chocolate carries the
Soil Association symbol. Their Mayo Gold chocolate also carries
the fair-trading symbol. The full range comprises dark and milk
chocolate, my current passion and their latest award-winning one,
hazelnut and currant dark chocolate, mint chocolate, Mayo Gold
(spiced orange) dark chocolate, milk chocolate Father Christmases
and Easter eggs. Dark, milk and Mayo Gold are also available as
30g bars. In addition, they produce hot chocolate and ice-cream.
A free twelve-page chocolate recipe leaflet, which includes recipes
from famous chefs, is available tel: 0171 243 0562. Their chocolate is also used in Village Bakery products (p. 218).

Organic Dried Beans and Other Pulses; Grains

Organic grains, beans and other pulses, once only available in
small quantities, are now commonplace. It's worth remembering
that organic soya beans and maize are the only kind guaranteed
not to be genetically modified.

Pulses include everything from haricot beans, chick-peas,
mung beans and split peas to the much prized creamy pale-green
flageolets and slate-grey Puy lentils. Most are imported from
America and Canada, but some come from Slovakia, Turkey and
elsewhere. The selection of grains is equally impressive: every kind
of rice, whole grains such as wheat and rye, as well as millet, buckwheat, popcorn and couscous and bulgur wheat plus excellent
organic polenta from Italy. Unusual grains include those from

South America like quinoa and amaranth seed; an ancient form of wheat, spelt, already mentioned in this book and useful for those with allergies to normal wheat; and kamut, which is even older than spelt. All are pleasantly nutty, and will be enjoyed by those who appreciate whole grains.

Grains in particular are major cash crops, in which, because they are intensively cultivated, pesticide residues are inevitably found. The two main victims are wheat (p. 211) and rice (p. 342), though residues in maize-based products are also very common. Rice is also a cause of environmental and health concerns for the farm workers involved in its production. Residues in pulses are generally extremely low.

Major brands The two major importers of organic pulses and grains are *Infinity Foods*, which have the most comprehensive range, and *Suma*, though smaller companies such as *Community Foods* and *Essential* deal in them also. All are wholesalers who sell on to retail outlets, either in bulk for the retailer to repack under his own label or prepacked with their own label.

Other brands include:

Biona Polenta, and various rices including brown risotto rice, Black Thai rice and wild-rice mix.

Eu Vita Precooked, ready-to-eat polenta.

Lima Wild Uruguay and Thai rice.

Morgenland A selection of pulses and grains including buckwheat, quinoa and popcorn.

Quinoa Real Specialise in fair-traded quinoa products from an organic farming co-operative in Bolivia, cultivated high in the Andes. Quinoa is a highly nutritious, agreeably nutty, gluten-free grain, native to the Andes and a traditional staple since the Incas. The range comprises quinoa mueslis, pastas, sandwich loaf, dried soups, plain and chocolate-covered rice cakes, pretzels (salted crackers), rice cakes and cookies.

Rapunzel A wide selection of pulses and grains including five kinds of lentils, wild and red Camargue rice, kamut and wood-dried green spelt.

Cooking with organic pulses and grains

From the culinary point of view you can expect to find two main differences between organically grown and non-organic dried pulses and grains. The first is appearance. Organic pulses are not uniformly shiny or cosmetically perfect; chick-peas, for example, are generally smaller and occasionally have a slightly wizened look, and you can expect variations in size, colour and shape in most beans. As any good gardener will tell you, this is perfectly natural. You will also find that, for instance, couscous, bulgur and polenta look darker and coarser. This is a good sign because – and here is the second difference – they tend to be nutty and more concentrated in flavour. My particular favourite, organic polenta, for example, tastes very different from the normal bland kind. The flavour differences of organic pulses are much less marked, though generally they seem to have a slightly fuller flavour and creamier texture. Soaking and cooking times are the same. By the way, the fact that organic dried pulses and grains are not cosmetically perfect does not mean that they should get away with being substandard. Inspect the packets carefully; they should not contain many broken beans or chipped grains, any debris, or any other signs of inferiority. Note also that brown risotto rice takes approximately twice as long as conventional risotto rice to cook.

Organic pulses and grains have the same shelf life as conventional ones; store in a cool, dark place.

Price guide: Generally, organic dried pulses and grains cost between one third more than and twice as much as non-organic lines, because of extra production costs, lower yields and the fact

---

fact

Conventional rice-farming accounts for 13 per cent of global pesticide use. An estimated 99.9 per cent of the OC lindane used in rice paddy fields in South India evaporates into the atmosphere.

Organic rice cakes

For anyone who cannot eat wheat, or who fancies a change, rice cakes are a popular crispbread and snack. Babies like them, too. All kinds are available – plain, salted and savoury; flavoured with sesame seeds; large and mini-sized, and with other grains such as buckwheat, corn and millet. Kallo and Lima are the major brands; others are De Rit, Evernat and Quinoa Real. Bonvita have introduced milk and dark chocolate ones.

that very few are grown compared to conventional output. However, all are cheap foods, and the extra per portion is minimal. As supplies stabilise, so prices are falling. Organic brown rice, for example, now costs only about 7–10 per cent extra in some stores. For a 500g packet, expect to pay 80–95p for organic rice and £2–£3 for speciality rices; and 80p–£1.95, depending on the type of bean. Organic wheat grain is very cheap, around 50p for 500g, couscous and bulgur wheat around £1.10–£1.40, and polenta around £1.50 for 500g. For more examples, see the chart on p. 31. Prepacked is more expensive than loose. Prices also vary from shop to shop. Bargains include Infinity Foods flageolet beans, and Suma tinned chick-peas, which cost less than their non-organic equivalent.

Organic Dried Fruit

A full range of organic dried fruit is available, including Italian citrus peel sweetened with maize syrup, pitted French prunes and intensely flavoured tropical dried fruit – mango, pineapple, papaya and banana. As you would expect, their flavour is generally excellent. You will also notice that organic dried fruit is darker; this is because none are sprayed with sulphur dioxide. To give you an idea of what else conventionally grown dried fruit may contain, one ready-to-eat brand of luxury mixed dried fruit included glucose syrup, salt, glazing agents, vegetable oil, glycerine, potassium sorbate, sulphur dioxide and tartaric acid. Also, unlike most conventional dried fruit, the organic sort is coated not with mineral oil but with organic sunflower oil, and chopped organic dried fruit is coated with organic rice flour. It's perhaps also worth pointing out that pesticide residues in conventional dried fruit mirror those found in fresh fruit. The WPPR have recently detected single residues, including OPs, in two-thirds of dried fruit samples and multiple residues in almost half.

Like nuts, organic dried fruit is often sourced from different areas from conventional dried fruit, and this has a bearing not only on their quality but also on their price. Organic dates, for example, primarily come from Israel and are much plumper and juicier (and more expensive) than the usual non-organic Iranian ones, while all organic currants are the Vostizza brand from Greece, which are the best you can buy. Apricots are another case in point. Though organic dried fruit is generally expensive compared to standard dried fruit, compare, say, unsulphured non-organic apricots with organic apricots and you will find there is only 15–20 per cent difference, yet the flavour is incomparably better. Organic sultanas are a bargain – a few pence extra, at most. Quality is consistently improving, and you should find little or no quality difference between organic and conventional dried fruit of the same grade.

Major brands
The major prepacked brands are *Infinity Foods* and *Suma*; many registered organic shops also pack their own. *Oxfam* sell fair-traded organic sultanas. *Nature's Way* sell prepacked dates, figs and raisins.

fact

Sulphur dioxide, E220, is routinely used as a preservative in dried apples, pears, cherries, prunes, mangoes, peaches, pineapple, fruit salad and candied peel, and can promote extreme allergic reactions in some people.

Imported brands

Rapunzel have an extensive range, including wild apricots, sour cherries, fruit salad, peach, mango, pineapple and candied lemon and orange peel. A new brand from America, *Made in Nature*, has a range of six prepacked dried fruits including Black Mission figs and pineapple pieces. Other brands include *Allos* (banana chips), *La Bio-Idea* (candied peel), *Morgenland* (dried bananas) and *TerraSana* (Pruneaux d'Agen).

Price guide: Prices range from around 75–80p for 250g of organic sultanas to around £1.50–£2 for 250g of dried apricots, apple slices and pitted prunes. Prices do vary according to outlet, so it's worth shopping around.

Freshly Made Organic Convenience Foods

Don't feel like cooking? Freshly made soups, state-of-the-art sandwiches and various ready-made organic meals can be had, and although as yet such convenience foods are very limited in availability, this is changing fast. Mail order meat-producers currently provide the best choice. Organic farm shops and shops specialising in organic food sometimes make their own, and often sell take-aways.

They include:

Bioline A new range of Soil Association certified frozen organic vegetarian ready-made meals – Vegetarian Lasagne, Chili con Carne, Macaroni with Cheese Sauce and Trio di Pasta Bolognaise, paprika and curry sausages, and vegetarian and cheese hamburgers – made in Belgium, distributed by Brewhurst and available in organic/wholefood and health food shops. The ready-made meals, sausages and burgers retail at £2.19, and are 100 per cent organic.

Carte Blanche Soil Association registered. A new fine foods catering company with a range of ready-prepared frozen meals fit to serve at any dinner party. The range currently includes Moroccan lamb with aubergines and dates, chicken with lemon and tarragon, twice-baked cheese soufflés, rich beef and tomato casserole with roasted root vegetables; and puddings and desserts including lemon, bread and butter pudding, and apricot and banana mascarpone tart. And all organic, too. Prices around £5.85 for main courses (450g) and £4.50 for desserts, each serving two. Available in selected organic/wholefood and fine food shops and delicatessens in the south-east and in Selfridges food hall, London. For mail order tel: 01763 849993.

Finemix Dips Supply tasty, fresh organic avocado, hummus, and avocado and hummus dips, perfect for dunking crudités and tortilla chips into, and ready-cooked Japanese-style organic brown rice with seaweed. Widely available.

Lekker Lounge A new London vegetarian catering company, based in W11, run by two keen cooks, specialising in special diets, including allergy-free, and organic meals and luxury cakes. Weddings, functions and dinner parties catered for. They cook with purified water and only certified organic ingredients are used in their organic dishes. Their sweet and savoury organic pies and pastries, organic muffins and Japanese macrobiotic snacks are on sale at Wild Oats (p. 81). Tel: 0171 792 8856.

The Quiet Revolution Soups Soil Association registered. Voted overall winner at the 1996 Soil Association Organic Food Awards and a winner again in 1997, the Quiet Revolution produce a range of highly praised vibrant fresh soups to exacting standards, which include chopping the onions by hand and using filtered water. They are sold in stylish 450ml plastic pouches, and have a shelf life of twelve days. Four soups are produced each season, with seasonal extras every month or so; they include Crunchy Carrot, Smashing Pumpkin, Summer Gazpacho, Mexican Vegetable and Luscious Leek. Available throughout the south-east and in Harvey Nichols, Bluebird and Selfridges food halls and through Organics Direct.

The Organic Sandwich Company Organic Food Federation registered. Sandwiches will never be the same again. Based in Wigan, but sprouting up in London and other major cities. The sandwiches are made with the Brilliant Bread Company's bread (p. 215) and are fully organic, including the black pepper. Fifteen different fillings are available, from cottage cheese and curried apple to chick-pea tikka and grilled vegetables with almond marinade. Priced around £1.79 and £1.99 if you live in the north, 20p more if you live in London. Special orders, around £2.30. Also available at Mad Hatter's deli in Liverpool; Holland & Barrett stores in Manchester; Planet Organic; Wild Oats; and several other shops in London.

Scottish Organic Foods Organic Farmers & Growers registered. A new dedicated organic food company providing single-portion complete meals containing 100 per cent organic ingredients. Meat is sourced from local farms, and UK fresh produce is used wherever possible. Meals come boxed, in sealed compartment trays ready to reheat in the oven or microwave, and can be bought chilled (shelf life, seven days) or frozen. The range currently comprises mixed bean and vegetable curry with spiced turmeric rice; penne pasta with mushroom, tomato and basil sauce; braised beef olives with sautéed leeks and potato purée; and ragoût of lamb in red wine and mushroom sauce with creamed parsnips and potatoes. A generous 400g portion per box, priced at around £3 for vegetarian meals and £4 for meat. Available nationwide through organic/wholefood and fine food shops, Out of This World, supermarkets, a few selected box schemes and mail order specialists, and from Planet Organic in London. For stockists tel: 01450 374746.

Others Evernat have a new range of soups – carrot, vegetable and tomato – in 500ml glass jars, to be found in the chilled section (shelf life, six weeks). Whole Earth produce ready-made chilled vegetarian pâtés, tempeh burgers, Seitan Casserole and Chilli Non Carne; plus frozen vegetables. Waitrose sell ready-cooked organic beetroot.

Mail Order: Swaddles Green Farm (p. 106) offer the most extensive range of meat and non-meat cooked dishes. The other meat-supplier offering a wide range is Graig Farm (see p. 104). Both also offer ready-to-eat pizzas and home-made chicken and beef stock cubes.

Organic Jams, Spreads and Marmalade

Commercial organic jams, spreads and marmalades are usually made from organic fruit and a natural organic sweetener, be it concentrated apple or other fruit juice or honey, and natural fruit pectin. This means they are healthier. It also means that they do not taste like ordinary fruit and white-sugar jams, and so are not to everyone's taste. They tend to be more concentrated, and the use of apple juice can sometimes produce an aftertaste not found in ordinary jams. Organic fruit spreads consists of mainly fruit, have a thick, soft texture, are suitable for diabetics and typically contain less than half the calories of conventional jams. They can be used in many ways: as a filling for cakes and pancakes, mixed with organic yoghurt as an instant dessert, made into sweet-sour sauces, or thinned down with a little extra fruit juice and laced with a dash of brandy as a fruit sauce to accompany ice-cream

The fruit content of organic jams and spreads varies, though most are higher in fruit than many conventional brands. Note, too, that the size of jars varies, and take it into account when comparing prices.

Major brands are:

Achillea Organic Italian preserves, made with 80 per cent fruit, 10 per cent malt and 10 per cent apple juice concentrate. The range comprises apple, apricot, bilberry and chestnut. 300g jars.

Allos A range of high-quality tangy, pure fruit spreads sweetened with neutral-flavoured agave syrup, which gives the spreads a vibrant fresh flavour, and set with natural pectin and lemon juice. The range comprises organic apricot, blackcurrant, cherry, strawberry and wild blueberry. 250g jars.

Crofter's Organic Conserves A recently introduced American range, with seven different flavours including Golden Apricot, Sicilian Blood Orange and Wild Blackberry. 283g jars.

De Rit Produce a range of deluxe organic fruit conserves sweetened with a mild wild honey and set with natural lemon rind pectin, some to Demeter standard. If you want a flavour most like conventional jams, try these. The range comprises apricot, strawberry and blackcurrant conserve, Demeter-registered cherry and plum conserve, marmalade, and Wild Forest and wild raspberry conserve. 400g jars.

Ekoland A recent addition, with the most extensive variety: apricot, blackcurrant, blueberry, blue plum, buckthorn, cranberry, elderberry, mixed berry, morello cherry and orange marmalade spreads. 250g jars.

Meridian Manufacture a range of high-quality all-fruit spreads containing only organic fruit, sweetened with concentrated organic apple juice set with lime pectin. The flavour is excellent, delicious with yoghurt. The range comprises apricot, blackcurrant, morello cherry, strawberry, wild blueberry and Seville orange. Recipe leaflets available. 284g jars.

Whole Earth Market a range of spreads sweetened with concentrated organic apple juice. They contain a proportion of water and are runnier than most. The range comprises organic apricot, cherry, strawberry and thin-cut orange marmalade. 300g jars.

Others 100 per cent apple and pear spread (Rapunzel).

Home-made organic jams and marmalades
A small range, of which two examples are:

Botton Village, North Yorks. tel: 01287 661 273 Demeter-registered. Make a range of jams, jellies and marmalades from organic fruit and organic raw cane sugar, for sale at the Food Centre shop on the estate, local outlets, Bumblebee wholefood shop in north London and other Camphill Village Trust centres. The range comprises apricot, blackcurrant, gooseberry, redcurrant, rhubarb and ginger, and strawberry jam; blackcurrant and redcurrant jelly, and Seville orange and grapefruit marmalade. The blackcurrant jam is superb. 340g jars.

Village Bakery Soil Association registered. A new range comprising blackcurrant, damson, gooseberry, plum and raspberry jams, and Seville orange and three-fruits marmalades made from organic fruit and raw cane sugar. 340g jars. Available by mail order.

Price guide: In general, organic jams and spreads cost around 40 per cent more than the equivalent conventional health-food jam or spread, around the same price as premium jams and less than luxury jams. Prices also vary depending on the manufacturer. Expect to pay around £1.70–£2.15 for 280–300g jars and around £2.50 for 400g jars. Home-made jams and marmalades vary from around £1.90 to £3.50 per 340g jar.

Organic Juices

Organic juices, made from organic fruit and vegetables, are delicious and are health drinks in their own right. They come fresh or concentrated, clear or thick, and range from the familiar apple and orange to exotic combinations. Many are imported, and all are certified. Pasteurised organic Florida orange juice, found in the chilled drink section of shops and supermarkets, is available in 1 litre cartons. A taste of the future, also from America, the first sparkling squashes are a world away from what most canned drinks are made of.

Once opened, bottled juices and cartons will keep in the fridge for three or four days, or longer for certain brands, though they are best drunk as soon as possible. Organic apple juice is cheaper than other organic juices, and some is made from different named varieties of apples. The thick, pulpy juices pressed from the whole fruit are more like a food, and best taken in small glasses and savoured slowly – which is what juice therapists recommend for any juice. Prune juice is surprisingly good.

Organic fruit and vegetable juices can also be used in cooking. Eden, for example, have produced two recipe leaflets for sweet and savoury dishes using their organic carrot, vegetable and beetroot juices, written by cookery expert Roz Denny. Write to PO Box 1059, Pulborough, West Sussex RH20 2YX.

Given the intensive use of pesticides on fruit, it's not surprising that residues are detected in some conventional fruit juices, including blackcurrant drinks, and in apple juice particularly. The 1994 WPPR report found that a quarter of UK-produced apple juice samples contained permitted fungicide residues, for example, and 10 per cent contained multiple residues. As explained in relation to baby food (p. 233), statistics show that infants especially, and toddlers and small children, who are all more susceptible to toxic chemicals than adults are, drink much higher quantities of juices, especially orange and apple; indeed, juices form a significant part of their diet. So try to give them organic when you can.

- Organic fruit and vegetable juices contain no artificial colourings or preservatives. The only preservative used is vitamin C.
- Most come in large – 700, 735 and 750ml – bottles; and 200ml bottles are also available; concentrated organic juices come in 375ml bottles.

Most I have tried have been excellent, with pure bursting-with-health flavours. The Florida chilled orange juice inevitably has that slightly flat pasteurised flavour if compared to the freshly squeezed sort. Varietal apple juices are really distinctive, and pear juices uniformly delicious. Add plain or sparkling mineral water to thick fruit juices, and you have a thirst-quenching drink.

Bottled fruit juices are excellent for breakfast, or diluted as non-alcoholic alternatives when entertaining. Vegetable juices are good lunchtime revivers – easier than making soup – or can be taken instead of a meal if you're feeling too tired to eat. Carrot juice, reckoned to be the most cleansing and revitalising juice, is delicious and the one to try first, while tomato juice is noted for its blood-purifying properties. Vegetable cocktail juices vary slightly in flavour depending on the mix, though are predominantly carrot and tomato. Clear beetroot juice is nothing like as strong as you would imagine. Therapeutically, it's rated second-highest to carrot juice and, like carrot, is recommended extensively in alternative cancer therapies. *Juice Therapy*, by Ray Hill, available from Sunshine Health Foods (p. 216), gives more information about the healing properties of organic juices and about how Biotta juices are made. Remember mail order organic wine companies also stock them.

Here is a selection of *major brands* and juices available:

Achillea Apple, apricot, cherry, grape, peach, pear, plum.

La Bio-Idea Apple, orange and red orange.

Biona Apple, orange, red grape, plum nectar; carrot, tomato, vegetable cocktail.

Biotta See p. 297.

Eden Beetroot, carrot and vegetable cocktail. The juices are flash-pasteurised in the bottle, which minimises nutrient losses to 1–2

Crone's apple-variety juices

Crone's, Kenninghall, Norfolk tel: 01379 687687 Soil Association registered. Produce award-winning single-variety organic apple juices such as Worcester, Russet and Cox, as well as delicious apple and pear blends and apple and sour cherry, pressed in their own cider press. All their fruit is UK-grown. They also produce organic pink grapefruit juice, and a range of traditional organic ciders and cider vinegar. Their juices can be bought direct from the farm by appointment, and are widely available in London, East Anglia, the Midlands and the south-east. They also supply farm shops.
Highly recommended.

per cent. The beetroot juice (clear and delicious) is fermented with lacto-fermenting bacteria, a process that gives it nutritional extras and is said to benefit intestinal flora, making it easier to digest and absorb nutrients and helping to increase resistance to intestinal infections. Widely distributed and stocked by major supermarkets. Recipe leaflets are available.

Evernat Apple, orange, grapefruit; carrot, vegetable.

Jacoby Demeter-registered apple and carrot, Children's, red grape, tomato, vegetable cocktail.

Rabenhorst Beetroot, carrot, grape.

Sedlescombe Vineyards Their 1066 brand comprises apple, pear, English grape, apple and blackcurrant, apple and grape. See p. 103.

Vitalia Beetroot, carrot, prune, red grape, white grape, vegetable cocktail.

Voelkel A high-quality Demeter-registered German brand run by a family firm involved in organic farming for generations. Their extensive range includes many mixed juices such as apple and pineapple; apple, blackcurrant and grape; and apple and mango. Plus single-fruit juices, Seven Dwarfs (children's) and Vital ACE juice. The bottles – small, medium and large – are filled to order, and arrive in the shops eight days, at most, after bottling.

Whole Earth Active Eight vegetable juice, Apple Magic (spiced apple) drink.

Others include apple (Aspell's and Peake's), lemon juice (Rapunzel), white grape (Jus'Louc), and red grape juice (Domaine de Brau).

Fruit juice concentrates
Concentrates are made by pressing the fruit, and filtering the juice to remove the solids; it is then clarified and refiltered, and finally

evaporated under a vacuum at 65°C, to drive off the water. The low temperature avoids a 'caramelised' or 'cooked' flavour and ensures a relatively fresh one. Care also needs to be taken by the manufacturer with apple concentrates, for example, to choose varieties with a good flavour and acidity. These two factors determine the quality of the finished product. Organic fruit concentrates are produced in exactly the same way as conventional ones. Some use bentonite, a natural mineral fining agent, instead of isinglass (derived from fish).

The *main brands* are:

Meridian Apple. They don't use isinglass to clarify their concentrates.

Morgenland Apple, pear, apple and blackcurrant, apple and cherry.

Voelkel Pear.

Biotta organic juices

A specialist, family-run Swiss juice company that has pioneered organic farming methods for over thirty years and has its own farms, plus others who grow specifically for it, in Switzerland, Austria and Israel. All crops (and soil) undertake rigorous laboratory analysis for purity. The fruit is pressed in as natural a way as possible, and the juices are preserved naturally by the addition of lacto-fermented whey, which also preserves the maximum amount of nutrients. They will keep for up to eight days in the fridge. The juices are commonly used in cure centres. Their range includes the specially formulated 'Breuss' vegetable juice, used in cancer therapy and as a dietary tonic, plus freshly squeezed orange and grapefruit juice.

Also

Camphill Village Trust, Botton, N. Yorks. tel: 01287 661250
Produce a range of organic juices and cordials for sale in their
shop and at local outlets. The range comprises apple, and apple
and pear, freshly pressed; apple and pear concentrates; and apple,
blackcurrant, pear, plum, redcurrant and strawberry cordials and
lemon squash. Just the thing to refresh your thirst when visiting
the area, their award-winning redcurrant cordial is especially
good.

Rock's Country Cordials, Loddon Park Farm, Twyford, Berks.
tel: 01734 342344 Have recently introduced a range of organic
cordials – orange, lemon, ginger and elderflower – certified by the
Soil Association, comprising purely organic fruit and sugar.
Cordials are made on the farm and retail at around £3.25 a bottle,
which makes three litres of squash. Available from the farm shop
and through health food shops nationwide. Excellent flavour,
though only for the sweet-toothed.

Sparkling drinks

As yet not generally available, but hopefully coming soon. *Santa
Cruz*, the organic arm of one of America's leading juice companies, R.W. Knudsen, have recently introduced their range of high-
quality organic carbonated drinks, comprising lemonade, ginger
ale, lemon and lime, orange and mango, tropical guava and raspberry lemonade. The drinks are made with carbonated filtered
well water, organic juices, cane juice and flavourings. The
company operates rigorous quality-control checks, testing its
products for purity, and the drinks are certified by an American
certifying body, QAI. More of their organic juice range is expected
to follow.

| fact | 'Comminuted' orange juices and drinks are made from the pulp and skin, where pesticide residues are frequently detected, as well as from the juice, and are reconstituted using tap water. |

Price guide: Most organic fruit juices are expensive, though prices are beginning to fall. Expect to pay £2.25–£3.50 for large bottles, £4.50–£5 for concentrates, and less for apple juices. One exception is Florida chilled orange juice, which sells at only 10p more than its conventional equivalent at around 99p per carton.

Organic Nuts and Seeds

If you try organic nuts and seeds, you will often find they have a better flavour. This is partly because they are sometimes sourced from different countries, and may be grown from different varieties. Organic almonds, for example, which come from Spain, have a darker, thicker and more bitter skin but a far richer, more distinctive flavour than the conventional bland almonds from California, and are to be especially recommended. It is the same with certain seeds. The most noteworthy are organic pumpkin seeds, from Hungary, not China – the Rapunzel brand, for instance, are darker-skinned, larger, plumper and far more delicious than your average pumpkin seeds. I find the same with African organic sesame seeds; but having chomped my way through several bags, I can detect little noticeable difference between conventional and organic sunflower seeds. There is sometimes, also, as so often with organic crops, more cosmetic variation, so do not expect them to be all the same size, shape or colour.

All organic nuts and seeds are grown without artificial fertilisers or synthetic pesticides, which means that yields are lower. Nor do they receive post-harvest treatments during shipment and storage, as is often the case with conventional nuts and seeds (peanuts, walnuts and pumpkin seeds are regularly treated with fumigants). Because supplies are very limited, they cost anything from 50 to 100 per cent more than conventional nuts and seeds. However, prices are gradually decreasing – see the chart on p. 31. As they are very light, the extra cost per portion of sesame, sunflower and pumpkin seeds is minimal, and these are good organic items to change to when you can.

TIP: Toasted organic hazelnuts, walnuts and sesame seeds all make an excellent salad dressing for salad leaves, as well as for vegetables such as cooked green beans, beetroot, cauliflower and broccoli. Toast and crush one tablespoon or so of the nuts or seeds with a little salt in a pestle and mortar, stir in organic olive oil and drizzle over the salad or cooked vegetables.

The two *major UK prepacked brands* are *Infinity Foods* and *Suma*; two others are *Community Foods* and *Essential*. The main imported brand is *Rapunzel*; another is *Morgenland*. Registered organic shops often buy in bulk for repacking. If you eat a lot of nuts and seeds, remember that both are much more economical when bought in large quantities. Excellent news is that there's a new range to look out for, *Nature's Way*, offering high-quality nuts (and dried fruit, coconut and popcorn), mostly organic, which come in foil packaging and at a single promotional price, 98p at the time of writing.

Something unusual to try, also recommended, is hempseed from a small company called *Hempseed Organics*. The seeds are crunchy and have a slightly buttery flavour, are brimming with essential fatty acids and amino acids and so are highly nutritious; they are good to snack on and to use lightly toasted, scattered over salads. Available in selected health food shops or direct through mail order tel: 0171 833 3178 E-Mail hempseed@En.apc.org together with a leaflet including recipes. New Earth tel: 01248 490239 E-mail mail@hemp.compulink.co.uk, another specialist hempseed company, also supply organic hempseeds and produce a range of organic hempseed products – cold pressed oil, hemp muesli and four different snack bars, including Hemp Flapjack and Chocolate 9bar – available widely. Interested to know more about how wonderful hempseed is? Contact New Earth's hempseed website on http://www.hemp.co.uk

Otherwise:

Nuts All available in different forms, including blanched, flaked and ground organic almonds and desiccated coconut. Rapunzel offer macadamia nuts, roasted and salted almonds, peanuts and pistachios, ground hazelnuts, coconut chips, pine kernels, mixed nuts and Trail Mix.

Seeds Alfalfa, hemp, linseed, pumpkin, sesame, sunflower. Rapunzel offer poppy seeds.

It's well worth pointing out that nuts and seeds do not last for ever – around nine to twelve months at most. How long they last depends on the oil content: the higher the oil content – it is particularly high, for example, in hazelnuts, Brazils, coconut and sesame seeds – the shorter the shelf life. Nuts have a shorter shelf life than seeds, and are particularly prone to rancidity. Both should be stored somewhere cool and dark – never in the light.

For pesticide residues in nuts and seeds, see Appendix 1, p. 342.

Price guide: Organic nuts range in price from around 70p for peanuts to £1.80 for whole cashews for a 125g packet, and around £1.80–£6.50 for a 500g pack. Pine kernels retail at around £3.50 per 100g. Organic seeds range from around 50p for sunflower seeds to £1.20 for pumpkin seeds per 125g packet, and around £1.70–£3.60 for a 500g pack.

Seeds for sprouting The seed is the 'vital' part of a plant, and where its inherent health is thought to be most potent. Organic alfalfa, cress, radish, mustard and sprouting mix are sold under the *Davert Muhle* brand.

Sprouted seeds Ready-sprouted organic seeds are widely available and cost very little more than the conventional equivalent. Look for them in the chilled cabinet of alternative supermarkets, and organic/wholefood/health food shops. Worth knowing is that alfalfa sprouts are much better value than conventional mustard and cress. Weight for weight you get far more for your money, they

> **fact** Some studies have shown that the seeds of crops grown conventionally lose their potency within three to four generations.

are more nutritious, and they are the only plant source of vitamin B12, so particularly important for vegetarians and vegans. They have a delicate flavour. Organic mung beans are sweet and crunchy.

Two popular brands of sprouted seeds are:

Aconbury Alfalfa, alfalfa and radish, chick-pea, mung bean, and mixed bean sprouts.

Skysprouts Alfalfa, alfalfa and radish, chick-pea, lentil, mung bean, and mixed bean sprouts.

Wheatgrass, the latest wonder health food, made from organic wheat sprouts and packed with essential vitamins and minerals, is said to boost the immune system. Available freshly juiced from Planet Organic, London.

Organic Olive Oil

Sadly, the image of olive oil as a 'pure' food produced by natural or traditional methods is no longer realistic. Most is produced from olives grown by modern methods dependent on chemical fertilisers and pesticides; whereas organic olive oil is pressed from olives grown naturally, using organic methods of cultivation. Often organic groves are in mountainous regions, where pests are less prevalent anyway, and where it is difficult to cultivate *except* by traditional methods. Though more olive groves are converting to organic production, especially in Spain, supply is still very limited: there are just a few French, Italian, Spanish and Greek organic olive oils, a good proportion of which are pressed in the traditional way.

Currently, all organic olive oils are extra-virgin, the highest grade you can buy, and are grown to the same set of standards throughout the EU. They are certified by one of the recognised organic certification bodies of the country in which they are grown, who inspects the groves and the production procedures and whose code number or symbol should be present on the label.

Broadly there are two types to choose from, everyday olive oils and premium ones:

Everyday olive oils Reasonably priced, and usually produced on a commercial scale in modern mills using organic olives from various growers. They are ideal for general cooking and dressings. Widely available brands are *La Bio-Idea* (Italian) and *Sunita* (Greek), plus *Meadowsweet*, *Midsummer* and *Suma* (no country of origin stated). Two other good-value ones are *Provence Regime* and *Rapunzel*. The most common brand, *Meridian* (Spanish), is exceptional value in that it is an award-winning premium oil but comes within the everyday price bracket, as does *Bio Aras* olive oil, both from Andalucía.

Premium olive oils Correspond to – indeed, in many cases are – estate-bottled conventional oils and command a similar high price. Most are produced by small growers who use traditional methods, which include picking the olives by hand and pressing the oil in traditional mills. Supply is limited. They should be used for dips and dressings, for salads, hot vegetables, pasta and risotto, and to pour over grilled meats and fish as a final enhancement.

They include *Mani* (Greek); *L'Estornell* and *Nuñez de Prado* (Spanish); *Romanico* (Catalan); *Oleificio Gabro*, *Campo*, *Il Casale*, *De Vito*, *Fattoria 'Roi'*, *La Terra E Il Cielo* and *Azienda Agricola S. Christiana* (Italian); *Ravida* (Sicilian); *Sadeg* and *Spectrum Organic* (Californian); *Mas de la Dame*, *Mas de Gourgonnier* (Provençal) and *Sphere* (French). Fortnum & Mason in London sell the only Demeter-registered olive oil, from *Fattoria Mose*, in Sicily, under their own label. *Seggiano* estate-bottled olive oil from a small group of growers near Sienna in Tuscany is made from a unique and ancient variety of olivastra olive, which produces a mild, delicate oil. The olives have always been grown without pesticides, are hand-picked and pressed in a traditional stone mill. The oil is expected to be certified organic in 1998.

Do organic olive oils taste different?

No. The flavour of all olive oils, whether organically produced or not, depends on the country of origin, the variety of olive, the climate, the acidity of the oil, how it is processed, and whether the oil is blended to suit a particular market. However, because organic olive oil is produced on a much smaller scale than the conventional kind, and often by small producers using traditional methods, many organic olive oils are individual oils with distinctive flavour notes.

Buying and storing: Olive oil is a matter of personal taste, so the first rule is to try different types to discover which ones you like. Remember that Greek, Spanish, French and Italian oils all have their own character, style and flavour, and that olive oils in dark bottles or in tins are protected from the light and will keep better than those in clear bottles.

The two guiding rules when buying olive oil are:

- Never buy oil that has been displayed under bright lights; light causes oxidation, which will make the oil deteriorate.
- Check the sell-by date; if possible, look for the harvest date – which will tell you when the oil was pressed – and buy the most recent vintage.

If stored correctly, olive oil has a shelf life of two or three years – though you will use it much sooner. As all organic olive oil is extra-virgin, neither processed nor heat-treated, you should store it carefully. Keep it somewhere cool and dark, and make sure you don't leave it on the table when the light streams in.

TIP: Extra-virgin olive oil may go cloudy and become solid in cold weather, and unfiltered oils will form a deposit in the bottom of the bottle.

Price guide: Producing organic olive oil is a precarious, costly, labour-intensive business that requires dedication. Given this, and the fact that all organic olive oil is extra-virgin, prices are not extortionate. Everyday oils currently sell at approximately £4–£5 per 500ml bottle, that is, at 30 per cent more than an equivalent conventionally produced oil. Premium oils, which are comparable to conventional estate-bottled oils, sell for around £8–£9 per 500ml bottle. As with the conventional kind, Greek and Spanish organic olive oils represent the best value for money. Italian and French organic oils are the most expensive. Look out for introductory promotional offers. Best-value oils are Bio Aras and Meridian. Also good value is Nuñez de Prado in 5 litre tins from the Oil Merchant (below), Mas de Gourgonnier in 5 litre tins from the Organic Wine Co. (p. 103), and L'Estornell olive oil sold loose from Bluebird, all in London.

Where to buy: Everyday organic olive oils are readily available from organic/wholefood/health food shops and alternative supermarkets. Premium olive oils are available from high-class food shops and specialist wine merchants and by mail order. Major supermarkets as yet stock very little, and in selected stores only. Sainsbury's and Booths in the north sell Meridian organic olive oil, Tesco sell Oleificio Gabro in their Italian Selection, Safeway are about to start selling organic olive oil at the time of writing, and Waitrose have just started.

Others Box schemes, home delivery and farm shops sometimes stock organic olive oil.

Mail order: The Oil Merchant tel: 0181 740 1335 is the country's leading olive oil specialist. Catalogue available and help and advice given. Stocks four organic olive oils, Mani, L'Estornell, Sphere and Nuñez de Prado. Take It from Here Ltd, freephone order number 0800 137064, supply 'Roi' Carte Noir and 'Roi' Biologica. The Organic Wine Company tel: 01494 446557 supply Il Casale Tuscan olive oil, and award-winning Mas de Gourgonnier Provençal oil in 1 litre and 5 litres. Organic olive oil is also available from Organic Health, Countryside Foods Ltd., Damhead Organically Grown Foods and Longwood Farm (pp. 98–106).

Producing organic olive oil
This first-hand account by Joachim I.F. Blok, an olive oil producer in Spain, tells how organic olives and olive oil are produced:

> In Spain most olive groves are in the south, especially in the Andalusian provinces of Sevilla, Córdoba and Jaén. Other main growing areas are Extremadura and Zaragoza, and there is a small production in Cataluña. The groves are generally situated in hilly areas

with little rainfall and generally poor soil. Olive trees are very tough and able to subsist on few nutrients and scarce rainfall. Olive groves also do a marvellous job of preventing soil erosion in these areas.

In conventional groves, herbicides are applied twice – once in early spring to prevent seeds germinating, and again a few months later to kill any vegetation that has begun to grow. Insecticides are used systematically for all types of possible plague in the olive grove. These are always used whatever the size of the plague may be. These products kill all useful fauna as well. The ground is principally fertilised with urea, and other chemical fertilisers.

In organic groves, ploughing is less deep so as not to alter the topsoil characteristics. If there is too much vegetation between the trees this is cut down, chopped up, and usually ploughed back into the soil as a fertiliser. Vegetation generally has to be cut back because of competition with the trees for scarce rainfall and nutrients, and in order to facilitate the work of the harvesters. Pheromone traps for insects are hung in the trees in order to ascertain the size of any possible plague. If the activity of any particular plague goes above tolerance levels, then specific pest-control products are used that are compatible with organic agriculture, that don't contaminate soil or water and don't harm most of the useful fauna. Fertilisation is done by sowing nitrogen-fixing vegetation in between the trees, which will then be ploughed back into the ground with other natural products such as guano and dolomite.

Cross-contamination with other olive groves is avoided by physical barriers such as a river, strips of non-agricultural land, mountains or even dense bands of trees around organic farms. This is essential for [organic] certification. Many farms find it impossible to convert to organic production because of the proximity and nature of their neighbours.

In our groves, Hojiblanca olives are primarily used, which yield the finest-quality oils: soft and sweet, but fruity. The olives are hand-picked off the trees and taken the same day to the mill before fermentation can begin, which destroys oil quality. There is rigorous washing of fruit and machinery and the lowest-possible temperatures are used while pressing. In conventional olive oil production these strict standards are not obligatory, and are rarely embraced.

Tasting notes

The following descriptions and tasting notes of some of the readily available organic olive oils mentioned in this section are from *The Olive Oil Companion*, written by olive oil authority Judy Ridgway, recently published by Little, Brown.

Fattoria 'Roi' From the one-hundred- to six-hundred-year-old groves in Liguria, produced by a small family firm established in 1900. The oil is pressed from Taggiasca olives in a traditional mill. 'Has a very attractive light almond aroma with apples and a touch of grassiness. The flavour is sweet and nutty with a light pepper and a little tart bitterness on the aftertaste. This is a very smooth, delicately complex and versatile oil.' For those who like mild olive oil, this is one of the most gentle you will find.

Mani From groves on the slopes of the Taygetos mountains, which run from Kalamata to Sparta in Greece. The oil is pressed from Koroneiki olives, harvested by hand. Half are pressed in the traditional manner, half by the cold centrifugal process. 'A very fruity oil with a flavour very reminiscent of pine resin. The aroma is all freshly mown grass and apple skins, and the flavour full of salad leaves and sweet-sour sorrel with only a touch of pepper.'

Meridian Organic From groves near Córdoba, Andalusia. The oil is pressed from Hojiblanca olives, harvested by hand and pressed using the cold centrifugal system. 'An aromatic lemony aroma, sometimes with a touch of tomato coulis. The flavour is smooth and lemony with a medium peppery finish.'

Nuñez de Prado From groves in Baena, Andalusia, produced by the Nuñez de Prado family since 1795. The oil is pressed from a mixture of Picudo, Hojiblanca and Picual olives, harvested by hand and pressed in the traditional manner in their own mill. Their premium oil, known as *flor* or 'flower' of the oil, is described thus by Judy: 'This wonderful extra-virgin olive oil has a very consistent aroma and flavour and varies very little from year to year. There is only a touch of pepper, with a lovely smooth, sweet aftertaste.' The oil available in large tins (which I use) has similar characteristics – expect a gentle, buttery oil.

Oleificio Gabro From groves in the Calabrian hills, produced by the largest private organic oil-producer in Italy. The oil is pressed from a mixture of 70 per cent Tondino and 30 per cent Grossa di Cassano olives, harvested by hand and pressed either traditionally or in centrifugal presses. 'A delicate but definite aroma of freshly crushed olives, grass and fruits like apples and even raspberries. The flavour is equally complex. It is full of fruit and nuts and, of course, olives with a light to medium pepper. The aftertaste is sweet.'

Sunita From groves in Mani. The oil is pressed from Kalamata olives in the traditional manner. 'Has a fresh apple aroma with grassy, lemony tones. The flavour is full and fruity with plenty of mown grass and bitter leaves like watercress. The pepper is deceptively light to start with, but builds up to quite a spicy finish.'

Organic Olives

Organic table olives are grown in the same way as those used for organic olive oil. In addition, they are not subjected to treatment with caustic soda – common in conventional olive-curing – but are cured entirely naturally with salt and water only. Most are Spanish and not yet sold loose, but in jars. *Bio Aras* is the main brand, with a range of black, green and stuffed olives retailing for around £1.50–£2.40 per jar. *Sunita* and *TerraSana* also do black olives (see list on page 318). Once opened, keep in the fridge. Alternatively, a good way to store them – and the best way for any loose olives you buy – is to drain off the brine and keep them in a small jar covered with olive oil.

Other Organic Oils

A complete range of other organic oils is available, including cooking oils, speciality oils and, from the USA, the latest state-of-

Designer health oils

These highly nutritious organic health oils, brimming with essential omega fatty acids, imported from the USA or Canada, could point to the latest food craze. There are several to choose from, each comprising a slightly different blend of oils extracted under special low temperature conditions to safeguard them from air, light and heat, and are hermetically sealed in dark bottles. All can be used for salad dressings or to pour over vegetables, or taken as a dietary supplement, and have, in the main, pleasant nutty flavours. They must be refrigerated and cost around £8–£9 for a small 250ml bottle. Available from health food shops, three well-known brands are:

Essential Balance A blend of flax, sunflower, sesame, pumpkin and borage oils.

Spectrum Naturals Produce flax, flax and borage, and hemp oils and a specially formulated Essential Max oil.

Udo's Choice Formulated by Udo Erasmus, a recognised expert and author on oils and fats, this is a blend of flax, sesame and sunflower oils with added vitamin E, and other essential nutrients.

the-art health oils. All are cold-pressed: this preserves the maximum nutritional value, which is considerable, and the flavour of the oils. It also means that, for example, a cold-pressed organic sunflower seed oil will not be bland and flavourless but will taste strongly of sunflower seeds, so allow for this in your cooking, keeping such oils for salad dressings rather than for frying. And because the flavours are positive, you need very little as a flavouring agent.

The precautions to be taken when buying and storing olive oil apply to these oils too.

Major brands are:

Emile Noël Pumpkin, rape seed and walnut oil.
Flora and Higher Nature Flax seed oil, a recent introduction, used for salads and uncooked dishes.
Meridian Safflower, sesame, sunflower oil.
Provence Regime Sesame, sunflower oil.
Rapunzel Have the largest selection, all in dark-brown bottles so as to exclude the light. Hazelnut, pumpkin seed, walnut oils; soya, safflower, sunflower, sesame; coconut fat.
Suma Sunflower oil.

Others Prospective Foods, Midsummer (sunflower oil); Kitchen Garden (soya and sunflower oil); Spectrum Products (sesame, safflower, canola).

Price guide: Organic safflower, sesame and sunflower oils are cheaper than organic olive oil, at around £2.25–£3.80 per 500ml bottle, while hazelnut, walnut, flax seed and pumpkin seed are more expensive, at around £6.50–£9 for a 250ml bottle.

Organic Pasta and Pasta Sauces

Pasta

Do not fear that your favourite kind of dried pasta isn't here – it is, and including stuffed tortellini. The range is staggering. Add to that an ever-increasing variety of non-wheat, gluten-free organic pastas and you probably have a wider choice than on most conventional shelves. New brands and varieties are constantly being added, both wholewheat and white.

The eating quality of organic dried pasta is exactly the same as that of other pastas; as with conventional dried pasta, the best, such as that of La Terra E Il Cielo, is made using traditional methods including slow drying, and is a little more expensive. Alas, no one is making *fresh* organic pasta – though I predict it won't be long. Note that although organic wheat pasta cooks and tastes exactly the same as conventional pasta, organic non-wheat pastas, produced primarily for those allergic to wheat or on gluten-free diets, taste entirely different – more like the grain they are made from – and most cook to a softer texture. It all depends on what you like. Food writer Annie Bell, for example, describes spelt pasta as pinkish in colour and quite fragrant and earthy, saying that it works best with rich vegetable sauces such as ratatouille, spinach or aubergine – though try convincing my husband, who would not sacrifice traditional pasta for anything. All organic pasta is made with certified organic durum wheat or other grains; and any other ingredients, such as the tomato and spinach in flavoured pastas, are also certified organic.

> **WATCHWORD:** Though it sounds organic, save for brown rice rigatoni and rice and ginseng spirals, Orgran, the Australian brand of speciality gluten-free pastas, is not organic.

Finally, if you are concerned about residues in conventional wheat, organic wholewheat pasta in particular may be a good idea; the last time it was analysed, in 1993, over a third of wholemeal pasta samples contained OP residues, as did over 15 per cent of both dried white and fresh pasta samples.

Major brands are:

Baby Organix Infant and toddler pasta shapes.

Biona Rice pasta.

Bionaturae An American brand of white pastas, including rigatoni and chiocciole.

Buonapasta A range of white pastas, including capelli d'angelo, farfalle, fusilli, maccheroni, penne, spaghetti and stellini (tiny star shapes for soup).

Campo From the Marche, Italy, a range of traditionally produced, high-quality pastas using home-grown freshly stoneground wheat, dried at low temperatures: 10 different wholewheat – including cavatappi (corkscrew) – 6 white and 6 speciality flavoured pastas, including spaghetti al peperoncino and spinach linguini.

De Rit Demeter-registered bio-dynamic pasta. Wholewheat macaroni, shells, spaghetti and spirelli.

Ecogrande A range of wholewheat and white pastas.

Eunature Wholewheat and white pastas, both available as fusilli, lasagne, macaroni, penne and spaghetti. Also, white tricolore fusilli.

Eu Vita A traditionally produced range of wholewheat and white pastas from Bologna, including maccheroni, coquillettes and penne rigate.

Everfresh Sell the Giovanni range of pasta: spaghettini with turmeric, tagliolini with basil and tortellini stuffed with mushroom or smoked tofu. The pastas are egg-free and are not dried but vacuum-packed; which means that they cook like fresh pasta, in three to five minutes.

Evernat Wholemeal spaghetti and penne, and tricolore fusilli.

La Bio-Idea Ten different sorts of wholewheat pasta shapes including lasagne verdi and wholewheat tricolore. Six different white pastas including gomitini ('little elbows') and tricolore twists.

La Terra E Il Cielo The widest range of standard and speciality wholewheat and white pastas, over twenty-five in total, produced using the traditional methods of the Marche region of Italy. Shapes include farfalle, orecchiette and alfabeti. Speciality pastas include buckwheat fettuccine, spaghetti with artichoke and spinach, carrot and beetroot puntine and three spelt pastas.

Lima Kamut penne and spaghetti.

L'Origine Demeter-registered children's pasta: wholewheat, wheat- and gluten-free, four-cereal, colourful, light pasta.

Organico Wholewheat and white spaghetti and penne; white fusilli and pasta shells.

Rapunzel A range of eleven pastas including non-wheat pastas such as spelt spaghetti, kamut macaroni, millet lumaconi and soya cornetti, and alphabet soup pasta.

Vita spelt Low-gluten pastas made with spelt: gomitini, spaghetti and spirals.

Price guide: The extra cost per serving for basic pastas is minimal. Traditionally produced organic pastas are cheaper than most up-market brands of conventionally produced pasta. Expect to pay around 90p–£1.50 per 500g packet for standard pastas, and up to £2.50 for speciality and non-wheat pastas. Look out for promotional bargains.

Organic pasta sauces

Organic tomato, mushroom, ragù and simple vegetable pasta sauces are easily made at home. But if you want to buy them ready-made, bottled vegetarian organic pasta sauces, including pestos, are on the shelves, and more are on the way. Those I have tried are of high quality and compare very favourably to conventional sauces of the same standard – though no bottled sauce can be expected to have the same appeal as a freshly made one. Inevitably, those imported from Italy, such as the excellent crema di rucola and pesto by '*Roi*', available by mail order (see p. 99), have the most authentic tastes. Tomato and basil sauces are generally a good bet. The American brand, *Muir Glen*, produces an extensive range of tinned fat-free pasta sauces including sweet pepper and onion, and roasted garlic.

   Others: Tomato and basil sauce (Campo, Eunature) and tomato, and tomato and mushroom sauces (Evernat); a variety of vegetable pasta sauces – artichoke, aubergine, mixed-pepper, pea, mixed-vegetable; Mediterranean pasta sauce (Cereal Terra); Giovanni mushroom and tomato cream sauce (Everfresh); garlic and herb pasta sauce (Meridian); basil, caper and mushroom sauce (Organico); children's and Tuscan pasta sauce (Rapunzel); Italiano and mushroom sauces (Whole Earth). Campo, La Bio-Idea, Rapunzel and 'Roi' all produce pestos.

Price guide: Prices and size of containers vary, and it pays to shop around when you can. Depending on size, they range from about £1.30–£1.95 for sauces and £1.50–£2.50 for pestos.

Snacks and Confectionery

There is very little organic confectionery; but the range of fruit and nut and seed bars, chocolate bars (p. 280) and other fruit sweets, though small, is growing. The same goes for savoury snacks. There isn't much available yet, but the exceptions are organic crisps and – especially – corn chips, where there is an embarrassment of choice. The latest arrival here is organic popcorn.

All those I have tried, including liquorice sweets, have been impressive: better flavour, less sickly, no artificial undertones, easier to digest and, in some cases, positively moreish. Organic crisps and corn chips are addictive.

Should you need any further encouragement here, it's worth pointing out, perhaps, that pesticide residues have been detected in, for example, 99 per cent of maize-based snacks in 1995. Residues also occur much more often in crisps made from stored as opposed to unstored potatoes – eleven times more when last tested in 1994, and in over three-quarters of the samples. Unfortunately, whether crisps have been made from stored or non-stored potatoes is not indicated on the packaging.

Almost all organic snacks and confectionery are imported. They include

Organic crisps Made with organic potatoes (skins left on), fried in unhydrogenated organic oil, seasoned with natural flavourings and sea salt; they have a nutty flavour.

    Major brands Evernat, Molen Aartje, Tra'fo. Flavours: plain, paprika; pickle (Tra'fo).

Organic corn chips, tortilla chips Made in the same way as crisps; there are loads to choose from, and they are easy to get hooked on, as are taco shells. Corn chips come in white, yellow or blue, plain or spicy, and in a wide range of flavours. Taste and prices vary, so it's worth trying several. The American Apache brand are made from stoneground organic corn, organic sunflower oil and sea salt. I find the Amaizin brand too salty.

Major brands Amaizin, Apache, Evernat, Margaritas, Mexi-snax, Molen Aartje, Rapunzel, Santa Cruz, TerraSana. Flavours include natural, basil and tomato, black bean and garlic, Cajun, chilli, French onion, Mexicana, sesame.

Other maize snacks, apart from taco shells (Apache, Terra-Sana), include corn puffs Provençal (Apache, Molen Aartje) and the long-awaited organic popcorn, flavoured with coconut oil and sea salt, from Nature's Way and also from Mayka.

> **WATCHWORD:** Mexi-snax produce both organic and conventional tortilla chips in virtually identical packs. Check the label – the organic version has the certification logo on the bottom of the packet.

Other snacks Bio Gouda crackers and pizza crackers (Rapunzel); corn cheese (Molen Aartje), puffed spelt chips, spelt pretzels and sticks (Mayka).

Price guide: Small bags of crisps and tortilla chips cost around 50p. Large bags of crisps around £1.35, large bags of tortilla chips range from 90p–£1.50, depending on brand and size. Popcorn retails at about 85p a bag.

Organic fruit, nut and seed bars Similar to conventional health food bars and just as power-packed. *Allos* have the largest and most exciting range, which includes marzipan, nougat and amaranth bars. *Evernat* have a new range of muesli bars including chocolate-coated hazelnut, and cinnamon and apple. *Shepherd Boy* sunflower fruit and nut bar is one of the most popular and is handy to slip into your pocket or handbag; other bars include Banana Fruitjack (*Tropical Wholefoods*), sesame and honey bar (*Sunita*), and the mightiest of them all, Hemp 9, a hempseed and chocolate sports nutrition bar by *Wholebake*, and other power-packed hemp bars from *New Earth* (p. 300).

Others Include fruit lollipops (Donna, Molen Aartje), various liquorice sweets (Bonvita), liquorice ropes (TerraSana), brown rice treats (Wallaby), coconut bars (Molen Aartje) and banana chips (Allos).

Price guide: These compare favourably to other high quality bars found in health food shops and cost from 40p–75p each. Organic lollipops can be yours for around 25p, and exotic candy bars for around 90p each.

The Store Cupboard A–Z

The list of tinned foods, condiments, dressings, and so on expands daily. Two of my personal favourites, organic tinned tomatoes and passata, are a revelation – they have a rich, fresh flavour nor normally found in tinned tomato products. The same goes for organic tomato purée. Organic mustard, too, is delicious – sweeter and with no harsh overtones. Organic tahini, tamari, stock cubes and cider vinegar are other worthwhile staples. Suma organic chick-peas canned in pure water are a bargain. Organic baked beans do not taste like Heinz; people either love them or hate them.

Beans (tinned) Various sorts including organic baked beans (Whole Earth, De Rit), chick-peas, haricots, red kidney beans (Suma); and a range of tasty spicy Mexican refried beans (TerraSana) – try these as a dip, with olive oil drizzled over, to serve with crudités or bitter salad leaves. They make a good instant lunch, too.

Condiments Range from chilli, curry and garlic paste and mint sauce (Kitchen Garden) to Mediterranean pastes for pasta and vegetables (Cereal Terra). Capers are available in olive oil (Cereal Terra, Rapunzel) or in salt (Cereal Terra). I have also bought wild capers, but do not think they are as good.

Fruit (tinned and in jars) Bottled fruit is popular on the continent, and makes an easy pudding. Organic fruits are usually bottled in a syrup made of water, organic fruit juice and apple concentrate. Morgenland is the main brand, with a range that includes everything from mango and sweet cherries to fruit cocktail. Others include apple purée (Bionova, De Rit) and peach slices (Rapunzel).

Mayonnaise Generally made with sunflower oil, egg yolk, vinegar and seasonings. Major brands are Bio Fan, Evernat and Fertillia, who also produce a low-fat mayonnaise.

Food from Japan

The Japanese take their organic food seriously. They were the first to set up subscription farming and are now becoming the largest per capita consumer of organic food. A wide range of organic Japanese soya bean products, used in macrobiotic diets particularly, are available in the UK, including all kinds of miso, pasteurised and unpasteurised.

A short list of what you can buy:

miso (various kinds), miso soup, saki, shoyu, tamari, tempeh (Clearspring); mugi, genmai miso, tempeh (Danival); barley mugi miso, tamari (Sanchi); bio shoyu, tamari (Manna, Rapunzel); miso (various kinds), miso mustard, horseradish (Source Foods); koji-amazake starter (Source Foods); frozen tempeh, plain, smoked, herb and garlic (Impulse Foods).

Also: noodles (Clearspring); brown rice vinegar (Western Isle); amazake rice pudding (3 varieties) (Clearspring); bio umeboshi plums (Clearspring, Manna); rice and umeboshi vinegar (Lima); gomasio (sesame and sea salt) (Lima, Rapunzel); saké (Clearspring); arame and hijiki seaweed (Clearspring).

Milk powder Organic skimmed-milk powder is available from Evernat.

Mustard Delicious, and available mild to extra-strong, and smooth, coarse or wholegrain. Evernat Dijon mustard remains my favourite all-rounder. Other good brands include Delouis, De Rit, Monki, Whole Earth and Tra'fo.

Nut dips, butters and spreads (in jars) Monki and Rapunzel have the widest selection, at over a dozen, which ranges from delicate pale-white almond and tropical nut butter to chocolatey carob nut spread. Others include carobella, orange and hazelnut spread (Molen Aartje), Halva Crème (Voegel) and various yummy chocolate spreads (Chocoreale, Rapunzel, Voegel). Tinned hummus is produced by Whole Earth.

Peanut butters Every child's favourite. The range continues to expand. Available as smooth or crunchy, with or without salt. Rapunzel peanut butters are stone-ground from freshly roasted premier-grade US blanched peanuts and triple-checked for aflatoxins (natural highly reactive carcinogens found in peanuts, and regularly monitored by official tests). Other brands include Essential, Evernat, Seyte, Suma, TerraSana and Whole Earth.

Tahini A must, available salted or unsalted, brown (from unhulled seeds) or white (from hulled seeds). Prices vary; Essential is usually the cheapest. Other brands include Lima, Rapunzel and Sunita.

Olives (in jars) Black and green olives, usually Spanish and packed in brine (Bio Aras, Sunita, Rapunzel, TerraSana), are the most common. Others include stuffed green olives (Bio Aras), Kalamata olives in olive oil, Manaki olives with herbs and lemon (Rapunzel) and black olive pâté (Cereal Terra, Rapunzel). Sunita also do black Nyons olives.

Pickled vegetables Beetroot and red cabbage (De Rit), gherkins (TerraSana) and sauerkraut (Bionova, De Rit, TerraSana).

Salad dressings Include American-style dressing (Whole Earth) and natural and flavoured vinaigrettes (Whole Earth, Fertillia).

Salsa dips Mild, piquant or fiery and all very tasty, usually tomato-based, excellent with tortillas, grilled meat and vegetables; a dollop is good, too, in tomato-based braised dishes or mine-strone-style soups. An ever-expanding field: major brands include Apache, Evernat, Mexi-snax, Rapunzel and TerraSana. From America, the Muir Glen range includes fat-free roasted garlic, and roasted garlic with cilantro (coriander) salsas.

Salt The organic sort is unwashed, unrefined sea salt from certi-fied unpolluted sources, harvested and evaporated using tradi-tional methods. Sea salts may contain added organic flavourings. The range comprises natural coarse and fine salt (Lima), Celtic whole sea salt from the Atlantic with the Soil Association symbol (Clearspring), herb salt (Laguna); and gomasio, a Japanese condi-ment of sesame seed and sea salt (Lima, Rapunzel).

Sauces Apart from bottled tomato sauce (see next page), there are hardly any as yet. De Rit produce a barbecue and spicy ketchup. Lima produce three stir-fry sauces, Bohème, Canton and Toscana. Muir Glen do tinned pizza sauce. For pasta sauces, see p. 313.

Soups All kinds, including freshly made (see p. 289). No packet, tinned or bottled soup can ever capture that fresh home-made flavouring but, that aside, those available taste of the real thing, and are excellent. The latest, Organic Café Gourmet soups, are to be commended. All have a long shelf life, around twelve to eigh-teen months.

Packet Barnhouse soups – a range of six, including barley and minestrone – contain no yeast or wheat. The organic vegeta-bles come from local growers and are processed as soon as they are harvested. Just Wholefoods produce six single-serving cuppa soups (less than 60 calories per serving), including carrot and coriander, and couscous, for 35p, also available as multipacks. There are also tomato, chestnut, vegetable and quinoa soups (Quinoa Real).

Tinned From Suma, five warming varieties: tomato, pea, spicy lentil, carrot and coriander, and swede and orange.

In jars From the continent, gazpacho (Cepad); minestrone, green pea, tomato, lentil, pumpkin (Vetera); vegetable, carrot, tomato, leek and potato (Organico). The excellent Organic Café

Gourmet soups (650g) contain two hefty portions, and come in six flavours including cream of mushroom, and green lentil and garlic.

Bottled Biofresh, made with organic vegetables, cream and Marigold organic bouillon. Carrot, leek and potato, tomato, and vegetable are available.

Powdered Produced by Nat Ali, a total of six including Japanese pumpkin, tomato and nettle.

Stock cubes and powdered stock Organic vegetable stock cubes are great and do not have a synthetic taste. As with all stock cubes, go easy: half is often sufficient. Major brands include Evernat, Friggs, Kallo, Rapunzel. Marigold powdered Swiss bouillon, now available as organic, has won high praise from both health guru Leslie Kenton and Delia Smith – 'an excellent store-cupboard standby' – and comes in a tin. Others include mixed-herb stock cubes (Friggs) and vegetable bouillon (Rapunzel).

Thickeners Maize starch for sauces and puddings (Rapunzel).

Tomatoes (processed) One of the most important items, and is the one item where you are spoilt for choice. The range increases constantly.

Ketchup Major brands are Eunature, Evernat, La Bio-Idea, Muir Glen, Whole Earth – and, from Rapunzel, Exotic Ketchup.

Passata Organic tomatoes and sea salt. Brands include Buonbio, Eunature, Everfresh, Campo, La Bio-Idea, Muir Glen and Organico. There's also concentrated passata (Campo, La Terra E Il Cielo).

Worth trying, too, is La Selva's polpa di pomodoro, bottled tomato pulp from Tuscany with an excellent fresh taste.

Purée Available in small and large sizes and has an extra rich flavour. Major brands are De Rit, Eunature, Muir Glen and Rapunzel. Try some.

Sun-dried In jars, plain (Rapunzel), or in olive oil (Cereal Terra, Rapunzel).

Tinned Excellent. For regular use, whole or chopped (Campo, Eunature, Muir Glen). Muir Glen also produce diced tomatoes with herbs and with garlic and basil.

Bottled La Selva (from Tuscany).

Vegetables A growing range of processed vegetables is available – from instant mashed potato (TerraSana) and dried vegetables (Rapunzel) to jars of pumpkin purée (Danival), ratatouille (Viver, Cepad, Danival), sliced beetroot and sweetcorn kernels (Bionova). Becoming popular are jars of Mediterranean-style products such as Sicilian aubergine in tomato sauce (Rapunzel), peperonata, tomato and vegetables, aubergine in oil with hot pepper (Achillea), aubergine and tomato, and Caviar d'Aubergine (Cepad). The ultimate luxury is artichoke hearts in olive oil (Rapunzel) and cream of artichokes (Cereal Terra). Others include aduki and vegetables (Achillea), and courgettes and brown rice (Cepad).

 Tinned French beans, peas, sweetcorn, baby onions, peas and carrots, red cabbage, beetroot (De Rit).

Vegetarian – burgers, dried meals, pâtés, textured vegetable protein (TVP) A small but increasing range of products includes bangers, burgers, Middle Eastern falafel and soya sausage mixes (Just Wholefoods, Joannusmolen). Also, vegetable biryani, chow mein with wholemeal noodle mix, Indian-style pilau with coconut and spices, and Mediterranean-style couscous with lentils – all dried packet meals (Just Wholefoods). There's a wide range of pâtés in tubes or jars, such as carrot, chestnut, mushroom and Provence Herb pâté (Urd); and Spicy Mexican, Tomato and Vegetable pâté tubes (Granovita). There are also three different-flavoured quinoa pâtés (Quinoa Real) and soya vegetable pâté (Herbert & Marot).

 TVP mince Major brands include Essential, Infinity Foods, Just Wholefoods. Curry-flavoured and savoury TVP is produced by Kitchen Garden.

 Vegetarian ready meals Hardly any. Cassoulet, Indian curry beans, seitan bali-style meals in jars (Vetera). Tinned ready brown rice (Whole Earth) sounds an extravagance, but came top in a tasting and is popular.

Vinegars All the major types of vinegar are available. Aspell's are a founder member of the Soil Association and have been producing organic cider vinegar since 1947. It is made from whole apples, not concentrate, and bottled unpasteurised. Cider vinegar is believed to be beneficial to health, particularly for arthritis sufferers. Other brands of cider vinegar include Biona and, from America, Bragg. Plus red wine vinegar (Campo), white wine vinegar (Rapunzel) and excellent balsamic vinegar (Bionaturae, Manicardi, Rapunzel). Oak-aged vinegar from Il Casale is available by mail order (p. 103).

Organic Soya Products

A range of organic non-dairy soya products – milk, tofu, tofu savouries, desserts – are available; all are made with non-genetically engineered soya beans and are suitable for vegans. Most will be found in the chilled section. Organic tofu burgers are surprisingly yummy – another good organic convenience food to add to your list, whether you are vegetarian or not.

Soya milk An alternative for those who cannot digest cow's milk, for vegans, or for anyone else who doesn't wish to drink cow's milk. Available at many retail outlets, including Safeway, Waitrose and the Co-op, in cartons, usually 500ml or 1 litre. Major brands are Bonsoy, Granose, Granovita, Provamel, Unisoy, Vitasoy; some have added calcium. Organic soya milk is guaranteed to be made from non-genetically modified soya beans.

Sweetened soya milk There are a few to choose from, including wheat-sweetened (Provamel), and with organic malt (Sunrise).

Flavoured soya milk Vitasoy produce Carob, Rich Cocoa and Vanilla Delite.

Soya Desserts Include vanilla Soya Dessert (Rev Riz), Original and Choco Dessert (Lima). Rapunzel produce a vanilla and chocolate pudding powder that makes up like custard.

Soya yoghurt The Elms Dairy produce plain and fruit.

Soya ice-cream and frozen desserts Swedish Glacé produce chocolate, pear, raspberry, strawberry and vanilla ice-cream. Maranelli make Frozen Soya Supreme.

Price guide: Organic soya milks range from around £1.10–£1.35 per litre carton, packet desserts from 50p per sachet to around £1.50 for 500g boxes, yoghurt around £1.75 and frozen desserts around £2.20 for a large 500g tub.

Tofu There are three major brands of organic tofu and tofu savouries. Plain tofu has a fridge life of three weeks; marinated tofu, two weeks; and fried tofu, five days.

Dragonfly Plain, smoked and deep-fried tofu. Seven varieties of tofu burgers, including smoky, spicy, mushroom and curry, and various tofu roasts.

Paul's Plain, marinated and fried tofu. Their wide range of savouries includes vegetable samosas, pasties, hot and spicy pies and mushroom and tofu rolls. These have a fridge life of five days.

Taifun A German brand of tofu savouries, very tasty. Plain, almond and sesame smoked and marinated tofu. Carrot and paprika terrine, smoked farmhouse terrine and six different sausages including frankfurters, cocktail, and the slicing sort.

Clearspring also produce plain organic tofu. In Edinburgh, The Engine Shed (p. 215) produce a range of organic tofu products including tofu and onion pies and tofu fruit whip, available through Sundrum Organics (p. 121) and Damhead Organically Grown Foods (p. 98).

Price guide: Organic tofu is generally good value and costs from around £1–£1.75, depending on size, brand and whether it is plain, smoked or deep-fried. Tofu burgers range from 85p–£1.95, depending on the brand and type. Sausages are £1–£1.25, while other products range from £1.50–£2.50 for the Taifun range and £1.65–£3.40 for Dragonfly's 500g-size tofu roasts.

See also vegetarian burgers and pâtés, p. 321.

Other non-dairy foods

Organic milk drinks and desserts made from grains are fairly widely available; you can also buy organic non-dairy margarines from Rapunzel, Munsterland and Fertillia. The most popular drink is Rice Dream, original and vanilla-flavoured, a naturally sweet drink made from brown rice imported by Clearspring. Lima make organic Rev Rice drink.

Rapunzel organic vegetarian margarine illustrates the difference between the organic and conventional approaches to making margarine. Rapunzel organic margarine contains no hydrogenated fats, transfats, milk protein, milk sugar or other animal ingredients, salt, added water or flavourings. It is made from 60 per cent organic sunflower oil, fair-traded organic palm and coconut fats to give the required spreading consistency, plus lemon juice, carrot juice as a natural colouring and soya lecithin as a stabiliser; and has a pleasant flavour.

appendix 1

pesticides:
residue and usage data

Vegetables

The following information, taken from the 1995 and 1996 WPPR reports, gives an indication of the probability of pesticide residues occurring in retail vegetables; OP residues were detected in all vegetables tested, except for courgettes. It also gives some idea of the number of different pesticides that farmers can use for each crop, though, as the pesticide usage data show (p. 328), in practice only a few are used on any individual vegetable.

As we cannot avoid them, whatever we think about pesticide residues it's important to keep them in perspective. On a reassuring note, remember that detection methods are very sophisticated and that amounts of residues detected are tiny. A measure of 0.1, for instance, which is quite large by some residue standards, means one hundredth of a milligram of residue found per kilogram of crop. Multiple residues means that two or more pesticides were detected in the same sample. Except where stated, residues found were below MRLs (maximum residue limits).

Broccoli No residues were detected in UK samples. OP residues were found in one-fifth of Spanish samples. Thirty-eight pesticides were sought and one (the OP chlorpyrifos) found.

Carrots Residues were detected in three-quarters of samples, and multiple residues (2 to 4 pesticides) in over a third. Residues were present in 5 out of every 9 UK samples. Twenty-one pesticides were sought and 8 found. In 1996, OP residues were detected in 10 per cent of imported samples.

Celery Residues were found in all except one sample, and multiple residues (2 to 5 pesticides) in half. They were present in over half UK samples and in over 90 per cent of imported ones. One hundred and three pesticides were sought, and 19 found. MRLs were exceeded in half of Israeli and almost half of the Spanish samples, and in one UK sample.

Courgettes No residues were detected in any samples, including UK ones, save for one Spanish sample. Forty-nine pesticides were sought and one found.

Cucumber Residues were detected in 2 UK and in half of imported samples, and multiple residues (2 to 4 pesticides) in a quarter. Thirty-eight pesticides were sought, and 6 found.

Leeks No residues detected (1996); nor were any detected the last time leeks were sampled, in 1993. Eleven pesticides were sought.

Winter lettuce The subject of ongoing scrutiny. In 1995, residues were detected in three-quarters of retail samples, and multiple residues (2 to 5 pesticides) in half; they were present in 80 per cent of UK samples. In 1995, 10 pesticides were sought and 9 found. No amounts above MRLs were recorded for imported lettuces.

Misuse of pesticides in UK winter lettuce, especially fungicides, has been a recurrent problem, and two growers have been prosecuted. Approximately 1 in every 5 UK samples exceeded MRLs. Six samples contained residues of non-approved pesticides, and 5 contained residues of the OP tolclofos-methyl in excess of 1mg/kg, indicating that pesticides may have been applied post-planting, which is not approved.

In 1996, 4 separate tests were done, the analysis of which takes up a page in the survey. Residues in retail samples had increased this time to 88 per cent, multiple residues to two-thirds, and residues in UK samples to 90 per cent. While no non-approved residues were detected, nearly 1 in 8 UK samples still exceeded MRLs. In a different test, UK retail lettuces fared much better, only one sample containing residues as compared to two-thirds of Spanish, though in a third test using wholesale lettuces it again soared to 90 per cent.

Potatoes As an important dietary staple, new and maincrop UK and imported potatoes are tested every year for a range of OP pesticides, fungicides and sprout-suppressants, though OCs are no longer sought. Over the last ten years or so, residues have been found in half the maincrop and in approximately one-fifth of new potatoes; multiple residues have been found in one-fifth of maincrop potatoes, with MRLs exceeded in some cases.

In 1995 residues were detected in almost half the samples, and multiple residues (2 to 4 pesticides) in almost a quarter. Over half of maincrop and 13 per cent of UK new potatoes contained residues. The majority of multiple residues were found in UK maincrop potatoes. Twelve pesticides were sought and 9 found (UK). The major ones detected were:

Chloropham (herbicide and growth-regulator): detected in a third of all maincrop potatoes, almost twice the proportion found in 1994 and 1993

Maleic hydrazide (growth-regulator): detected in 12 per cent of maincrop potatoes, 3 times the percentage found in 1994 and 1993

Tecnazene (sprout-suppressant): detected in a third of all maincrop potatoes

Thiabendazole (systemic fungicide): detected in almost a quarter of all maincrop potatoes

In 1996 the situation was very similar, though the levels of the 4 major pesticides had fallen slightly and no residues were reported in imported samples. Aldicarb (p. 348), which had first been found in relatively large amounts in one sample in 1994, was being detected at lower levels in a small number of samples.

Spring greens No residues detected (1996). All were UK samples. Thirty-seven pesticides sought.

Sprouted seeds No residues detected in samples of cress or bean sprouts (1996). Thirteen pesticides were sought.

Tomatoes A greater number of pesticides were being sought; lower reporting levels resulted in a fivefold increase since 1993. In 1995, residues were detected in over half the samples, and multiple residues (2 to 4 pesticides) in over a quarter. They were present in two-fifths of UK samples and in almost two-thirds of imported samples. Thirty-six pesticides were sought and 9 found.

Finally, as part of the Total Diet Survey, residues were detected in one-fifth of composite samples of green vegetables, and in 46 per cent of composite samples of other vegetables.

What sprays, which crops?

The following information, taken from various *Pesticide Usage Survey Reports* published by the Ministry of Agriculture, gives an indication of the extent of pesticide sprays used on and around various crops.

Outdoor crops

Pesticide usage generally reflects the area of crops grown, though the latest data (1995) show relatively higher usage on onions and leeks, carrots, parsnips, celery and brassicas. Insecticides, herbicides and fungicides are all used extensively and are often all applied to the same crop. The use of each has increased since 1991, by 17–27 per cent of the area treated, though rates of application are generally lower. Insecticides are the most important group. Crops, or the land they are grown on, can expect to receive one to several applications of different pesticide formulations, including repeat spraying. In terms of the weight of active ingredients used, overall far more herbicides and fungicides are used than insecticides – though this is not necessarily true for individual crops.

Although their use has declined and rates of application are lower, OPs are still the most extensively used insecticides, accounting for 40 per cent of the total insecticide-treated area, followed by synthetic pyrethroids and then carbamates. The three most widely used insecticides are cypermethrin, the OP demeton-

S-methyl and pirimicarb. Other extensively used OP pesticides are triazophos and dimethoate.

Biological control is minimal, accounting for less than 1 per cent of pesticides used, though there was a 28 per cent increase in the area treated between 1991 and 1995.

Brassicas This group includes cabbages, cauliflowers, Brussels sprouts, broccoli and kale. In 1995, these received an average of 4 insecticide sprays, 2 herbicides and 1 fungicide. Molluscicides (against slugs) were also used. The 2 insecticides most used were the OP demeton-S-methyl and cypermethrin. Insecticide, herbicide and fungicide use had increased substantially since 1991.

Carrots, parsnips and celery In 1995, these received an average of 4 insecticide sprays, 3 herbicides and 2 fungicides. Insecticide use was most extensive on these crops, with almost all receiving 4 applications of 4 active substances. The area treated with OPs had declined by 44 per cent since 1991, while the use of synthetic pyrethroids had increased fourfold. The OP triazophos was still the major insecticide used. Fungicide usage also doubled between 1991 and 1995.

Cucurbits This group includes courgettes, marrows, pumpkins and other squashes. In 1995, these received an average of 1 herbicide spray and 1 fungicide. Fungicides were the major pesticide group used. The soil sterilant dazomet was also used for 1 per cent of the area treated. Insecticides were used less in this group, and only half received herbicides, which were used more for pre-planting and clean-up treatments. The main insecticides used were pirimicarb and the OP demeton-S-methyl.

Lettuce, endive etc. This group includes Chinese cabbage. In 1995, these received an average of 5 insecticide sprays, 2 herbicides and 2 fungicides. Use of insecticides was most intensive in this group. The soil sterilant, dazomet, was used for 1 per cent of lettuces. The use of OPs had decreased by 44 per cent since 1991. The three major insecticides used were pirimicarb, cypermethrin and the OP demeton-S-methyl. Molluscicide usage had increased by almost 13 times since 1991, while herbicide usage had increased slightly.

Onions and leeks This group includes salad onions. In 1995, these received an average of 1 insecticide spray, 5 herbicides and 2 fungicides. Herbicides were used more intensively on these crops than on others. A third were also treated with the growth-regulator maleic hydrazide, and a sprout-suppressant was used on dry onion bulbs. Use of insecticides had more than doubled since 1991: the ones used most were deltamethrin, cypermethrin and aldicarb, plus the OPs triazophos and chlorpyrifos. Use of fungicides also increased substantially between 1991 and 1995.

Peas and beans In 1995, these received an average of 1 insecticide spray and 2 herbicides – herbicides were the most important group of pesticides used. Processors' requirement that peas be grown without the use of fungicides has resulted in their use decreasing dramatically. Insecticides used included the OPs dimethoate and demeton-S-methyl, and cypermethrin.

Potatoes A major arable crop, potatoes receive repeated treatments of pesticides. Fungicides are the main group used, primarily to control blight. In 1994, crops received an average of 6.5 applications of fungicides, 2 herbicide and 2 insecticide sprays. Molluscicides and sulphuric acid were also used, the latter as a foliage desiccant. In some cases, seed treatments were applied and maleic hydrazide was used as a growth-regulator. Dithiocarbamates (EBDCs) were the major fungicides used and paraquat the major herbicide. The major insecticide was pirimicarb; the OPs dimethoate and heptenophos were used widely. Potatoes grown for seed are also sprayed extensively: in 1994, crops on average received 5 fungicide sprays, 4 insecticides and 2 herbicides.

Root crucifers This group includes turnips, swedes and radishes. In 1995, these received an average of 3 insecticide sprays, 2 herbicides and 1 fungicide. Molluscicides were also used. The most widely used insecticide was the OP chlorfenvinphos. Other important pesticides were the systemic carbamate, carbofuran, the OPs chlorpyrifos and dimethoate, and cypermethrin.

Sweetcorn In 1995, this received an average of 2 insecticide sprays and 2 herbicides, but no fungicides. Herbicides were the major pesticide group used. Insecticide usage had almost doubled since

1991, though weights of substances used had declined, reflecting lower application rates. The OPs demeton-S-methyl and dimethoate were the most important pesticides used, followed by the OP triazophos and pirimicarb.

Post-harvest treatment of vegetables in store: Onions, beetroot and white cabbage are commonly stored after harvest. In 1995 all samples of white cabbage received a post-harvest application of the fungicide iprodione, two-thirds receiving an additional application of carbendazim fungicide or metalaxyl systemic fungicide.

Potatoes in store: Over 4 million tonnes of maincrop potatoes are stored each year, the great majority of which are treated with pesticides, primarily to prevent sprouting. In 1994, 70 per cent of those stored on farms received an average of 1.7 applications of pesticides, while 87 per cent of those in merchant stores received an average of 3 applications. The main pesticides used are the herbicide and growth-regulator chlorpropham, followed by the fungicide and growth-regulator tecnazene and the systemic fungicide thiabendazole applied primarily as a fumigant or spray, or in the case of tecnazene, also as dust. Tecnazene is also used far more extensively on farms than in merchant stores. Between 1992 and 1994, the tonnage of potatoes treated in store increased by 10 per cent, and the weight of active substances applied, by 37 per cent; tecnazene use decreased by 8 per cent.

Vegetable seed treatments: Fungicides or fungicide mixtures are often applied to seeds before they are sown. Crops which are usually treated in this way are brassicas, peas and beans, onions and leeks, carrots, sweetcorn and, to a lesser extent, lettuces. Fungicides used include benomyl, captan, carbendazim and iprodione. Except in the case of lettuce, vegetable seeds may also receive insecticide treatments. The 1995 data showed that this included the OC lindane on some brassica, root crucifer and carrot seeds, and the OP chlorpyrifos on pea and bean seeds.

In 1994, a third of seed potatoes were treated with pesticides, applied as a fumigant or spray, the main ones used being 2-aminobutane and the systemic fungicides, thiabendazole and imazalil.

Indoor crops

In contrast to outdoor crops, with the exception of lettuce and celery, biological control is now a major means of controlling protected crops, especially tomatoes and cucumbers, and pesticide use has fallen substantially. Fungicides are still the most important group of pesticides, especially for lettuces and cucumbers, while the use of soil sterilants, herbicides and molluscicides is now very limited. Acaricides are also used, particularly on tomatoes and cucumbers.

In 1991, the latest data available, biological control accounted for 52 per cent of the area treated. Soil sterilants accounted for only 1 per cent of the area treated but for 71 per cent of the total weight of active ingredients, with methyl bromide and chloropicrin accounting for 71 per cent of soil sterilants used. OPs were the most important insecticides, followed by synthetic pyrethroids and carbamates, the three main ones used being cypermethrin, the OP heptenophos and pirimicarb. Growth-regulators were used for ripening tomatoes.

Cucumbers Cucumbers present a similar picture to tomatoes, with biological pest control now a major factor; fungicides are the most used group of pesticides, while the use of soil sterilants, especially methyl bromide, has declined, due in part to the increased use of rockwool as the growing medium. In 1991, the major insecticides in use were the OP dichlorvos, nicotine and the synthetic pyrethroid, deltamethrin. However, unlike with tomatoes, the amount of OPs used had increased sixfold in 1991 compared to 1981. The OC lindane was also in use.

Lettuce Most indoor lettuce is grown in soil, so herbicide use is more extensive than with tomatoes or cucumbers. Generally, the use of pesticides on lettuce, including OPs and soil sterilants, has declined substantially. In 1991 fungicides accounted for 62 per cent of the area treated, insecticides for 29 per cent, herbicides for 4 per cent, molluscicides for 3 per cent, and soil sterilants, methyl bromide and dazomet, for 2 per cent. Fourteen times more fungicide was used than insecticide. The main insecticides were cypermethrin, pirimicarb and, at the top of the list in terms of weight, the OP heptenophos. The OC lindane was also in use, and other

OP pesticides in extensive use included demeton-S-methyl, oxydemeton-methyl and dimethoate.

Mushrooms Pesticide use has halved since the 1980s, and the reduction has been more significant in mushrooms than in any other crop, particularly as regards the use of OCs and OPs, which has fallen by over 90 per cent; though the use of fungicides and soil sterilants – namely, chloropicrin, methyl bromide and dazomet – increased substantially between 1991 and 1995. Biological controls are also being introduced. The sterilising of equipment and compost accounts for a proportion of pesticide usage. The pesticides can be applied in various ways: sprays, drenches, fogs and space treatments are the main ones, followed by granules, liquid irrigation, and dips or washes (5 per cent). In terms of the total weight of active substances applied in 1995, disinfectants accounted for the greatest part, fungicides for 10 per cent and insecticides for 2 per cent. Over a third of insecticides and the majority of fungicides were applied to crops directly. The main insecticides used were diflubenzuron, the OP diazinon and (by weight) dichlorvos, and the pyrethrins resmethrin and permethrin. A small amount of the OC lindane was in use in 1995, as a fabric treatment (buildings etc.) and as a direct application to crops.

Peppers As with tomatoes and cucumbers, biological controls are used extensively, accounting for three-quarters of the area treated in 1991, while fungicides, insecticides and acaracides all accounted for approximately the same weight (4–5 per cent) of active ingredients used. The major insecticides in use in 1991 were pirimicarb, cypermethrin, and the OPs heptenophos and dichlorvos. There was limited use of herbicides and soil sterilants.

Tomatoes Indoor tomatoes are grown in soil, rockwool or hydroponically in a nutrient solution. Biological control is now the major form of pest control, account for 76 per cent of the area treated in 1991, though OPs, lindane and other pesticides were also used. Though in decline, fungicides are still used extensively. In 1991, the principal fungicides used included chlorothalonil, iprodione, and dichlofluanid. Growth-regulators to enhance the setting of fruit have been replaced by bumblebees!

Fruit

The following information, like that on vegetables in the previous section, comes from the 1995 and 1996 WPPR reports. It gives an idea of the likelihood of pesticide residues occurring in the fruit you buy. OP residues were detected in all fruits sampled.

Eating-apples In 1995, residues were detected in three-quarters of samples, and multiple residues (2 to 5 pesticides) in over a third. They were present in over half of UK and in over three-quarters of imported samples. One hundred and one pesticides were sought, and 14 found. In 1996, the OP chlorpyrifos was detected in all but one of UK retail samples, and in two-fifths of samples of imported eating-apples.

Apricots Residues were detected in over three-quarters of samples, and multiple residues of 2 pesticides in one-sixth. Seventy-three pesticides were sought and 8 found. Because relatively high levels (17mg/kg) of one EBDC fungicide were found in one sample, and apricot purée is eaten by infants, a risk assessment was carried out for infants which showed that the ADI was slightly exceeded in this case.

Bananas Residues are mainly detected in the peel rather than in the pulp, and are usually fungicides. In 1996, they were present in 80 per cent of samples – three times more than when last tested in 1993 – and multiple residues (2 or 3 pesticides) were found in just over a quarter. Twenty-three pesticides were sought and 4 found. Two samples from Guatemala reached MRLs. There was also a threefold increase in one pesticide, due in part to a lowering of reporting levels.

Gooseberries Residues were detected in two-thirds, and multiple residues of 2 pesticides in two-fifths of UK samples. Twenty-five pesticides were sought and 6 found.

Grapes Residues were detected in two-thirds of samples and multiple residues (2 to 5 pesticides) in one-third, from grapes taken from 12 different countries. Ninety-nine pesticides were sought and 22 found.

Kiwi fruit Residues were detected in over half, and multiple residues of 2 pesticides in some samples. Forty-eight pesticides were sought and 3 found.

Oranges When carrying out tests, the whole fruit is used, including the skins. In 1995, residues were detected in all samples and multiple residues in over 90 per cent, from oranges taken from 9 different countries. Up to 9 multiple residues were found, occupying three pages of data. Two samples from Cyprus contained residues of an OP insecticide double and 4 times that of the MRL. Ninety-nine pesticides were sought and, incredibly, 87 found.

Peaches and nectarines Residues were found in half of the samples and multiple residues (2 to 4 pesticides) in one-sixth. Ninety-three pesticides were sought and 6 found.

Eating-pears Residues were detected in all but 1 UK and 1 imported sample, and multiple residues (2 to 6 pesticides) in half. Four UK samples contained residues of pesticides not approved for commercial use on pears. Ninety-nine pesticides were sought and 16 found.

Soft fruit Over half soft fruit – sometimes more – including currants, raspberries and loganberries, is likely to contain residues. In 1996 a survey was carried out of UK pick-your-own soft fruit from a grower where misuse had previously been shown. Residues were detected in over half the samples and multiple residues (2 to 5 pesticides) in almost a quarter. Fifty-five residues were sought and 10 detected. Other recent tests on individual soft fruits have shown:

Blackcurrants (1994) Residues detected in two-thirds of samples, and multiple residues in just over a half.

Raspberries (1993) Residues detected in one-third of samples, and multiple residues in some.

Strawberries (1994) Residues detected in over 90 per cent of samples, and multiple residues in about a sixth. In 1996, another test conducted as part of the EU monitoring programme showed residues in only a third of UK and in under a sixth of imported retail samples.

Finally, the Total Diet Survey of 1996 revealed that residues were found in five-sixths of composite samples of fresh fruit, and multiple residues in just over half.

What sprays, which crops?

Pesticides are used more on fruit than on vegetables; a wider variety is used, and they are applied more often. OPs are the most extensively used insecticides on both soft and top fruit. The latest data recorded, 1992 for top fruit and 1994 for soft fruit, also showed some use of the OC lindane on some crops.

Top fruit

Orchard crops, including apples, pears and stone fruits, have a long growing season, and are routinely repeat-sprayed in order to protect them from pests and to ensure cosmetically attractive good-quality fruit. Apples and pears are the most intensively treated, with Cox's apples being the most repeatedly sprayed crop.

Generally, pesticide use has decreased considerably since the late 1980s, particularly as far as rates of application are concerned. In 1992, the latest data available, fungicides accounted for 60 per cent of the total area treated, insecticides for 17 per cent, herbicides for 11 per cent, and growth-regulators, used primarily on apple and pear crops, for 8 per cent. The most extensively used were dithianon fungicide, the OP insecticide chlorpyrifos, and amitrole and simazine herbicides. The OC lindane was applied to 2 per cent of crops, being used on Cox's and Bramleys, and on cider apples and perry pears. Though application rates decreased, usage of OPs between 1987 and 1992 increased.

Biological control is minimal – less than 1 per cent of all pesticides used – and is confined to apple and pear crops.

Apples In 1992, Cox's received an average of 13 fungicide sprays, 5 insecticides, 2 herbicides, 1 acaricide and 3 growth-regulators, with 96 per cent of the area grown receiving some pesticide treatment utilising 40 active ingredients. OPs accounted for two-thirds of the area treated, with chlorpyrifos the main one used. Carbyl was also widely used. Other dessert apples show a similar pattern, crops receiving an average of 12 fungicide sprays, 4 insecticides, 2 herbicides, 1 acaricide and 2 growth-regulators in 1992. Pesticide use on culinary apples is slightly less, with Bramleys the most extensively treated crop, in 1992 receiving an average of 11 fungicide sprays, 5 insecticides or acaricides, 2 herbicides, and 2 growth-regulators.

Pears Here pesticide usage is considerable, though slightly less than with apples. In 1992, crops received an average of 9 fungicide sprays, 3 insecticides, 1 acaricide, 2 herbicides and 2 growth-regulators. Diflubenzuron, and the OPs chlorpyrifos and pirimiphos-methyl, were the major insecticides used.

Cider apples and perry pears Though usage is significant, these are far less intensively treated than dessert apples and pears, with half the area grown receiving no pesticide treatments in 1992 and crops receiving an average of 4 fungicide sprays, 2 insecticides or acaricides and 1 herbicide. The major insecticides used were the OPs pirimiphos-methyl and chlorpyrifos, and the OC lindane.

Stone fruits In the UK, these primarily include plums and cherries, but also apricots and quinces as well as cobnuts and filberts. Generally, pesticide use is much less intensive on these than on apples or pears. In 1992, over 80 per cent of plums and cherries were treated, while almost half the area of the others grown received no pesticide sprays. In 1992, plums received an average of 4 sprays, comprising 2 insecticides, 1 fungicide and 1 herbicide; and cherries received 3 sprays, comprising 1 insecticide, 1 fungicide and 1 herbicide, while the rest received on average 1 fungicide and 1 herbicide.

Post-harvest treatment of fruit in store: Though usage has decreased since the late 1980s, particularly as regards pears, the majority of apples and a significant proportion of pears receive pre-storage treatment, in the form of a dip or drench. Antioxidants, especially on Bramleys, and fungicides, are used on apples, and fungicides are used on pears. In 1992, the latest data available, 88

per cent of Cox's and Bramleys and 38 per cent of pears were treated. The major antioxidant used was diphenylamine, and the major fungicides were carbendazim/metalaxyl and benomyl. Vinclozin, which is not approved for use in the UK on pears, was also recorded for a tiny minority of crops, but accounted for less than 1 per cent in weight of the active ingredient.

Soft fruit

Pesticide usage generally reflects the area of crops grown, though the latest data available (1994) show that it is much higher for blackcurrants used for processing than for other soft fruits. Insecticides, herbicides and fungicides are used extensively and applied to 80–90 per cent of the area grown. Fungicides are the most important group, the two most extensively used being dichlofluanid and chlorothalonil. Insecticides are used most extensively on raspberries, herbicides on strawberries, and fungicides on vines and blackcurrants. The two most used herbicides are simazine and paraquat. Acaricides are used primarily on blackcurrants, and molluscicides primarily for strawberry crops.

In 1994, the number of spray rounds applied to crops varied from about 5 for redcurrants and whitecurrants to up to 10 for vines and blackcurrants grown for processing. The number of active substances used varied from 9 for redcurrants and whitecurrants to 13 for strawberries, 17 for vines and 20 for blackcurrants grown for processing.

Pesticide use showed a relative increase between 1990 and 1994, though rates of application were declining (reduced weight of pesticide per given area treated). The use of the OC lindane increased by 14 per cent, OPs decreased by over a third, and molluscicides increased by 19 per cent. The area treated with soil sterilants more than doubled, and there was a threefold increase in the weight of active substances used, primarily methyl bromide (for more information on the use of methyl bromide, see p. 144).

Biological control is minimal for soft fruit, confined to a minority of strawberries and raspberries.

Blackcurrants In 1994, blackcurrants grown for the fresh market received an average of 4 fungicide sprays, 2 herbicides, 1 insecticide and 1 acaricide. Those grown for processing received an average of 6 fungicide sprays, 3 herbicides, 3 acaricides and 1 insecticide. OPs accounted for 6 out of 9 pesticides used and, excluding tar oil, accounted for 96 per cent (by weight) of active substances used. Fenitrothion was the major OP used.

Other bush fruits Red and white currants receive fewer pesticides than blackcurrants. In 1994, crops were treated with an average of 3 fungicides, 2 herbicides, 1 insecticide and 1 acaricide. Gooseberries received on average 4 fungicides, 2 herbicides and 1 insecticide. OPs, especially chlorpyrifos and fenitrothion, were the most extensively used insecticides. Pirimicarb was also used extensively for currants. Molluscicides and a growth-regulator were used for some gooseberry crops.

Raspberries In 1994, raspberries received an average of 4 fungicide sprays, 2 herbicides and 2 insecticides. Acaricides and molluscicides were also used. The two major insecticides, accounting for 70 per cent of applications, were the OP fenitrothion and chlorpyrifos. The OC lindane was also used on some crops.

Other cane fruits In 1994, blackberries received an average of 4 fungicide sprays, 2 herbicides and 1 insecticide, while hybrid berries – tayberries, loganberries, boysenberries etc. – received an average of 3 fungicide sprays, 2 herbicides and 1 insecticide. The OP fenitrothion and chlorpyrifos were the major insecticides used. The OC lindane was also used on some crops.

Strawberries In 1994, strawberries received an average of 5 fungicide sprays, 3 herbicides and 1 insecticide. Molluscicides and soil sterilants were also used. Two insecticides, the OP chlorpyrifos and pirimicarb, accounted for almost 70 per cent of applications, chlorpyrifos being used twice as much as pirimicarb. The OC lindane was also used on some crops.

Vines In 1994, vines received on average 8 fungicide sprays and 2 herbicides. Fungicides are the major group of pesticides, accounting for 88 per cent of the total area treated and employing 15 active substances, while insecticides are used very little and account for 1 per cent of the area treated. Cypermethrin was the only insecticide recorded.

Arable Crops

Arable crops include wheat, barley, oats, rye, potatoes, peas and beans, and sugar beet. Since the mid-1980s there has been a significant increase in the number and range of fungicides applied to many arable crops, particularly cereals, pulses and potatoes, and a major increase in the use of insecticides and growth-regulators on cereals. The use of newer pesticides which are active at lower rates of application, and repeat-spraying at reduced or low-dose rates, are two major trends, especially in the case of fungicides and herbicides, leading to a reduction in weight of pesticides used. Tank mixing of mixed-spray formulations has also increased.

Taken overall, the 1994 data, the latest available, indicate that herbicides and desiccants accounted for 34 per cent of the total area treated, fungicides for another third, seed treatments for 14 per cent, insecticides for 10 per cent, growth-regulators for 7 per cent and molluscicides for 2 per cent, though there is considerable variation within each crop group. Wheat, for example, accounted for 38 per cent of the area cultivated but 54 per cent of the total pesticide area treated. Herbicides were applied to at least 85 per cent of all arable crops, averaging 2 applications, and fungicides were applied to 67 per cent, also averaging 2 applications. Just over half set-aside land received one application of herbicide. The main insecticide groups used were pyrethroids, followed by OPs and carbamates, the use of OPs on cereals having increased since 1992. In 1994 the OC lindane was used on some cereals for seed treatment, and on sugar beet and linseed. Growth-regulators are used mainly on cereals.

Cereals

Wheat The use of pesticides on wheat has intensified since the early 1980s, and the use of fungicides, insecticides and growth-regulators has also increased significantly. In 1994, wheat crops received an average of 2 fungicide sprays, 2 herbicides, 1 insecticide and 1 growth-regulator. The main fungicide used was chlorothalonil, the main herbicides included isoproturon and fluroxypyr, and the main insecticide was the OP dimethoate. Other insecticides used extensively were cypermethrin, pirimicarb and the OPs chlorpyrifos and triazophos. Nearly 5 tonnes of the OC lindane were used on 4 per cent of the area treated, primarily as a seed treatment.

Other cereal crops Winter barley shows a similar pesticide usage pattern to wheat; other cereals receive slightly fewer treatments, with spring barley getting least; in 1994, on average these crops received 1 fungicide and 1 herbicide spray. OPs were used extensively, and over half a tonne of lindane was used, primarily as a seed treatment, on 17 per cent of the spring barley area treated.

Sugar beet

Sugar beet is a major arable crop, used in the production of sugar and also as animal feed. Herbicides account for half the total area treated, insecticides for 11 per cent and fungicides (excluding seed treatments) for 4 per cent. In 1994, sugar beet was treated, on average, four times with herbicide, primarily repeat low-dose spraying, and once with insecticide; the fungicides used are relatively limited – primarily sulphur. The main insecticides used were pirimicarb, deltamethrin and the OP heptenophos. Over 7 tonnes of lindane were used on 27 per cent of the area treated.

Cereals in store:

Post-harvest treatment with pesticides is common. They are mainly applied prophylactically to grain stores and equipment before the grain is stored, in the form of sprays and occasionally fogs, but may also be applied as admixtures to the stored grain, usually in the form of dust but also as a fumigant or as sprays. OPs, notably pirimiphos-methyl and etrimfos, are by far the most extensively used pesticides. Methyl bromide is now a major fumigant used by contractors.

The latest data available on grain stored during 1995 show that on an estimated 17.5 million tonnes stored, 15.8 tonnes of pesticides were used – 17 per cent as fabric treatments to buildings and 29 per cent as admixtures. Compared to 1991, this was an overall increase in pesticides used. Most of those used as grain treatments, accounting for 71 per cent, were applied to wheat; the main pesticides applied were the OPs pirimiphos-methyl and etrimfos, and methyl bromide. Overall, only 9 per cent of stored grain was given an admixture, though admixtures accounted for

69 per cent of the total weight of active substances applied to grain. A small amount of the OC lindane, 55 tonnes, was employed by some farmers as a smoke in fabric treatments.

Rice

Residues in rice tested in 1996 were significantly up from 1994: they were detected in two-thirds of white and over three-quarters of brown rice samples, with 9 per cent of samples exceeding the MRLs for inorganic bromide. The increase was partly due to another pesticide being added to the list of those usually sought and which was subsequently found.

Nuts and Seeds

Like any other crop, conventional nuts and seeds are grown with extensive use of pesticides, and a variety of residues are common. Systemic pesticides, which act by entering the plant and moving around it, probably get into the developing nuts and seeds before the outer shell has formed. UK data published in the late 1980s showed that three-quarters or more of the almonds, walnuts, pistachios and peanuts tested, and all the Brazil nut samples, were affected. In addition, most of the sunflower seeds and half of the sesame seeds tested contained traces of inorganic bromide, indicating the use of methyl bromide as a fumigant. The 1994 WPPR report describes a similar picture, with most tree nuts and peanuts containing pesticide residues. Multiple residues also occur – in some peanut butters, for instance. Lindane is the most prevalent residue detected in UK rape and linseed. Though we don't often eat these two in their natural state, rape seed is used extensively in cattle feed and as a vegetable oil.

Dairy Produce

Milk Residues have become a permanent feature of our milk supplies. Over the last decade OC residues have been found in 40 per cent of samples, and multiple residues in 2 per cent; in 1995, almost half the samples tested contained residues. Though levels have systematically fallen, traces of banned highly toxic OCs – hexachlorobenzene, dieldrin and DDT – have been consistently present, and are still being found. Because they are in the environment and have such a long life, organic milk cannot absolutely be guaranteed to be free of these. The other OC pesticide found commonly in milk, lindane, still used by some conventional farmers, especially to produce sugar beet, but never by organic farmers, reached record levels between July and December 1995, with nine samples tested containing lindane in excess of their MRLs, thought now to be possibly due to the exceptionally hot, dry summer. Further extensive monitoring has been carried out since, and levels have now returned to 'normal'. No other groups of pesticides are sought, so it is impossible to say whether other residues exist or not.

Butter Butter is only periodically tested, so information is scant. As with milk, OC residues in general, and lindane in particular, are found in some samples. This is to be expected, as OC residues collect in fat. In 1993, for example, they were present in half the samples. Interestingly, lindane seems only to appear in UK samples. In 1996, following raised lindane levels in milk during 1995, the WPPR report revealed that almost three-quarters of UK butter samples contained traces of lindane, though this is exceptionally high and is not expected to be repeated. In addition, over 10 per cent of imported samples contained traces of DDT.

Cheese As with butter, the data are scant, but OC residues, including lindane, are detected in a small minority of samples. In 1994, for example, they were present in 7–16 per cent of samples, which included goat's and ewe's milk cheeses. As expected, the high levels of lindane in cow's milk in 1995 were reflected in some cheeses made at that time, with well over a third of samples analysed in 1996 containing residues, 9 per cent of which were above the MRL, the highest level recorded in one sample being

4 times that limit. The WPPR Total Diet Survey for 1996 also indicated cheese to be a likely or possible source of DDT.

Eggs Pesticide residues are not usually identified, though OC residues can occasionally find their way into eggs. In 1992, traces of lindane and DDT were recorded in some samples, and again in eggs analysed as part of the 1996 WPPR Total Diet Survey.

Meat and Fish

Meat

Here, we can breathe slightly easier – though current data do not give us the whole picture. Because the major pesticides regularly found in meat are OCs, which collect and remain in fat, the WPPR monitors residues – including those in meat products and in infant food – only in the fat part of meat samples. Consequently it is impossible to say, from the published results, whether or not pesticides are present in lean meat, but they are thought to be extremely low if present at all.

The two most commonly detected OCs in meat and poultry fat are DDT and lindane. Imported New Zealand lamb seems to be the worst offender, with residues occurring in over a third of samples, sometimes more. Chinese rabbit, where MRLs have been exceeded, is another. Otherwise, residues usually occur in a minority of samples tested, and only a tiny proportion have been found to include both of these OCs. In all cases, levels of OCs above MRLs are rare. OP residues are also monitored, but are not detected. In future, residues which are not generally fat-soluble and could be present in lean meat are likely to be monitored.

The general consensus, then, is that there is far less potential cause for concern about pesticide residues in meat than, say, in fresh produce; if you are at all concerned, a sensible precaution would be to leave the fat. The 1995 WPPR report detected the OC lindane in just over a quarter of UK beef samples, in 3 per cent of UK chicken and pork, and in 14 per cent of all pâté samples. Only one sample of UK lamb was tested, and no residues were found.

Traces of OCs were also detected in just under 10 per cent of meat-based UK-produced infant foods.

Sheep-dipping: The dipping of sheep in OP insecticides to combat sheep scab and head- and blow-fly strike has become a major environmental hazard, as well as a considerable health risk for farmers, many of whom have suffered the classic symptoms of OP poisoning, and also for people who work in the wool industry. In an effort to eradicate scab, sheep-dipping was compulsory from 1976 to 1992 and is still practised by around half of farmers. Some 20 million gallons of sheep-dip are used every year. Disposal is not regulated, and there have been many recorded cases of sheep-dip polluting waterways, either directly or indirectly through soak-aways, or being illegally discharged directly into streams, harming invertebrates and crustaceans. Sheep-dip is also spread direct on to land. Organic farmers do not use them.

Scab has to be controlled by law, and farmers risk prosecution if their animals are found to have it. In response to concerns over the use of OP sheep-dips, synthetic pyrethroids, namely cypermethrin and flumethrin for scab, and deltamethrin for fly control, are increasingly being used. Unfortunately, though less hazardous to humans than OPs, these are considerably more toxic to aquatic life, including trout and fresh-water shrimps, and are causing more, not less, pollution in waterways. Cypermethrin is banned under Soil Association standards, but flumethrin and deltamethrin are allowed where necessary, should other methods fail. Standards are currently being revised to incorporate stricter controls, including those concerning disposal. Currently only a very small proportion of organic farmers have had to use these chemicals. A new product, moxidectin, has recently been introduced, which, if proved effective, could solve the problem.

Fish

This is probably something that you would prefer not to read about, but it illustrates the dilemma we are beginning to have to face about one of our best and most enjoyable natural foods. OC residues, such as lindane, DDT, dieldrin or hexachlorobenzene, are regularly found in the body fat and livers of 'wild' fish – and, sadly, this puts a question mark over the otherwise blemish-free health profile of fatty fish. In 1996, half the tested samples of imported non-indigenous fish and of some imported shellfish contained DDT. High levels have also been recorded in North Sea fish, including whiting, mussels and eels; and relatively high concentrations have been found in dab, cod and plaice – though, as we eat only the white flesh, presumably the risk is lessened. OCs also survive processing. The 1995 WPPR report, for example, detected them in three-quarters of the samples of UK-produced fish-oil products and in most eels, including jellied eels. In another independent test, OC residues were detected in all but one retail sample of fish-oil dietary supplements (mostly cod liver oil).

Residues of toxaphene, used as a pesticide in cotton production, but widely banned in Europe and extremely toxic to fish, have been detected in North Sea herring and mackerel, while residues of malachite green, used extensively in trout-farming as a fungicide and parasiticide, are regularly found in trout and are being monitored. Residues of tecnazene, a pesticide normally associated with stored potatoes, have been found in farmed fish and also in fishcakes. On the brighter side, no OP residues were found in either farmed salmon or farmed trout in 1996.

Antibiotic Residues in Meat, Eggs and Fish

Extensive routine and prophylactic use of antibiotics, either as growth-promoting agents or in disease management in conventional animal husbandry, is likely to be the next 'hot potato'. Antibiotics are necessary because of the intensive way the animals are reared and because of the economic necessity for them to reach their required weight as quickly as possible. Because of the long-term implications for health, and to safeguard their future effectiveness, the Soil Association has called for a ban on their routine use.

Antibiotics are routinely used to control diseases such as mastitis, respiratory conditions, enteritis and foot rot. As growth-promoters, they improve the conversion of feed in the intestine by neutralising certain bacteria, thereby enabling the animal to put on more weight without laying down more fat. Antibiotics are mixed into feed rations and used as growth-promoters for pigs, poultry and reared game, and for calves, beef cattle and intensively reared lambs. Rigorous testing for antibiotics and for other veterinary medicines, including synthetic hormones in meat, is carried out annually by the Veterinary Medicines Directorate (VMD), and residues occur in less than 1 per cent of over 30,000 samples tested. In a few isolated examples, however, residue levels can be over a hundred times greater than permitted.

The concern is not so much that antibiotics are an immediate danger to health – the amounts detected are tiny compared to the doses given in human medication – but that increasing bacterial resistance to antibiotics and the development of 'superbugs' immune to them present a growing problem to which the routine, as opposed to the specific, use of farm antibiotics may be a contributory factor. Another potential threat is that there are no new antibiotics in the pipeline to replace the life-saving drugs to which resistance is developing – and so what will happen then? Avoparcin, used as a feed additive in the poultry industry, was banned by the EU in March 1997 because of fears that it may be linked to a growing bacterial resistance to vancomycin, a last-resort antibiotic used in human medicine. The UK voted against the ban, though the Ministry of Agriculture has now established a working group to assess the problem of antibiotic-resistant micro-organisms in food. New studies conducted in Germany and Holland have found vancomycin-resistant bacteria present in farms using avoparcin, but not in farms which did not. German researchers have also found vancomycin to be widely present in frozen chicken, and the first recorded case in the UK of vancomycin resistance contracted directly from livestock treated with antibiotics happened recently when a poultry worker broke his leg at a chicken-processing factory.

Eggs Routine use of antibiotics in feed is standard in almost all egg-producing systems other than organic ones. Though not allowed to be used in laying hens, coccidiostats are conventionally used to control diarrhoea and dysentery in chicks; coccidiostat residues are frequently detected in eggs, their presence usually attributed to contamination with other feed or with droppings. In 1996, for example, the VMD report on veterinary residues found that approximately 1 in 8 and 1 in 10 samples contained traces of two commonly used antibiotics.

Fish Antibiotics are used widely in farmed fish, and are regularly monitored by the VMD. Generally detected in a minority of samples, when there is a problem remedial steps are taken which usually result in lower levels being detected the year after. Residues of ivermectin, an antibiotic used to control parasitic worms but which is not authorised for use in fish – except as a component of fish feed in certain circumstances – were previously detected in up to 10 per cent of salmon samples.

The British Dirty Dozen

The following pesticides are those currently used on UK crops – sometimes extensively – which appear on one or more of the following internationally recognised lists of harmful chemicals: the Pesticides Action Network (PAN) list of the most harmful pesticides; the World Health Organisation (WHO) list of acutely toxic pesticides to humans; the UK Red List (RL) of chemicals whose toxicity, persistence and bioaccumulation qualify them as major environmental pollutants; and the US Environmental Protection Agency (EPA) human carcinogenity pesticide evaluation list.

Aldicarb (herbicide): PAN; WHO Class Ib, Extremely Hazardous.

Captan (fungicide): EPA, probable human carcinogen (sufficient evidence of carcinogenity from animal studies).

Cypermethrin (synthetic pyrethroid insecticide): EPA, possible human carcinogen.

Demeton-S-methyl (OP insecticide): WHO Class 1b, Highly Hazardous.

Dichlorvos (OP insecticide): RL; WHO Class 1b, Highly Hazardous; EPA, possible human carcinogen.

Endosulfan (OC insecticide): RL.

Lindane (OC insecticide): PAN; RL; EPA, probable or possible human carcinogen.

Malathion (OP insecticide): RL.

Paraquat (herbicide): PAN.

Simazine (herbicide): RL; EPA, possible human carcinogen.

Triazophos (OP insecticide, used extensively on carrots, parsnips and celery): WHO Class 1b, Highly Hazardous.

Zineb (EBDC fungicide): EPA, probable human carcinogen (sufficient evidence of carcinogenity from animal studies).

NOTE: Methyl bromide is not listed but is a major ozone depleter. The OP, chlorpyrifos (brand name Dursban in the USA), used extensively in the UK, has recently been the subject of a highly critical report by the EPA, citing chronic and acute health problems resulting from its use.

Source: The List of Lists, published by the Pesticide Trust.

appendix 2

box schemes:
select list

This list, arranged alphabetically by county, city or region, has been compiled from entries selected from *The Organic Directory* and *Where to Buy Organic Food*. It comprises box schemes, a few home delivery services (HD), and shops offering a box scheme. Remember that some box schemes offer only seasonal services, and some are local while others deliver to a wide area, extending into surrounding counties; and that some shops act only as box-scheme collection points. For London box schemes, see pp. 119–120.

england

Bedfordshire
Rosehaven Organics, Gamlinghay, Sandy
tel: 0118 9650142
Berkshire
Ellis Organics, Sonning Common, Reading
tel: 01734 722826
Garlands Farm Shop, Gardeners Lane, Upper Basildon
tel: 01491 671556 (p. 142)
The Kulika Trust, Warren Farm, Rectory Rd, Streatley
tel: 01491 872149
Tolhurst Organic Produce, Whitchurch-on-Thames,
Reading tel: 0118 9843428 (p. 117)
Birmingham
Organic Roots, King's Norton tel: 01564 822294 (HD)
Organic Roundabout, Hockley tel: 0121 551 1679 (p. 119)
Bristol
The Better Food Company, Barrow Gurney
tel: 01275 474545 (p. 121)
The Green Wheel, St George tel: 0117 9559264

Buckinghamshire
>The Organic Trail, Stony Stratford, Milton Keynes
>>tel: 01908 568952

Cambridgeshire
>Earthly Goods, Huntingdon tel: 01480 812004
>Naturally Yours, Ely tel: 01353 778723 (p. 97)
>Organic Connections, Wisbech tel: 01945 773374 (p. 118)
>Waterland Organics, Reach tel: 01638 742178

Cheshire
>Oakcroft Organic Gardens, Malpas tel: 01948 860213

Cleveland
>Camphill Village Trust, Larchfield Community, Hemlington
>>tel: 01642 596892

Cornwall
>A. & N. Health Foods, 62 Fore St, Saltash
>>tel: 01752 844926
>Carley's, 34–36 St Austell St, Truro tel: 01872 77686 (HD)
>Cusgarne Organics, Cusgarne nr Truro tel: 01872 865922
>>(p. 194)
>Good Nature, 2 Esplanade, Fowey tel: 01726 832110
>Stoneybridge Organic Nursery, Tywardreath,
>>Par tel: 01726 813858 (p. 89)
>Tregannick Farm, Drakewells, Gunnislake
>>tel: 01822 833969

Cumbria
>Allergarth, Roweltown, Carlisle tel: 016977 48214
>Appleseeds, 59 Market St, Ulverston tel: 01229 583394
>Kan Foods, 9 New Shambles, Kendal tel: 01539 721190
>Sundance Wholefoods, 33 Main St, Keswick
>>tel: 017687 74712
>The Village Bakery, Melmerby tel: 01768 881515 E-mail:
>>Admin@village-bakery.com. (p. 218)

Derbyshire
>Market Wholefoods, The Shambles, 1A Mellor Rd, New
>>Mills, High Peak tel: 01663 747550
>Organic Health, 139 Ilkeston Rd, Marlpool, Heanor
>>tel: 01773 717718 (p. 82)

Devon
>Highfield Farm Shop, Topsham, nr Exeter
>>tel: 01392 876388 (p. 87)
>Lower Turley Farm, Cullompton tel: 01884 32234

Marshford Organic Nursery, Northam, Bideford
  tel: 01237 477160 (p. 87)
Northwood Farm, Christow, Exeter tel: 01647 252915 (p.
  116)
Riverford Organic Vegetables, Buckfastleigh
  tel: 01803 762720 (p. 117)
St Maurice Nurseries, Plympton, Plymouth
  tel: 01752 335580

Dorset

Down to Earth, 18 Princes St, Dorchester
  tel: 0135 268325
Gold Hill Organic Farm, Child Okeford, Blandford tel:
  01258 860293 (p. 88)
Longmeadow Organic Vegetables, Godmanstone,
  Dorchester tel: 01300 341779
Tamarisk Farm, West Bexington, Dorchester
  tel: 01308 897784

Durham

Molly's Wholefood Store, Framwellgate Moor, Durham
  City tel: 0191 3862216
Organic Growers of Durham Ltd, Walworth, Darlington
  tel: 01325 362466

Essex

The Happy Caterpillar, 92 Leigh Rd, Leigh-on-Sea
  tel: 01702 72982
Pilgrims Natural, 41–43 High St, Halstead
  tel: 01787 478513
Traders' Fair, 10 High St, Old Harlow tel: 0279 450908

Gloucestershire

Camphill Village Trust, Oaklands Park, Newnham
  tel: 01594 516063
Health-wise, 27 North Walk, Yate tel: 01454 322168
Slipstream Organics, Cheltenham tel: 01242 227273

Hampshire

Northdown Orchard, South Litchfield, Basingstoke
  tel: 01256 771477
Sunnyfields Organic, Marchwood, Southampton
  tel: 01703 871408 (p. 89)

Herefordshire

Abundance Produce, Little Birch, Hereford
  tel: 01981 540181

Flights Orchard Organics, Ledbury tel: 01531 635929
Ledbury Wholefoods, 82 The Homend, Ledbury
tel: 01531 632889
Prospect Organic Growers' Farm Shop, Bartestree,
Hereford tel: 01432 851164 (p. 88)
S.C. & S.M. Hall, Hopleys Green, Almeley
tel: 01544 340689

Hertfordshire

Cook's Delight, 360–364 High St, Berkhamsted
tel: 01442 863584 (p. 81)
Down to Earth, 7 Amwell End, Ware tel: 01920 463358
Fairhaven Wholefoods Ltd, 27 Jubilee Trade Centre,
Letchworth tel: 01462 675300 (HD)
Full of Beans, 3 Church St, Sawbridgeworth
tel: 01279 726002

Humberside

Green Growers, Nafferton, Driffield tel: 01377 255362
Wheelbarrow Foods, Barrow-on-Humber
tel: 01469 530721

Isle of Man

Garey Margee, Andreas tel: 01624 8805329 (day), 878480
(eve)

Isle of Wight

Godshill Organics, Godshill tel: 01908 840723
(p. 81)

Kent

Canterbury Wholefoods, 10 The Borough, Canterbury tel:
01227 464623 (HD)
Luddesdown Organic Farms, Luddesdown, nr Cobham tel:
01474 813376
Ripple Farm, Godmersham, nr Canterbury
tel: 01227 730748
Yalding Organic Gardens (HDRA), Yalding, nr Maidstone
tel: 01622 814650

Lancashire

Growing with Nature, Pilling, Preston tel: 01253 790046
(p. 116)
The Organic Way, Bradley Fold, Bolton tel: 01204 795590
Red Rose Organics, Helmshore, Rossendale
tel: 01706 226189

Leicestershire

Chevelswarde Organic Growers, South Kilworth
  tel: 01858 575309

Current Affairs, 19A Loseby Lane, Leicester
  tel: 0116 2510887

Tur Langton Organic Stores, Carpenters House, Tur
  Langton, Kibworth tel: 01858 545226

Lincolnshire

Barrow and Goxhill Organic Growers, Barrow-on-Humber
  tel: 01469 530721

Holbeach Wholefood, 32 High St, Holbeach, Spalding tel:
  01406 422149

Spice of Life, 4 Burghley Centre, Bourne tel: 01778 394735

Liverpool

Organic Direct, Unit 6, Greenland St tel: 0151 707 9008

Greater Manchester

Home Farm Deliveries, Longsight tel: 0161 224 8884

Limited Resources, Hulme tel: 0161 226 4777
  (p. 118)

Mossley Wholefoods, 11 & 13 Arundle St, Mossley,
  Thameside tel: 01457 837743

Sunflowers Wholefoods, 34 Beech Rd, Chorlton-cum-
  Hardy, Trafford tel: 0161 881 6399

Merseyside

A. & G. Organics, Formby, Sefton tel: 01704 831 893

Abbotts Vegetable & Herb Garden, Birkenhead, Wirral
  tel: 0151 608 4566 (p. 253)

Norfolk

Camphill Communities, Thornage Hall, Holt
  tel: 01263 861481

Evergreen Farm, Gressenhall, Dereham tel: 01362 860190

Green City Central, 42–46 Bethel St, Norwich
  tel: 01603 631007

Old Hall Farm Organic Garden, Burgh next Aylsham,
  Norwich tel: 01263 732772

Sesame Wholefoods, 11 Matlock Rd, Norwich
  tel: 01603 433908

The Stables, Gresham, Norwich tel: 01263 577468

Northamptonshire

Daily Bread Co-operative Ltd, The Old Laundry, Bedford
  Rd, Northampton tel: 01604 21531

Northumberland

The Green Shop, 54 Bridge St, Berwick-upon-Tweed tel:
01289 330897 (p. 84)

North East Organic Growers' Co-op, Bedlington
tel: 01665 575785

Nottinghamshire

Awsworth Nurseries, Cossall tel: 01159 442545

Hiziki Wholefood Collective, 15 Goosegate, Hockley tel:
0115 9505523

Oxfordshire

Frugal Food, 17 West Saint Helen St, Abingdon
tel: 01235 522239

Meat Matters, Letcombe Regis, Wantage
tel: 01235 762461 (p. 96)

Serena Howard, 21 Market Place, Chipping Norton tel:
01608 642973

Shropshire

Broad Bean, 60 Broad St, Ludlow tel: 01584 874239

Shropshire Hills Organic Produce, Clungunford, nr Craven
Arms tel: 01588 660255

Somerset

Arcadia Organics, Claverham tel: 01934 876886

Ceres Natural Foods, 42 Princes St, Yeovil
tel: 01935 28791 (p. 98)

Merrick's Organic Farm, Langport tel: 01458 252901
(p. 116)

Oake Bridge Farm, Oake, Taunton tel: 01823 461317

Radford Mill Farm, Timsbury, Bath tel: 01761 472549 (p.
169)

Staffordshire

Food for Thought Wholefoods, 57 Tamworth St, Lichfield
tel: 01543 253726; also shop 6, Market Hall, Market
St, Burton-on-Trent tel: 01283 510423

The Good Food Shop, 475–477 Hartshill Rd, Hartshill,
Stoke-on-Trent tel: 01782 710234

Weston Wholefoods, Milwich, Stafford tel: 01889 505567
(HD)

Suffolk

Barleycorn Wholefoods, Barsham, Beccles
tel: 01502 715637

Hillside Nurseries, Hintlesham, Ipswich tel: 01473 652682

Longwood Farm, Bury St Edmunds tel: 01638 717120 (p. 106)

Surrey

Carshalton Friends of Organic Farmers, 62 Cambridge Rd, Carshalton Beeches tel: 0181 395 5390; Epsom Downs Friends of Organic Farmers, 73 Shawley Way, Epsom Downs tel: 01737 359620. Both collection points.

Greenshoot, 22A Crown Lane, Morden, Surrey tel: 01483 203179

Octavia's Organics, 7 Prices Lane, Woodhatch, Reigate, Surrey tel: 01737 244155

Organic Home Deliveries, Worcester Park tel: 0181 337 1853 (HD)

The Pumpkin Patch, 10 High St, Banstead tel: 01737 371007

East Sussex

Ashurst Organics, Plumpton tel: 01273 891219

Beaumont's, Outlook Avenue, Peacehaven tel: 01273 585551; The Organic Centre, 363 South Coast Rd, Telscombe Cliffs, Brighton (p. 82)

Harvest Supplies, Chuck Hatch, Hartfield tel: 01342 823392

Scragoak Farm, Robertsbridge tel: 01424 838420 (p. 89)

Trinity Wholefoods, 3 Trinity St, Hastings tel: 01424 430473; Finbarr's Wholefoods, 57 George St, Hastings tel: 01424 443025. Both collection points.

West Sussex

Flint Acres Farm, Bury Gate, Pulborough tel: 01798 831036

Michelle Hanford, Henfield tel: 01273 493241

Wayside Organics, Oving, Chichester tel: 01243 7797126

Willow Nursery, Barnham tel: 01243 55852

Warwickshire

Grange Cottage Herbs, Nailstone, Nuneaton tel: 01530 262072 (p. 253)

The Henry Doubleday Research Association, Ryton Organic Gardens, Ryton-on-Dunsmore, Coventry tel: 01203 303517 (p. 83)

The Wholefood Shop, St Andrew's Church House, Church
St, Rugby tel: 01788 567757

West Midlands

The Small Green Company, Stourbridge, Dudley
tel: 01384 396384

Wiltshire

Pertwood Organics Co-op, Hindon, Salisbury
tel: 01747 820763

Worcestershire

Greenlink Organic Foods, 9 Graham Rd, Malvern tel:
01684 576266 (p. 84)

Oxton Organics, Fladbury, nr Evesham tel: 01386 860477

N. Yorkshire

The Food Emporium, 25 Front St, Acomb, York
tel: 01904 781993

Goosemoorganics, Cowthorpe, Wetherby, Leeds
tel: 01423 358887 E-mail
Postbox@Wethfoe.demon.co.uk.

The Green House, 5 Station Parade, Harrogate
tel: 01423 502580

Mustard Seed Good Food Shop, 1 Skinner St, Whitby tel:
01947 601608

Simply Organic, Barlby, Selby tel: 01757 708540 (p. 89)

Standfield Hall Farm, Pickering tel: 01751 472249

S. Yorkshire

Beanies, 205–207 Crooks Valley Rd, Sheffield
tel: 01142 681662

Fieldgate, Fishlake, Doncaster tel: 01302 846293

Natural Delivery Wholefoods, Brough, Bradwell, Sheffield
tel: 01433 620383

W. Yorkshire

Bradford Wholefoods, 78 Morley St, Bradford
tel: 01274 307539

Brickyard Farm Shop, Babsworth, nr Pontefract, Wakefield
tel: 01977 617327

Eve's Organics, Todmorden tel: 01706 817672

Half Moon Wholefoods, 6 Half Moon, Huddersfield
tel: 01484 456392

scotland

L. & M. Allison, Forglen, Turriff, Aberdeenshire
tel: 01888 568501

Bean Machine, Greatridgehall, Kelso tel: 01573 460346 (HD)

Bellfield Organic Nursery, Strathmiglo, Fife tel: 01337 860764

Damhead Organic Farm Shop, Edinburgh, Lothian
tel: 0131 4451490 (p. 98)

E.P.O. Growers, Glasgow tel: 01389 875337

I. and A. Lambie Organic Growers, Thornhill, Stirling
tel: 01786 815367

Organic and Free-range Meats Ltd, Farmshop, Jamesfield, Fife
tel: 01738 850498 (p. 97)

Parkgate Organic Nursery, Parkgate, Dumfries, Dumfries &
Galloway tel: 01387 860391

Pillars of Hercules Farm, Falkland, Cupar, Fife
tel: 01337 857749

Sundrum Organics, Auchinleck, E. Ayrshire tel: 01290 552020
(HD) (p. 121)

Colin J. Ward, Bridgefoot, Newmachar, Aberdeenshire
tel: 01651 862041

Wheems, South Ronaldsay, Orkney Islands tel: 01856 831537

wales

Green Cuisine, 87 Westville Road, Penylan, Cardiff tel: 01222
498721 (p. 121)

Medhope Organic Growers, Tintern, nr Chepstow,
Monmouthshire tel: 01291 689797

Only Organics, Rhiston, Montgomery, Powys tel: 01588 620109

Primrose Farm, Felindre, Brecon, Powys tel: 01497 847636

Pumpkin Shed, St David's, Pembrokeshire tel: 01437 721949

Spice of Life, 1 Inverness Place, Roath, Cardiff
tel: 01222 487146

Whitebrook Organic Growers, Llanvaches, Newport
tel: 01633 400406

Useful
Addresses

The Banana Link, 38–40 Exchange Street, Norwich, Norfolk
    NR2 1AX   tel: 01603 765670
Environment and Health News, P.O.Box 1954, Glastonbury,
    Somerset BA6 9FE   tel: 01767 627038
The Food Magazine, the Food Commission (UK) Ltd, 5–11
    Worship Street, London EC2A 2BH   tel: 0171 628 7774
Genetix Update, P.O.Box 9656, London N4 4JY
    tel: 0181 374 9516
The Green Guide for London, 3A Tyndale Lane, London
    N1 2UL   tel: 0171 354 2709
The Green Network, 9 Clairmont Rd, Lexden, Colchester, Essex
    CO3 5BE   tel: 01206 546902
Greenpeace, Canonbury Villas, London N1 2PN
    tel: 0171 865 8100
Henry Doubleday Research Association, Ryton Organic
    Gardens, Ryton-on-Dunsmore, Coventry CV8 3LG
    tel: 01203 303517
The International Federation of Organic Agricultural
    Movements, Okozentrum Imsbach, D-66636, Tholey-
    Theley, Germany   tel: +49 6853 5190
The Organic Directory, Green Earth Books, Foxhole,
    Dartington, Totnes, Devon TQ9 6EB   tel: 01803 863260
The Pesticides Trust, Eurolink Centre, 49 Effra Rd, London
    SW2 1BZ   tel: 0171 274 8895
SAFE Alliance, 94 White Lion Street, London N1 9DF
    tel: 0171 837 8980
The Soil Association, Bristol House, Victoria Street, Bristol
    BS1 6DF   tel: 0117 9290661
What Doctors Don't Tell You, 4 Wallace Rd, London N1 2PG

tel: 0171 354 4592
Women's Environmental Network, Aberdeen Studios,
22 Highbury Grove, London N5 2EA   tel: 0171 354 8823
Worldwide Fund for Nature UK, Panda House, Weyside Park,
Godalming, Surrey GU7 1XR   tel: 01483 426444

UK approved certification bodies for organic food
Bio-dynamic Agricultural Association, Woodman Lane, Clent,
Stourbridge, West Midlands DY9 9PX   tel: 01562 884933
Irish Organic Farmers' and Growers' Association,
56 Blessingham Street, Dublin 7, Ireland
tel: 00353 1830 7996
Organic Farmers & Growers Ltd, 50 High Street, Soham, Ely,
Cambridgeshire CB7 5HF   tel: 01353 720250
Organic Food Federation, The Tithe House, Peaseland Green,
Elsing, East Dereham, Norfolk NR20 3DY
tel: 01362 637314
The Scottish Organic Producers' Association, Milton of Cambus,
Doune, Perthshire FK16 6HG   tel: 01786 841657
The Soil Association Marketing Company. As above
UKROFS, Room 320C, c/o Ministry of Agriculture, Fisheries
and Food, Nobel House, 17 Smith Square, London
SW1P 3JR   tel: 0171 238 5915

Sources

The information in this book has been drawn from a wide range of sources. Occasionally, if especially appropriate, I have given the source at the end of the text, but I should like to acknowledge here all major sources to which I am indebted. Any interpretation of facts and figures is, of course, my responsibility, not theirs. All books and journals cited have been extremely useful, and are to be recommended as further reading.

Directories
Where to Buy Organic Food, the Soil Association, new edition 1998, available from the SA direct: the booklet I most recommend to anyone who wants to find their nearest stockist or who wants to source organic food; *The Organic Directory*, Clive Litchfield, Green Earth Books, 1996 (new edition, 1998); *The Green Guide for London*, Green Guide Company; *Food Lovers' Guide to Britain*, Henrietta Green, BBC Books, 1997 (new edition, 1998).

Organic farming, environment, health
Living Earth, *New Farmer and Grower*, *Environment and Health News*, journals; *The Killing of the Countryside*, Graham Harvey, Jonathan Cape, 1996; *The Environment Handbook*, published by What Doctors Don't Tell You.
Also
Various literature supplied by the Soil Association, including *Standards for Organic Food and Farming*; *the Organic Farmers' and Growers' Standards for Organic Food and Farming*; literature supplied by the Bio-Dynamic Association and Elm Tree Research Centre; private paper on organic vegetables by Lisa Saffron; information supplied by the Ministry of Agriculture, Fisheries and Food, including Food Safety Information bulletins; various papers presented at the International Federation of Organic Movements conference, Oxford, September 1997.

Pesticides

Pesticides News, journal of the Pesticides Trust; excellent, informative and factual; *Pesticides in Your Food*, Andrew Watterson, Greenprint; *P Is for Pesticides*, Dr Tim Lang and Dr Charlie Clutterbuck, Ebury Press; *Our Children's Toxic Legacy*, John Wargo, Yale University Press: a major scientific reference work; *Network News*, newsletter, Green Network.

Also

Chocolate Unwrapped: The Politics of Pleasure, Cat Cox, Women's Environmental Network; *Pesticides, Policies and People*, Peter Beaumont, the Pesticides Trust; *The Pesticide Hazard*, Barbara Dinham, Zed Books; various Pesticides Trust publications; *Just Green Bananas*, booklet, Banana Link; *How Green Are Our Strawberries?*, briefing paper, Kerry Rankine, SAFE Alliance; *Pesticides: The Myths and the Facts*, booklet, Fresh Fruit and Vegetable Information Bureau; various literature supplied by the Worldwide Fund for Nature; 'Chemical mixtures and synergism', private paper, by Dr Vyvyan Howard; briefing papers on oestrogen mimics, supplied by Green Network.

Genetic Engineering

Various briefing papers supplied by Greenpeace; *Genetix Updates*.

General

The Food We Eat, Joanna Blythman, Michael Joseph. This is the book I have referred to constantly when dealing with the production of food.

Others

The Food Magazine, journal, the Food Commission; *Baby Food Watch*, Drew Smith, HarperCollins; *The ABC of Healthy Eating for Babies and Toddlers*, Janette Marshall, Hodder & Stoughton; Sainsbury's *The Magazine*, October 1997, 'The organics revolution'.

Ministry of Agriculture, Fisheries and Food publications

Working Party on Pesticide Residues annual reports, Veterinary Medicines Directorate annual reports (1995–6, 1996–7), Pesticide Usage Survey annual reports. All models of clarity, and representing the most up-to-date factual information on pesticide usage and monitoring.

Index

An asterisk * indicates that a mail order service is operated. For a further list of box schemes and home delivery services, see Appendix 2, p. 351.

General Index

the shopper's guide to organic food

sperm counts, declining 127, 188
spices *see* herbs and spices
spinach 123–4
spirits, organic 102–3
sprays, use of
    fruit 336–7, 338–9; vegetables
        328–31, 332–3
spreads, organic 291–3
squashes 133, 136
St Helena, fish from 208
standards, organic 2–3, 18–24
    for imported foods 22–3; for
        manufactured foods 21–2
starting to buy organic food 57–60
strawberries 142, 145, 335, 339
subscription farming 124
sugar 243–5
sugar beet, pesticides used 341
sulphur dioxide 287
supermarkets 29–30, 61–71
    alternative 71–5
Sweden 132, 148
swedes 136
Swiss chard 136
syrups, non–sugar 243, 244, 245

tahini 318
tea 256–9, 260–62
    fair–traded 260–61; flavoured 258;
        green 258; Japanese 258; mail
        order 102, 262; organic brands
        258–9, 261; price guide 261–2;
        where to buy 70, 262
textured vegetable protein (TVP) 321
tinned food 316–22
tofu and tofu savouries 323
tomato ketchup 320
tomatoes 126, 137, 145, 328, 333
    processed 320
turkey 200–201

UK Register of Organic Food
    Standards (UKROFS) 3, 19–20, 25,
    180

veal 192
vegans, products suitable for 322–4
vegetable juices 70, 293–6, 297
vegetables
    availability of 124–5, 130; box
        schemes 107–80; buying 129,

130; flavour 127–8; frozen 124,
    137; looks vs. health 125–6; mail
    order 99–100; nutritional
    superiority 126–7; organic
    123–40; pesticides used 58,
    123–4, 131–3, 325–33; pickled
    318; post-harvest treatment 9,
    331; price guide 137; processed
    and tinned 321; seed treatments
    331; shelf life 128–30; where to
    buy 68, 130, 137
vegetarian dishes 321, 323
    freshly made 288–90
venison 204
vinegars 321–2
vitality, and organic food 4, 6
vitamins, in organic produce 126

water supplies, effect of pesticides
    11–12, 42–4, 45
watercress 139
waxed fruit 143
wheat
    conventional 224, 225; organic
        226–7
wheatgrass 302
wholefood shops 78
wild boar pork 194
wildlife, effect of pesticides 42
wines, organic 70, 102–4
Working Party on Pesticide Residues
    (WPPR) 4, 344

xenobiotics 238

yoghurt 68, 164–9

~ 370 ~